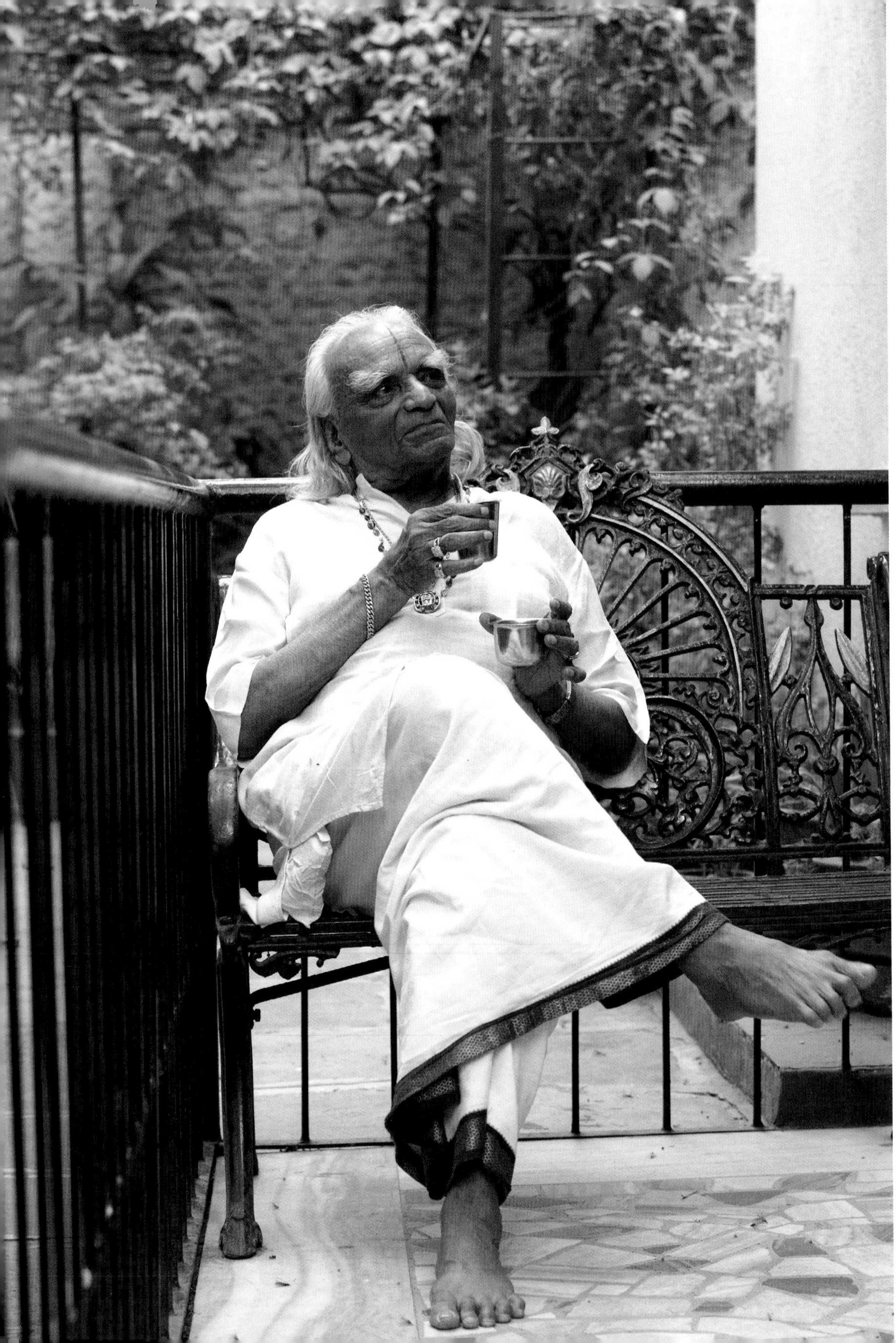

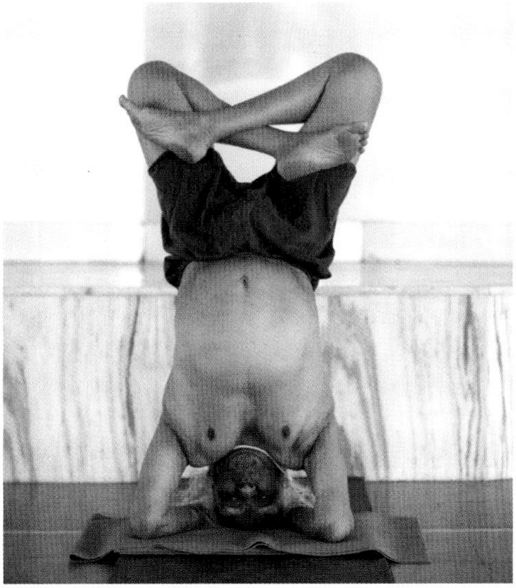

BKS IYENGAR

YOGA WISDOM AND PRACTICE

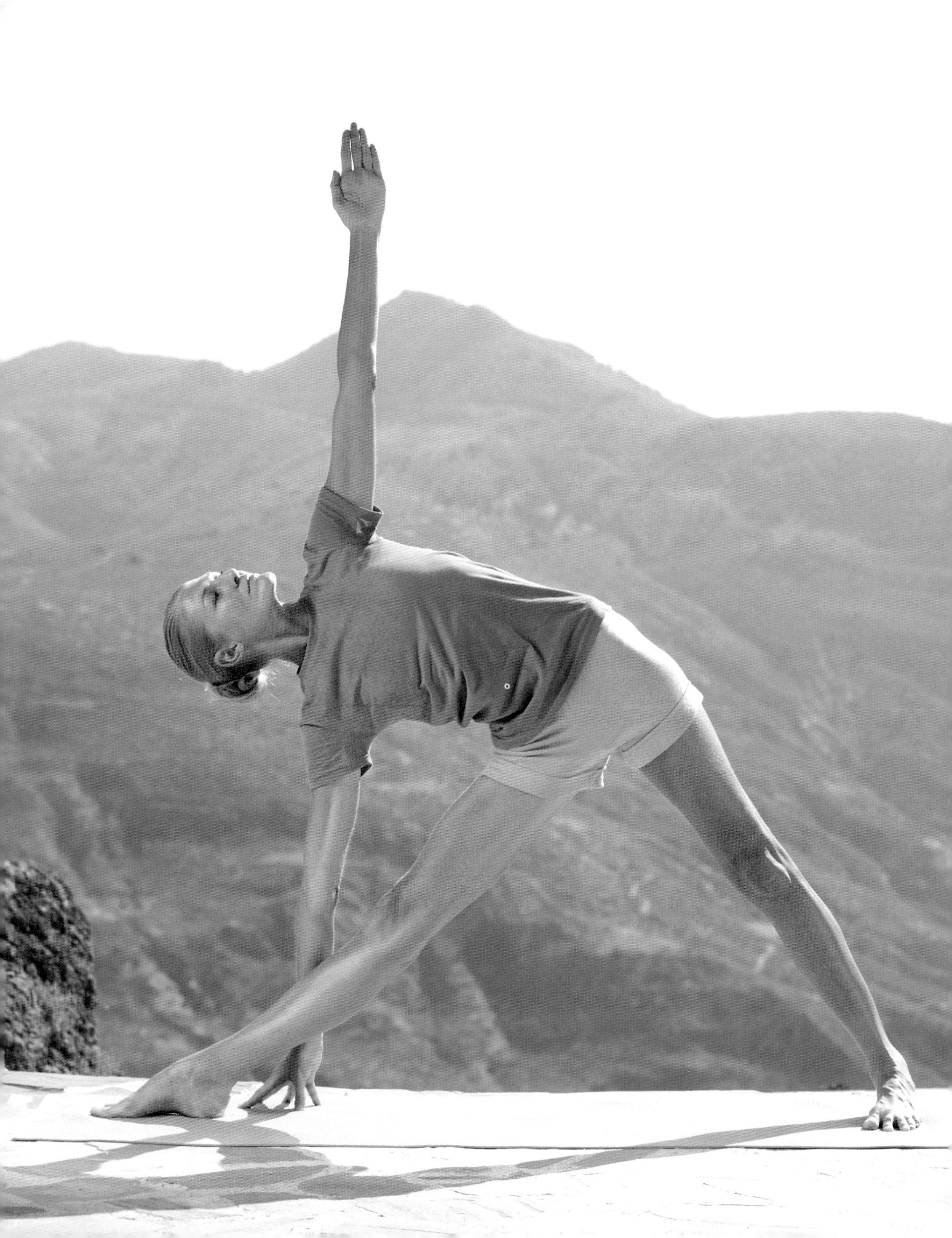

BKS IYENGAR

YOGA WISDOM AND PRACTICE

DK

DK

London, New York, Melbourne, Munich, and Delhi

Project Editor Susannah Marriott
Senior Editor Jennifer Latham
Senior Art Editor Susan Downing
Designers Nicky Collings, Mandy Earey, Ruth Hope, Helen McTeer
Managing Editor Dawn Henderson
Managing Art Editor Christine Keilty
Art Director Peter Luff
Publishing Director Mary-Clare Jerram
DTP Designer Sonia Charbonnier
Production Editor Ben Marcus
Production Controller Alice Holloway
Photography John Freeman

First published in Great Britain in 2009 by Dorling Kindersley Limited 80 Strand, London WC2R 0RL Penguin Group (UK)

2 4 6 8 10 9 7 5 3 1

Caution

This is not a book for beginners – it is best to learn asana and pranayama with a properly trained, experienced Iyengar yoga teacher, and to practice them sequenced as advised by your teacher. While performing asana, do not hold your breath; breathe normally throughout. Heavy or erratic breathing indicates strain. Timings indicated are only a guide. Always come out of a pose if you feel strained or if holding it becomes problematic.

A CIP catalogue record is available from the British Library

ISBN 978-1-4053-3550-8

Colour reproduction by MDP, England
Printed and bound in Singapore by TWP

Discover more at
www.dk.com

Contents

Foreword

By Yogacharya B.K.S. Iyengar

Yoga Wisdom and Practice is filled with gems extracted from the eight volumes of my *Aṣṭadaḷa Yogamālā*, covering yogic knowledge (*vidyā*) and experienced wisdom (*buddhi*) for those who love and live in yoga. Yoga came to me by chance. It soon made me accept it as a choice. Practising day in, day out to absorb and maintain the subtle transformations brought about by each *āsana* and each breath, I re-acted and re-adjusted in each *āsana* to experience the zenith – a single state of uninterrupted flow of attention and awareness.

We are all born with inquisitiveness. This makes us seach for ways to live this God-given life with honour and dignity. Though I initially practised *āsana* and *prāṇāyāma* using the body and mind compartmentally, later I began to associate (*saṁyoga*) these differentiating movements to integrate (*saṁyama*) every part of the gross body with an even flow of energy. Such an intensive internal penetration of intelligence towards the causal body through the suble inner body encourages the dormant consciousness to spread and touch the frontier of the soul – the inner layer of skin. Thus, yoga uses the body – the container – to touch the content – the soul. In order to make the soul "ring its bells" within each cell, I had to stay in each *āsana* for a long period. Though I was explicitly involved in *āsana* and *prāṇāyāma*, I knew in my heart of hearts that the other petals of yoga were implicitly involved and operating.

The body is finite and mortal, but the soul is infinite and eternal. I worked the soul (*jivātma*) to engulf its frontier – the body – by using the five elements of nature with their infrastructures, namely, earth, water, fire, air, and ether with smell, taste, form, touch, and vibration. Thus balanced evenly, the body is divinely united with the divine Soul as a divine union.

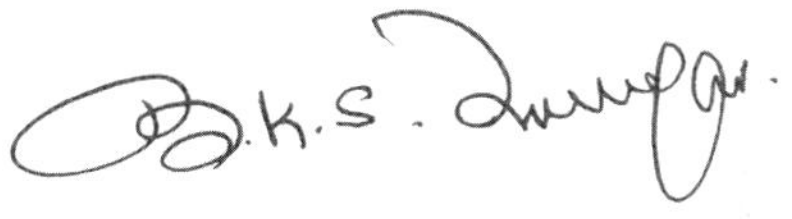

28 December, 2008
Pune, India

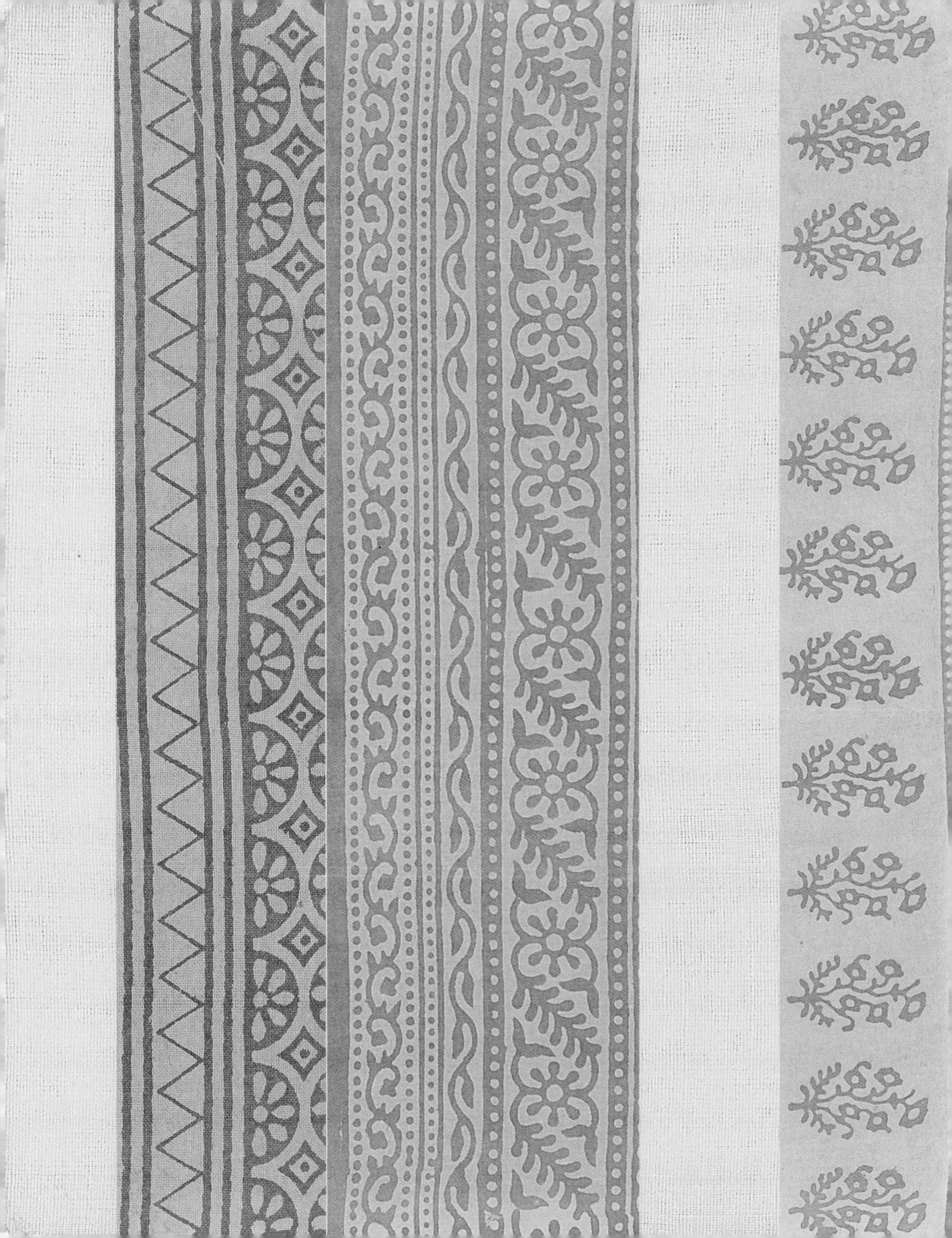

Reflections on My Life

"The interest in yoga came not from the love of yoga, but for the sake of earning my livelihood."

How Yoga Transformed Me

"Yogic discipline lifted me from a sub-human level and made me a man of confidence, sincere in my efforts, hardy and honest, clear in my thinking, and clean in my conscience.... Now I am the proudest man on earth, as I carry the message of yoga along with many of my pupils, in the form of physical health, mental poise, intellectual clarity, and spiritual solace for millions and millions of people all over the world.

I was born during the world influenza epidemic of 1918, in a village called Bellur, situated in the Kolar District of Karnataka State, India. The actual date of my birth is 14 December 1918, Saturday night at 3 a.m.... As my mother was in the grip of influenza, there was little hope of my survival, but the hands of God spared both of us. Nevertheless, I was born sick, with thin arms and legs, a protruding stomach, and a heavy head. My appearance was not prepossessing and my physical weakness caused me despair.

As sorrow and pain follow each other like a chain, my health began deteriorating with bouts of illnesses like constant malaria, typhoid and, as doctors suspected, tuberculosis of the lungs. All these brought me almost close to the jaws of death. I became a burden to myself and to my brothers and sisters. When I was on the threshold of turning nine years, my father breathed his last, leaving a vacuum in our family. No one in the house could guide me to gain health. My studies were affected as I was forced to spend more days in bed than at school....

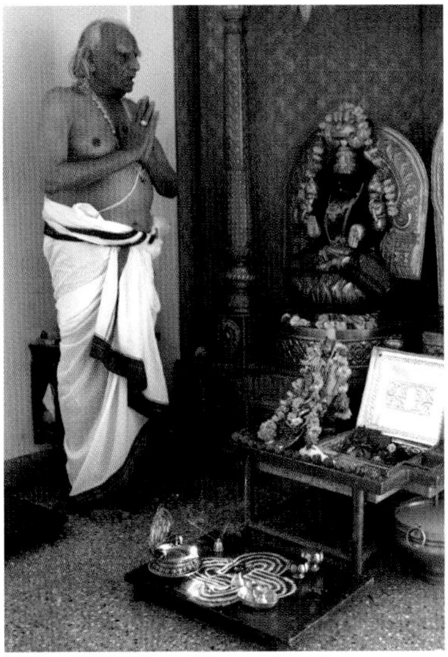

Destiny decreed B.K.S. Iyengar's role when his family deity Lord Venkateswara told him, in a dream, of his vocation. He thanks the lord daily at the shrine in his home.

The turning point in my life came for the better in March 1934. My *guru,* Shri T. Krishnamacharya, was my brother-in-law. He was married to my elder sister. Before his marriage, he was staying in Varanasi studying various *darśanas.* From there he went to Nepal and learnt yoga under a great master known as Shri Ramamohana Bramachari. He was a married man. After his return...he was running yoga seminars at various places. The Maharaja of Mysore...hearing of my *Gurujī*, opened a *yoga´ sālā* in the Jaganmohan Palace of Mysore and patronized that school. He appointed my *Gurujī* to teach there.... In 1934, the Maharaja sent my *Gurujī*, with his pupils, to visit Kaivalyadhāma at Lonavla and Bombay [now Mumbai]. He broke his journey at Bangalore on his way to Bombay. As I was having my summer holidays, he asked me whether I could go to Mysore and stay with my sister until his return. As I had not seen the city of Mysore and had heard of the palaces and lush gardens, I willingly said 'yes' to his suggestion. He gave me money to buy the ticket to go to Mysore.... He began teaching me *āsana,* to improve my health. Having rested on a bed for years, my body had become so stiff that I could hardly bend down and extend my arm to reach my knees. As my brother-in-law had implanted the seed of yoga in me, I began to address him as *Gurujī.*

continued

Though I was struggling hard in yoga, I was not sure that it would do me any good, as my body was not responding. I stayed with my *guru* for two years. In the beginning, he did not show much interest in teaching me, possibly due to my weak physical condition. After one year had passed, one day a young but advanced student who was staying with him left forever, without informing *Gurujī*. This made my *guru* turn his attention on me to make me practise yoga daily, both morning and evening. He also became very stern, which built a fear complex in me. So, I had to do yoga as demanded by him. The hard practice of yoga, walking every day from house to school, from school to house, from house to *yogaśālā*, from *yogaśālā* to house, as well as doing my homework, brought about severe aches and pains, and added fatigue to my weak physique. This physical exhaustion was affecting my mind and study became so difficult that I fell asleep whenever I sat for my homework. Though I was practising yoga, *Gurujī* did not explain to me any of the principles or subtleties of yoga. Circumstances forced me to do as commanded by my *guru*.... In 1936, the Maharaja of Mysore sent my *guru* with a few pupils, including me, on a lecture-cum-demonstration tour of Northern Karnataka, which then belonged to the Bombay Presidency. A number of people, including ladies, wanted to learn yoga and they requested *Gurujī* to start classes for them.

In those days, women were shy of practising yoga and were not ready to stand in front of grown-ups and elderly men. As I was the youngest of the group, my *Gurujī* asked me to conduct classes for the ladies and they gladly accepted me as their teacher. Thus, the seed of teaching yoga that was implanted in me has now grown into a mighty gigantic tree, spreading its branches in all the six continents of the world, for yoga to stay and grow healthily for centuries to come....

In 1937, the Deccan Gymkhana Club of Pune invited my *guru* to send an instructor to teach yoga for six months.... As I knew a bit of English, *Gurujī* thought of me and ordered me to go. I accepted it as I was looking for freedom from fear. I met the Club members who asked me to teach in various colleges, schools, and physical education centres. This was quite a heavy responsibility for my age. Those who were coming to the classes were older in age, bigger in size, and more cultured in their behaviour. For me it was a great delight to enter the college premises to teach yoga, when I had not even completed school education. I was weighing about 32 kilos [about 5 stone] and my chest measured only 22 inches [56 cm]. It increased by half an inch [about 1 cm] only after inhalation.

The first humiliation I faced was when the college students laughed sarcastically at me when looking at my figure. Ironically, their behaviour made me face them boldly and accept the challenge. The second weakness in me was the language. I was neither good in English, nor in my own mother tongue, let alone the language of the land, Marathi. The third weak point was that I had no theoretical knowledge or practical experience. I was without any qualification, but was forced to call myself a yoga teacher. I was faced with the option of acquiring second-hand knowledge from books or to practise vigorously, with determination to gain first-hand information through subjective experience. I opted for the latter and began practising ten hours a day to master what little I had learnt from my *guru*.... My hard practice caused agony to my body, to my nerves, to my mind, and even to my self. I was tossed from one side to the other; sometimes the body refused to co-operate and at other times the mind would not bear the pain. This way my body and my mind oscillated. My energies were sapped and mental fatigue set in. If I did not try, the self within grew restless: if I tried, failure brought on dejection. Very often, exhaustion brought me to the point of collapse. I could neither eat nor drink with comfort. Sleep was almost impossible due to pain and failure causing restlessness in my body and mind. Even easing myself had become a problem. Though I continued practising yoga for years, dejection and doubt tormented me, and my mind found no rest except in renewed effort. Each day was an ordeal, but God's grace forced me to make one more attempt for every failure. As I had no guide, I made enormous mistakes but I learnt discrimination from observing my own errors.... Slowly, I began to feel that my body was growing in strength, my restless, agitated mind was gaining stability. Though I started with the practice of yoga in 1934 it was only in 1946 that an innate interest in yoga arose in me.

I had a dream. I saw the Lord in a dream. Our family deity Lord Venkaṭeśwara (commonly known as Bālāji) smiled at me and blessed me in a dream. I was told by the Lord that I had no other vocation but to practise and teach yoga. The Lord blessed me with one hand and with the other hand gave me a few grains of rice. The benevolent Deity told me that from now on I should not worry about my physical survival. This dream gave me hope to continue my practices. The same night my wife too dreamt of Devi Lakṣmi, who gave her a coin, saying that She was returning the said amount She had borrowed from me long long ago. The very next day pupils called on me for lessons and from then on, my stars have been always ascending and the grace of God continues to be upon me. ”

From "How Yoga Transformed Me", Aṣṭadaḷa Yogamālā *Volume 1, pp15–20.*

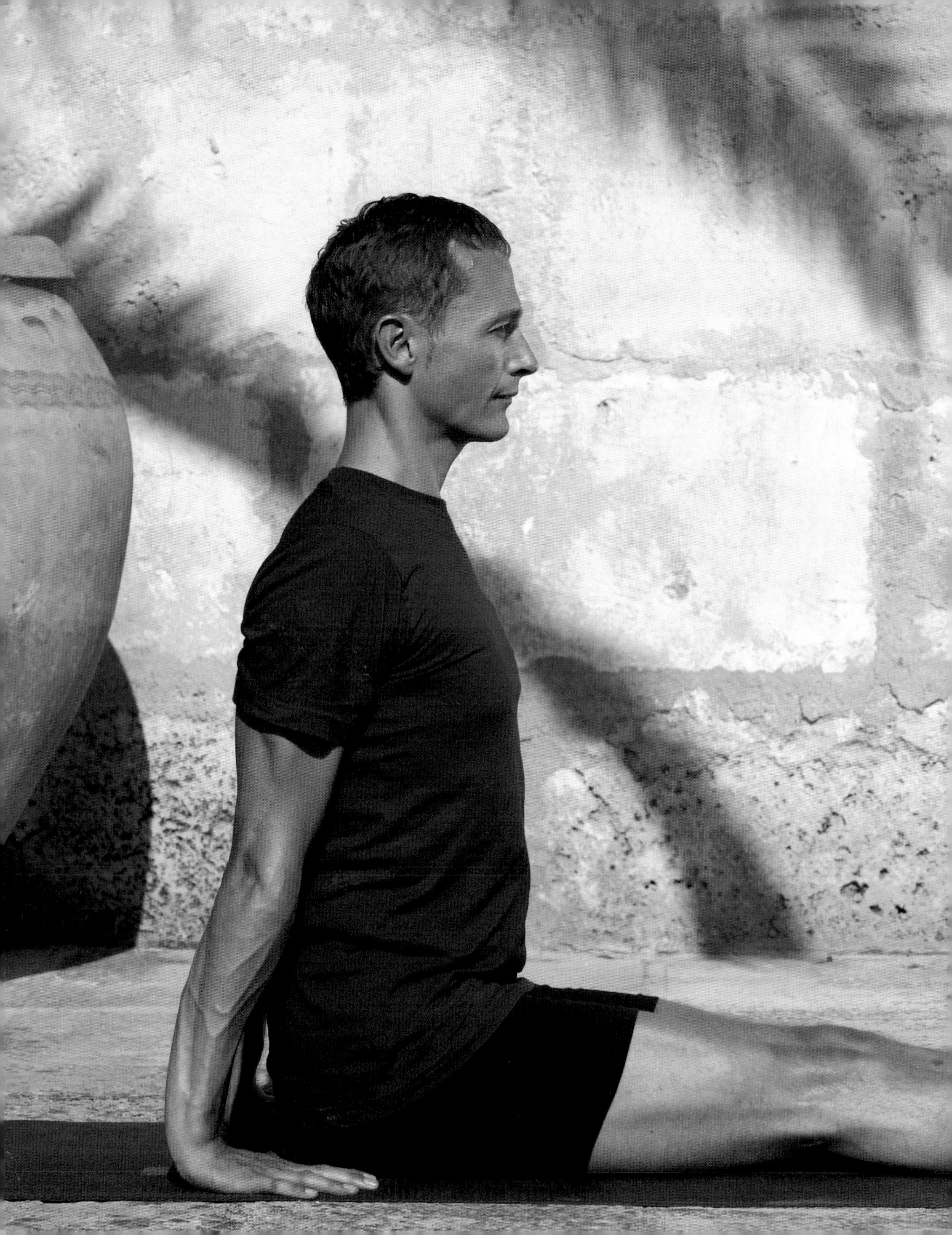

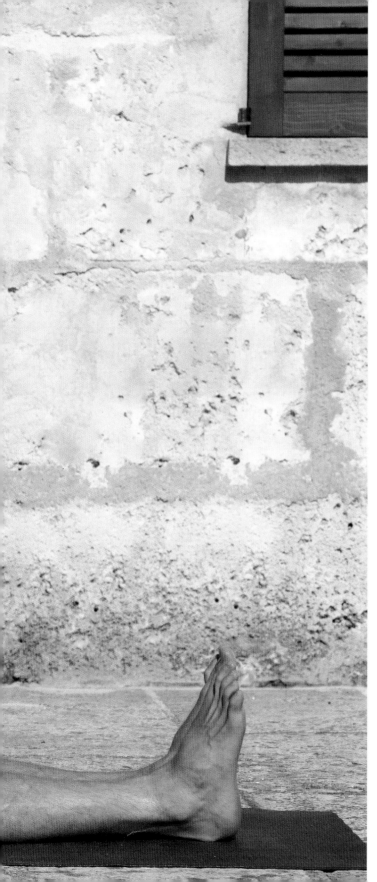

Dandasana

Staff Pose

"I could not sit straight like him [my *guru*] at all, because of all the backbends in my early days. My spine used to curve backwards if I sat straight. I had no power to resist. Naturally, without resistance I could not sit straight.... Others would have given up, but I never did."

Sit with your legs outstretched, feet together. Take the backs of your thighs and knees down. Extend into your heels and press them down, stretching your toes up. Press your palms beside your hips, fingers pointing forwards. Roll your shoulders back and down, straighten your arms, and lift your spine. Lift your abdomen and lower ribs, take your dorsal spine in, then lift and open your chest. Look ahead, aligning the back of your head with your sacrum. Hold for 20 seconds before relaxing.

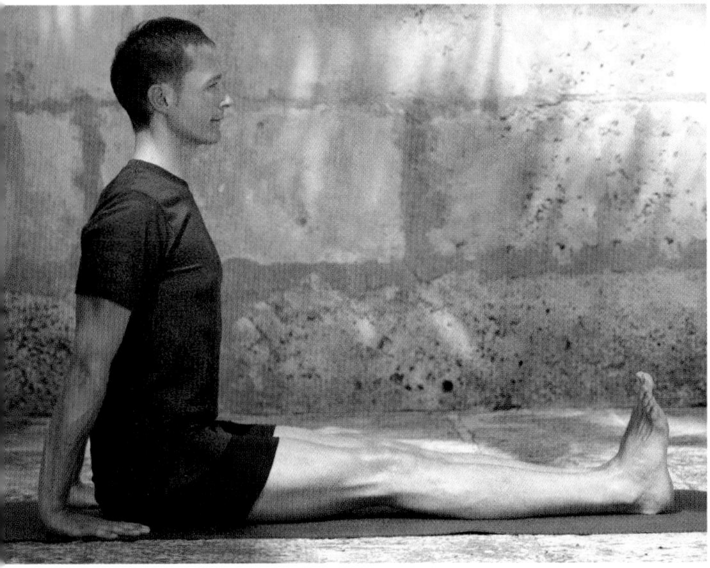

1 Sit in Dandasana (see pages 14-15). Do not disturb your left leg as you begin step 2.

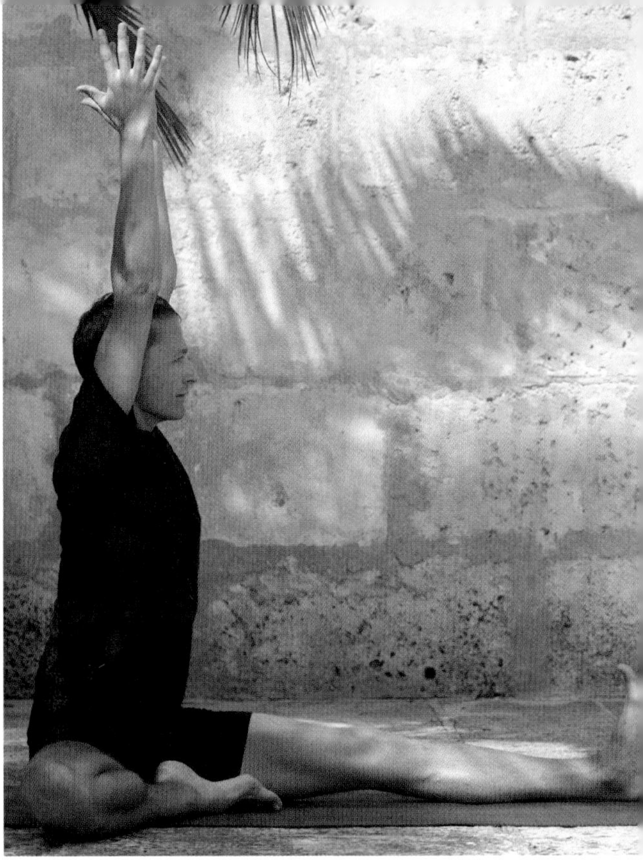

2 Bend your right leg and place the sole against the top of your left thigh. Press your right knee away and stretch your arms overhead, palms facing each other.

Janu Sirsasana

Head-on-knee Pose

"I was doing too many backbends...; one day I made up my mind to do forward bends like *Jānu Śīrṣāsana* – I could not stay in it even for a few minutes. My spine and back muscles became sore and I couldn't bear the soreness when I used to do forward bends. It was as if somebody was using a sledgehammer on my back. Then I determined that if I could do backbends, I should learn to do forward bends too. Since then, I keep a day for forward bends and my pupils follow the same routine."

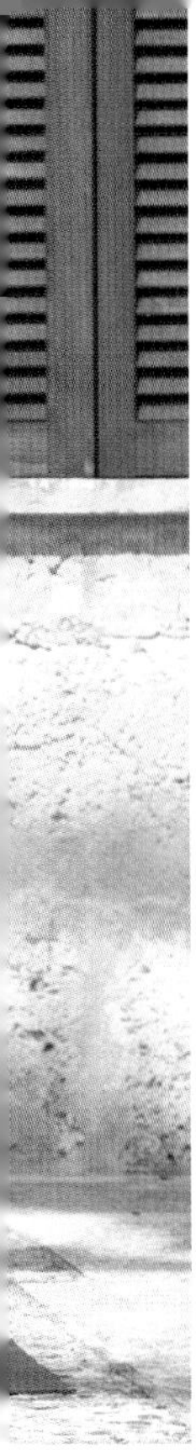

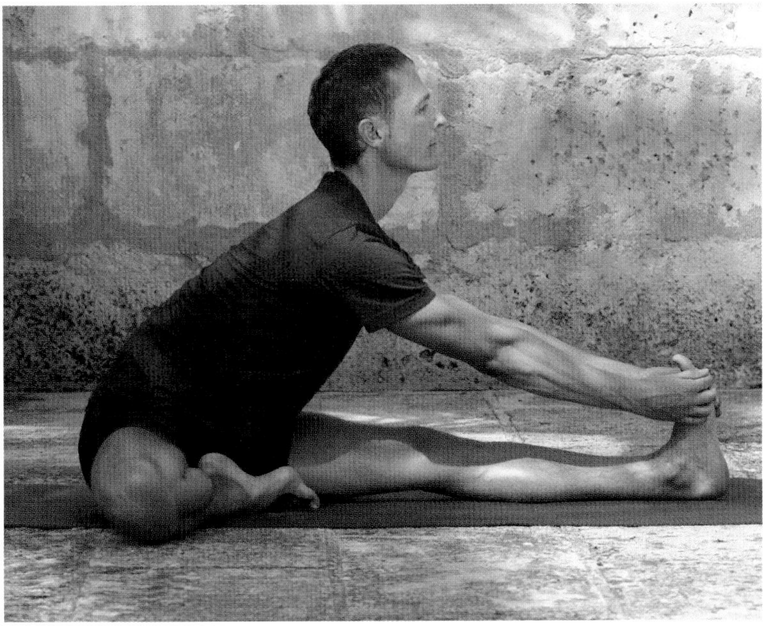

3 Exhale, extend forwards from your hips, stretch your hands towards your left foot and catch it. Keep the leg fully outstretched.

4 Extend your sternum further to bring your forehead, nose, lips, and chin to your leg. Hold for 30–60 seconds. Inhale to Dandasana, repeat to the right, and finish in Dandasana.

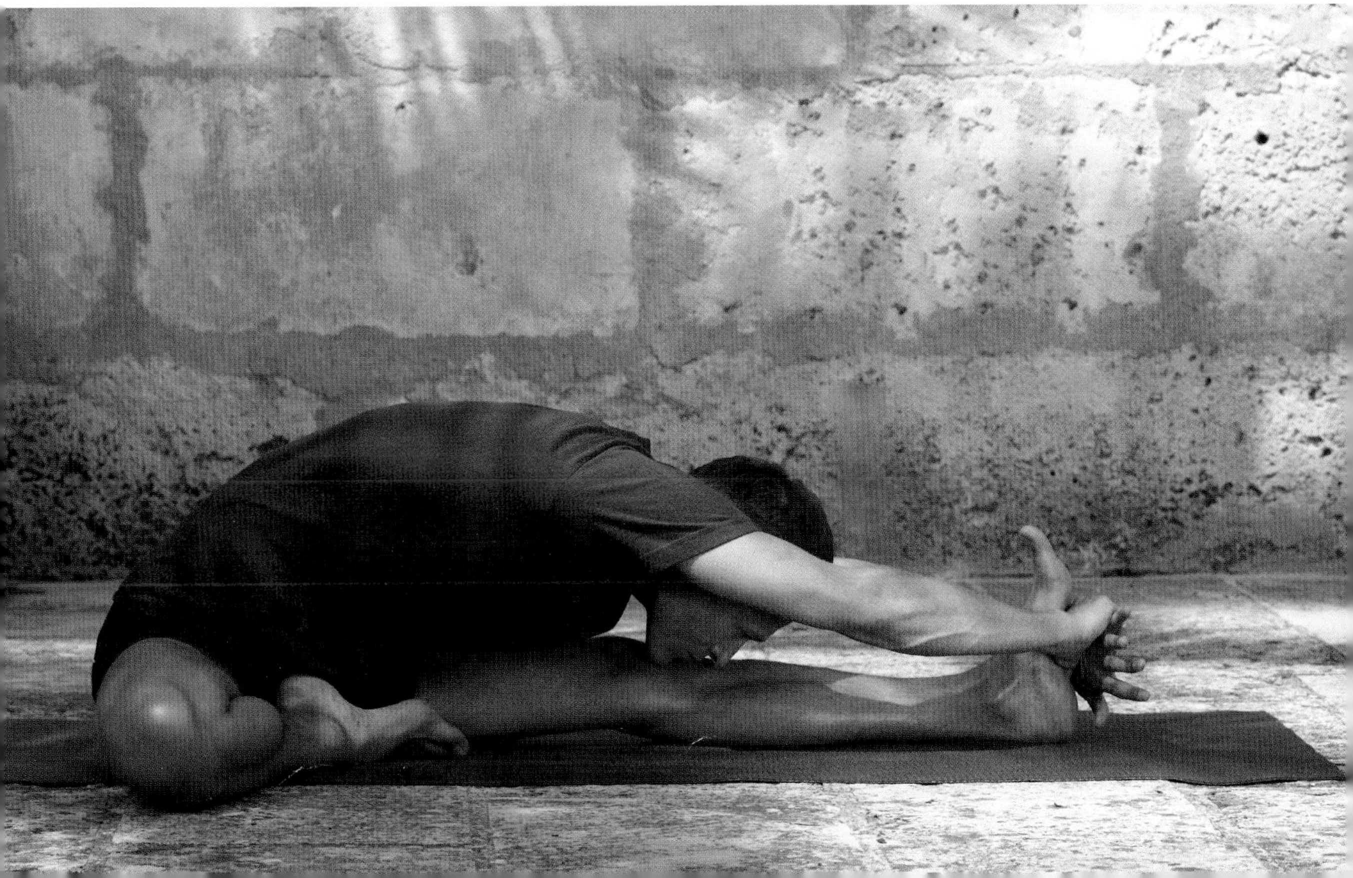

"Guruji sowed the seed, but it took a long time to grow. Now it has spread like a gigantic tree. It has conquered the world."

My Guruji

"I was a non-entity, but *Gurujī* made me a hero. I was at the nadir in this subject. I climbed the tree of yoga step by step. Perhaps *Gurujī's* eagle eyes made me think and re-think. Indirectly he taught me how to be totally aware. Today, I feel happy at heart and satisfied that I served my *guru.* There are three ways to serve the *guru:* one is to serve him physically, the second financially, and the third to impart the knowledge that was acquired from him. I served him in all the three ways.

Gurujī was a gifted man, with a very high intellectual calibre, powerful physical prowess, and an unfaltering memory. I am sure he would have won the title of 'Mr. Universe,' if he had stood for such a contest. He was naturally gifted with a well-built body, proportionately muscular, expressing tremendous strength and vigour.

He was also a master of *Āyurveda*. He used to prepare *Āyurvedic* medicines and herbal oils such as *lehyams* and *tailam* at home, which were very effective when used on his patients. But he never gave any clues to how they were mixed and prepared.

Besides mastery in the fine art of music, he played Karnatak classical music on the *veeṇā*. *Gurujī* was also a wonderful cook.... I used to call his preparations *Madhupākam* – it was like honey. He was a first-class gardener. He used to grow flowers and vegetables at his house in Mysore. He would sow any seed and by his magical touch the plant would flourish.... He was precise in whatever work he did; whether cooking or cutting wood; singing *vedic* hymns or playing the *veeṇā*. He would not tolerate any compromise or slackness with precision. He demanded the same from all of us. His moods and modes were very difficult to comprehend and often unpredictable. Hence, we were always alert in his presence. He was like a great Zen master in the art of teaching....

You may not be knowing that after his marriage he got a job in a coffee plantation in the Hasan district of Karnataka. He used to dress differently, wearing half-pants and half-sleeved shirt, socks and shoes, a hat on his head, and a stick in his hand. It was unimaginable to see a man dressed in such a manner, who had studied *Ṣad-darṣanas* (the original texts of six schools of thought in Indian philosophy)....

In 1931, he left the plantation job and began giving lectures on philosophy. Shri Sheshachar, a lawyer of Mysore, invited him to give a talk on the *Upaniṣads* in the town hall of Mysore. The event proved to be a turning point in his life. A hidden scholarly personality, in that garb of half-pant, half-sleeve shirt, hat, socks and shoes, was unearthed. His discourses on the *Vedas, Upaniṣads*, and yoga attracted the elite of Mysore. The news of this scholar and his scholarly debate reached the ears of the then Maharaja of Mysore, His Highness Shri Krishnaraja Wadiar IV. The Maharaja was attracted by his knowledge and personality and became his student in order to understand the scriptures and yoga....and gave him the recognition of *Āsthāna Vidwān* – the intelligentsia of the palace. From a plantation worker, *Gurujī* had become an *Āsthāna Vidwān* and a *Yogāchārya*. ”

From "My Gurujī – Shriman T.Krishnamacharya", Aṣṭadaḷa Yogamālā *Volume 1, pp51–61.*

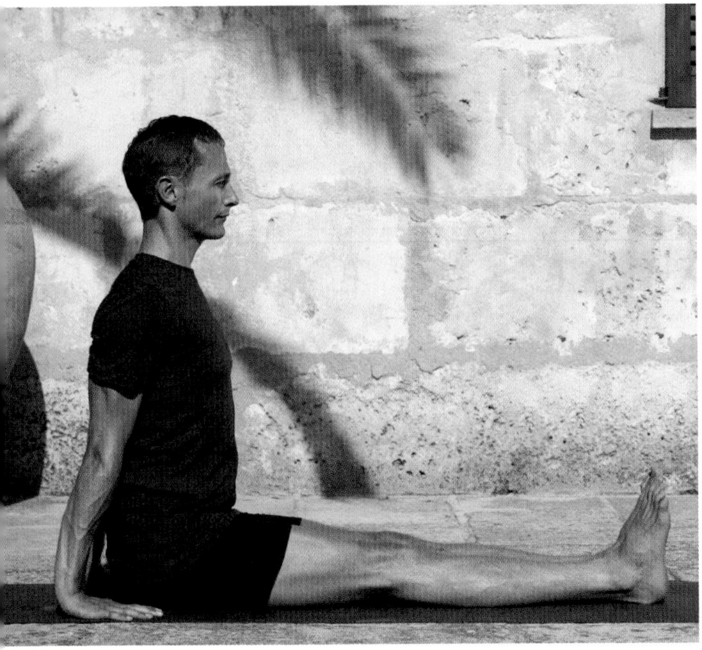

1 Sit in Dandasana (see pages 14-15).

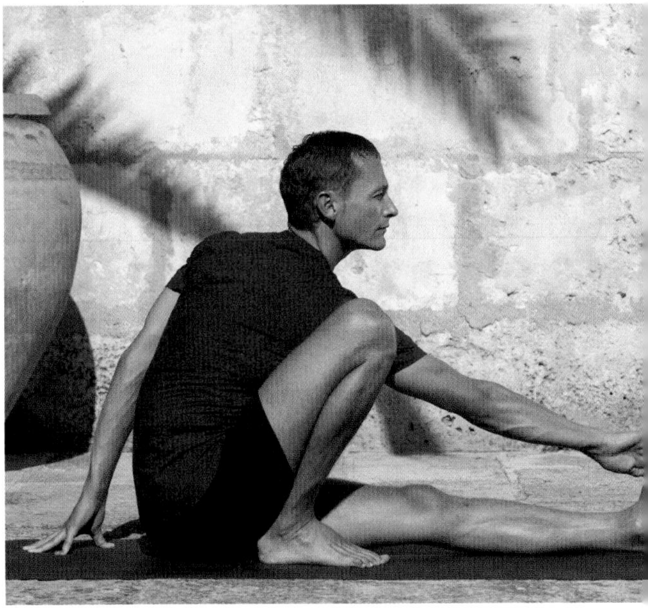

2 Bend your right knee and place the heel in line with your right buttock, toes pointing forwards. Stretch your right shoulder forwards until the armpit touches the inner bent knee. Extend your right arm forwards.

Marichyasana I

Asana I Dedicated to the Sage Marichi

"If the practitioner weighs the front, back, and side trunk with equidistance to the core of the being, along with parallel adjustments of the spinal muscles, shoulder blades, muscles of the arms, grips of the wrists and legs, I say he is close to the *ananta samāpatti*, i.e., embracing the Soul evenly from all sides of the body, directing towards the Soul as if all parts of the body are completely mingled to the core."

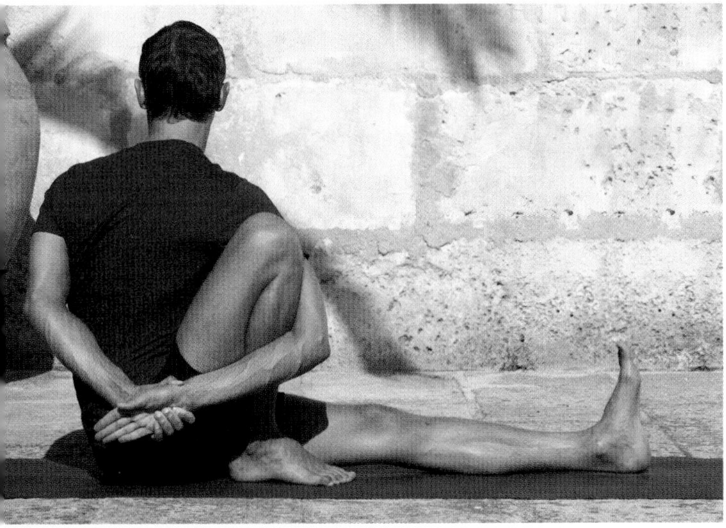

3 Exhale, wrap your right arm around your bent shin and thigh, then reach back towards your waist. Take your left arm behind your waist and clasp your right wrist with your left hand, or vice versa, palm facing outwards. Keep your bent leg perpendicular to the floor.

4 Turn your trunk to face forwards. Exhale, make your back concave, take your chin towards your left shin, and try to rest your forehead. Hold for 20-30 seconds. Inhaling, lift your trunk, release your hands, and straighten your right leg back to Dandasana. Repeat on the other side. Finish in Dandasana.

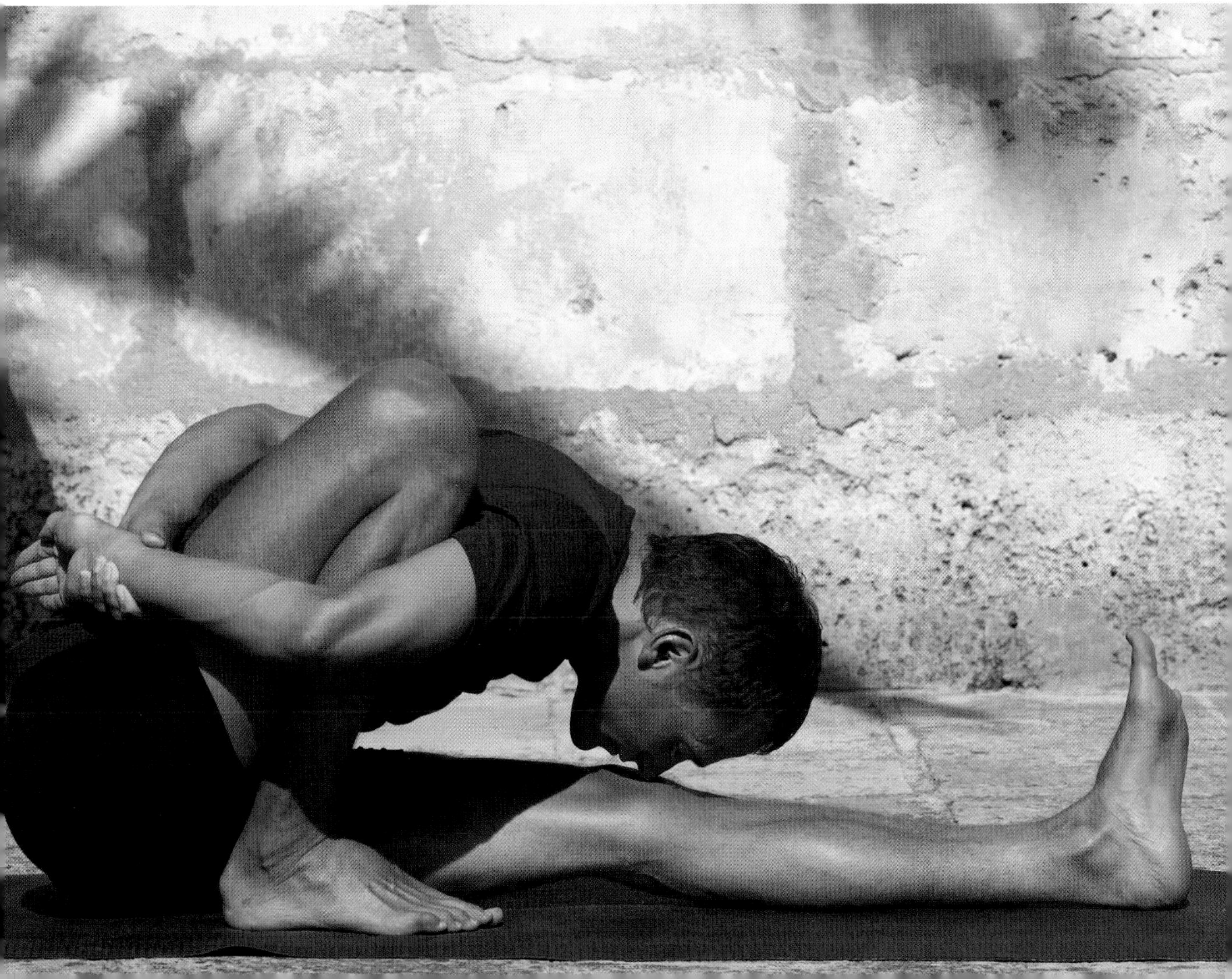

"Whenever she found time, she not only practised yoga for herself, but she helped me too. She was always ready to assist and adjust in different asana so that I could master them."

The Light on My Yoga

"My wife, Ramaa, was born on November 2nd, 1927, at Anekal, 20km away from Bangalore.... Our marriage took place on July 9th, 1943, when Ramaa was sixteen and I was twenty-four. After four months of marriage, we started our life in Pune in November 1943, when I got a contract to teach yoga in Perugate, at the Bhave School for Girls for a period of six months. When she arrived in Pune she had only her *mangalsūtra,* the wedding necklace tied by me at the time of our marriage, and nothing else. I had nothing in my possession to make her live with ease or comfort....

Each day I used to get up very early in the morning for my yoga practices. Ramaa, too, was up at the same time to prepare coffee, which was the only nourishment for both of us. Though the word 'yoga' was unknown to her, she used to observe my practices with interest and without any interference. As she was too young, she did not know what yoga stood for, and she never ventured to ask what I learned or what yoga teaching was meant for. However, as time went by, she evinced keen interest in practising the art with me. I started teaching her daily while practising myself and she became not only my pupil, but a partner in my profession. As she made progress in her practices, I taught her how to assist me, for me to improve

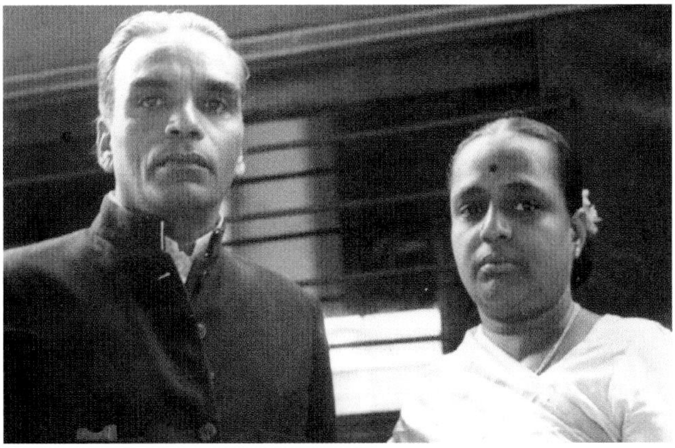

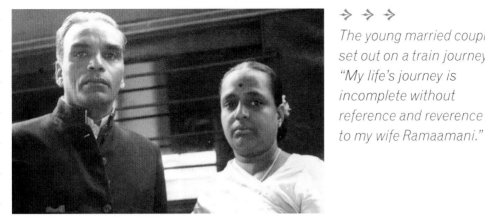

The young married couple set out on a train journey: "My life's journey is incomplete without reference and reverence to my wife Ramaamani."

my methods. This in turn helped me to excavate the potentials of the art hidden deep in my heart. My instructions and guidance to her to help me during practice made her to become a good teacher. This enabled her to independently teach the lady students from my group....

I had already mentioned that earlier we both had dreams the same night in 1946. The dreams came true, which indicated bright days ahead. People started enquiring for lessons. With the blessing of God, fortune favoured us, our domestic life became secure and our suffering decreased, and by His grace our wants were fulfilled. We had not imagined that our life at home as well as in the field of yoga would make such good and great progress. As time passed, we slowly understood each other, and lived happily, mentally and spiritually. We adored each other. With a strong feeling of togetherness, we discussed with each other and worked out that her interest in life must be to take care of our children, and mine to pursue my practices and teaching without any hindrance so that life may go on smoothly. I was everything to her and she was everything to me. We shared the love of the divine through each other. Ramaa

continued

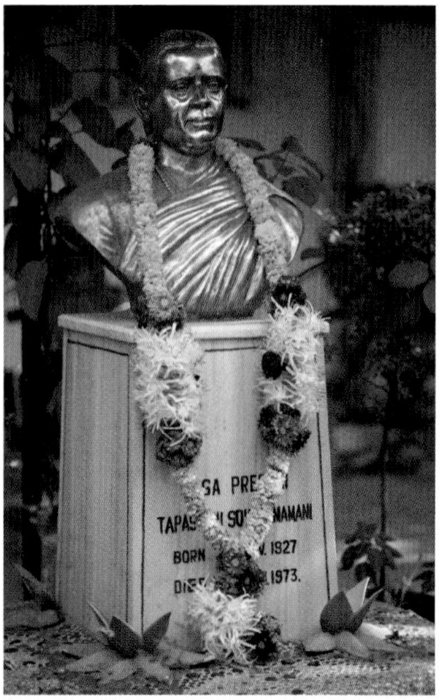

The Ramaamani Iyengar Memorial Yoga Institute was built in memory of Guruji's beloved wife, funded by donations from friends, pupils, and admirers. This is her memorial there.

was the personification of patience and magnanimity. She was simple, generous, and unostentatious. She was kind to one and all. She had great forbearance, even towards people who did not wish her well. She was quiet, serene, peaceful, and remained unruffled in adverse circumstances. She took everything in her stride coolly. With love, joy, and devotion, she looked after those who came to her for help or advice. She served all with friendliness and compassion, extending to them both her hands....

Hospitality, kindness, and self-sacrifice were very much in her blood. She treated her maidservants and the sweepers of the street as if they were members of her family. During festival days, she used to reserve their share of food, lest they should be overlooked. Her feelings and thoughts were virtuous and she never wished ill of anyone. Such was her disposition. Her love was unique, she had a heart full of compassion and people called her *Ammā,* which means 'mother'. Her physique was big, her mind great, and her soul noble....

Ramaa suddenly became weak after performing the *Bhūmi Pūjā* on land purchased by us for our proposed new house on January 25th, 1973. On Friday January 26th, 1973, I had her admitted to a nursing home so that she might rest and recover from fatigue. I was with her for a few hours. As she showed signs of recovery, I came home, since I had to go to Bombay the next day. I had left for Bombay to conduct yoga classes as usual. On the Sunday, January 28th, 1973, at four o'clock in the morning, my pupils Shri Madhu Tijoriwala and Shri Barzo Taraporewala came to the hotel where I was staying. I had been restless the whole night and I was already up when they knocked on the door. They asked me to proceed to Pune, saying that they had a message from my son that my wife was in a serious condition.... As I entered the premises, I saw many of my pupils and people and knew that everything was over. I calmly comforted my weeping children, telling them not to weep for their mother, who was a pious soul. From then on I was both their mother and father. As the news spread that Ramaa embraced mother earth, people from all walks of life, known and unknown, thronged the house, as if it were a temple, to pay their homage to the departed soul. Pupils who had come from South Africa for lessons witnessed her body being laid to rest. Messages poured in from all parts of the world, expressing their grief and sorrow. She embraced death with the same graceful serenity with which she had lived – with patience and forbearance.

What a noble lady my wife was! She knew her death was approaching. That night my two daughters, Sunita and Suchita, had a sitar recital. She did not want to disturb them nor had she stopped me from going to Bombay. Noticing the time when the concert would be over, she asked the doctors at the nursing home to phone Dr. Pabalkar, our neighbour, who had a telephone. It was three o'clock in the morning when my son Prashant and daughter Geeta went to see her. She asked them to go home immediately and to light up the lamps to our deity and to come back soon with the other children. All the children could not go, as no transport was available at that odd hour. She just asked them why they did not bring the other children. She said to Prashant and Geeta that her duties and responsibilities were coming to an end and she would be departing in a few moments. She did not want to die on the bed of the nursing home. She wanted to be closer to mother earth and lie on a carpet on the floor but the doctors did not permit it. So she sat reclining. Placing the children's palms in hers, she blessed them and told them to bear the future responsibilities on their own. She breathed her last like a great *tapasvini* who knew of her death beforehand. Her soul merged with the Universal Divine Soul. ”

From "Ramaa – The Light on My Yoga" (courtesy Timeless Publishers, USA).

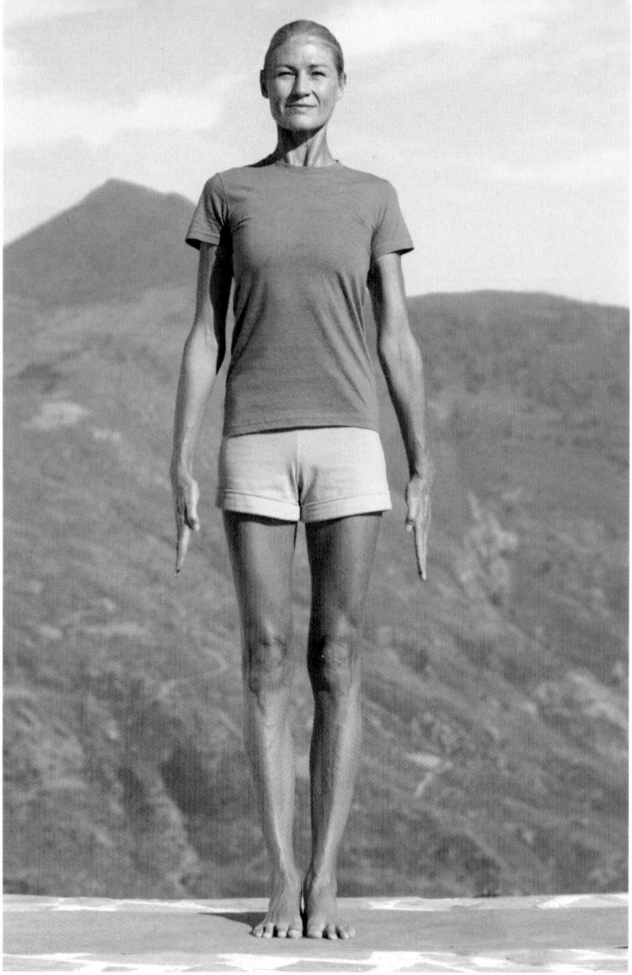

1 Stand with your feet together, toes, heels, and ankles properly aligned. Press down your heels and spread the mounds of your toes. Extend your toes forwards, balancing evenly between the front and back of both feet. Tightening your knees and thighs, suck them in, then pull them up. Draw in your hips, lengthen your inner tailbone, and lift your abdomen. Extend your spine. Align your arms with your sides, palms in. Lift your sternum, taking your shoulders back and shoulderblades in.

Tadasana

Mountain Pose

"If I have to do *Tāḍāsana*...it often happens that one leg appears strong, attentive, steady and straight whereas the other leg remains inattentive. One can feel that one leg is in a passive, non-violent state and the other is in a violent or aggressive state. Hence, it becomes necessary to balance the two legs evenly so that one will not be able to differentiate between activity and passivity, or violence and non-violence.... Secondly, if you keep the legs unevenly, the mind remains unstable. Establish alignment in the body; align the muscles, joints, and intelligence, energy and attention."

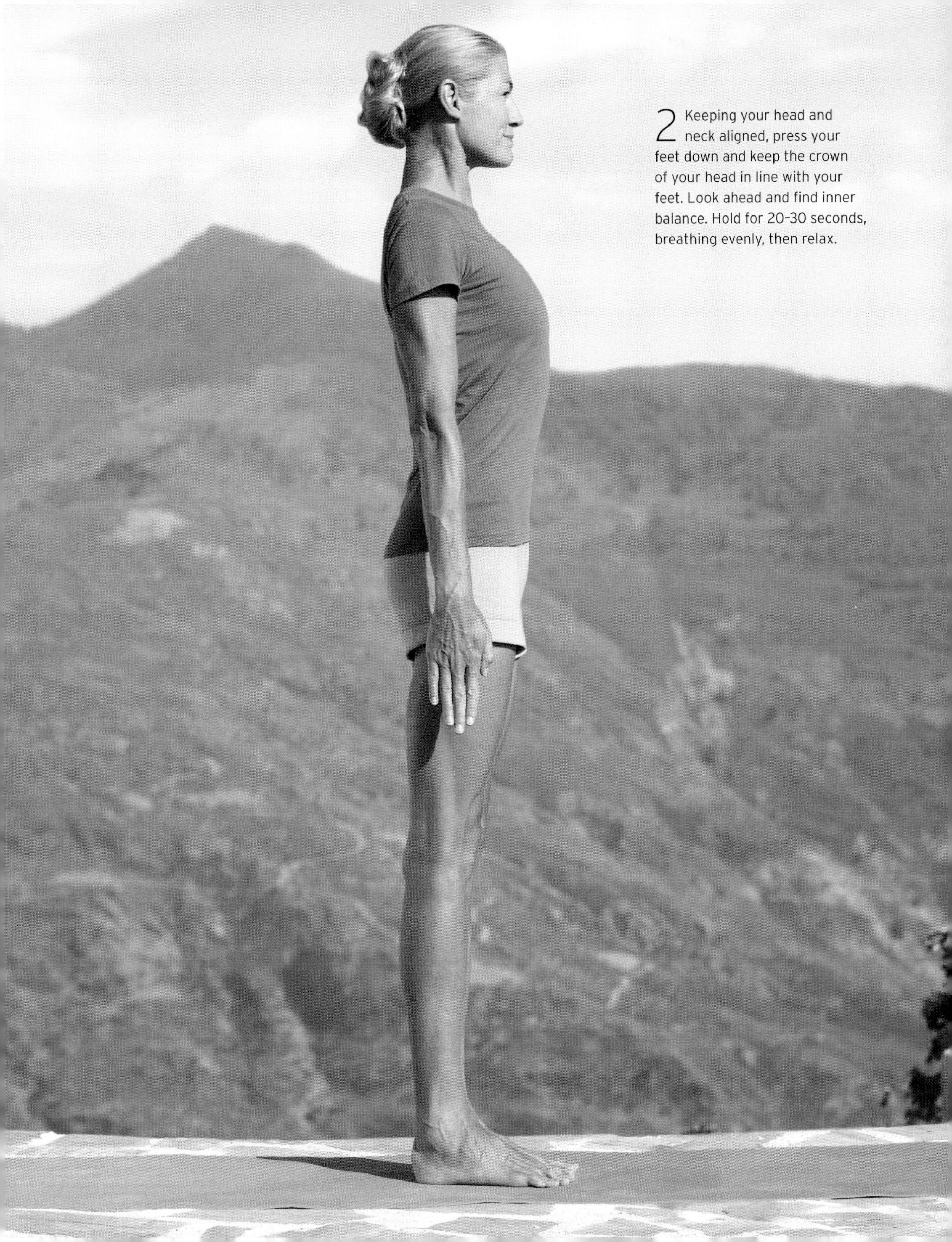

2 Keeping your head and neck aligned, press your feet down and keep the crown of your head in line with your feet. Look ahead and find inner balance. Hold for 20–30 seconds, breathing evenly, then relax.

"In every posture, the body, the mind, action and motion as well as each breath of the physical, physiological, mental and intellectual sheaths have to be evenly balanced."

How the Iyengar Method Evolved

"I knew I should present yoga in such a way that even people who had done it before would know they were hearing something new for the first time. That made me revolutionize the subject. The idea struck me in 1937, but did not fructify for several years.

In 1944 I began getting clues from my hard work, realizing the normal way *āsana* should be done this way rather than that way. I started realizing the importance of linking external actions with the inner-body, the mercurial mind, and the sharp intelligence. My inward journey began there. Then I tried to find the correct way to work in each and every *āsana*. Between 1937 and 1944, my teaching was completely immature. The advantage was that I was young. Vanity was in the pupils and in me. If I had to prove my superiority, naturally I had to express my vanity more. The only way I could do this was through my practice of yoga. I could see that my own pupils were doing better than me, and that gave me a clue that if they could do well, I should do better. I was always thinking ahead of them, looking for clues from the best of the class. I used to look at each limb separately. I first used a prop in 1948 when I was not getting *Baddha Koṇāsana* at all. I started using bricks, the heavy stones which were available in the street. But the idea to use props on a large scale and in a systematic way really struck me in 1975, when the Institute came into existence, and I was planning what to put into it.

It wasn't until then that the idea struck me that alignment is the most important thing. Yoga is alignment. This word was there theoretically, but no one explained what it meant. Almost all were saying that *āsana* are only physical and have nothing to do with the spiritual.... I began to look at photographs of people, drawing lines between their way and my way of doing it, chest to chest, hand to hand, elbow to elbow. The *āsana* were performed, but the position of the body was not aligned. In head balance, the head was in one place and one leg was straight and the other leg was turning. I wondered why there was this difference. Where was that alignment that yoga talks about when it says one has to be balanced? Where was the equilibrium or balance – *samatvam?*

In order to know what alignment is, it is important to realize that the central portion of the body is the median plane in each and every part. If you take your finger and divide it down the middle, you get the median plane. When we stretch, are we in the median plane on either side, or are we overstretching from the median plane on one side and understretching on the other side? If there is overstretch somewhere, there must be understretch elsewhere. The median plane is the god: it is what brings you to the art of precision. From the outer part, inner part, front part and back part – you always have to measure how much you are extending from the median plane. There is no overstretch; you are balanced exactly in the middle.

Later, with this alignment of the skeleto-muscular body, I began to align my mind, intelligence, and consciousness, which made me look within. This new frame of study and observation made me engulf all the instruments of the self and made the very self occupy the body – its frontiers – as *citta prasādana* and *ātma prasādana*. ”

From "The Search in Alignment Led Me to Experience the Inner Mind", interview by Carol Cavanaugh, first published by the IYTE Review, *January 1982. Published by* Yoga Journal, *July/August 1982.*[o]

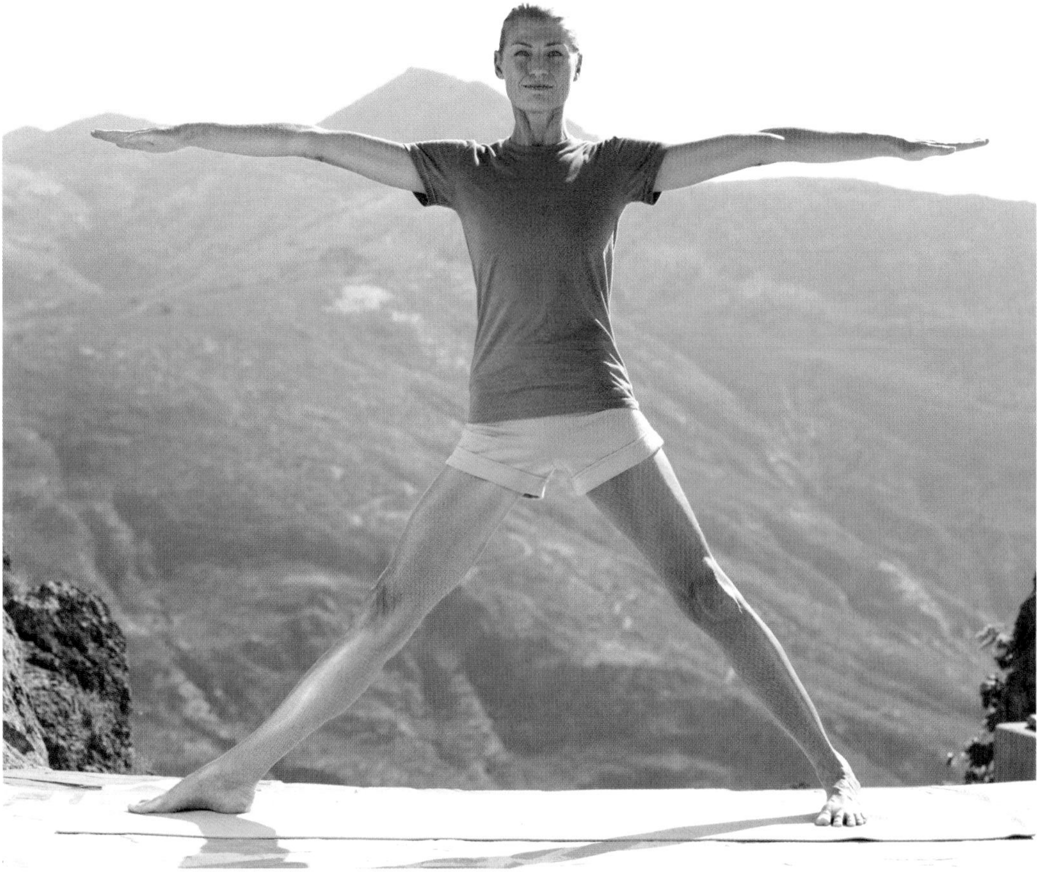

1 From Tadasana, jump into Utthita Hasta Padasana (see pages 108–109). Turn your left foot in slightly and your right leg and foot 90° to the right. Keep your arms outstretched. Look ahead and open your chest.

Utthita Trikonasana

Extended Triangle Pose

"If I turn my right foot out in *Trikoṇāsana*, and left foot inward, I see whether the width and length of my right foot is equal to the left or whether the left is affected to become short. This way I started adjusting my body, dividing the body from the centre of the legs to understand clearly. At the early stage, it seemed to be a limbering process, but later I found that I am not only digging into the body but my intelligence too. This penetration removed the weeds that were in my body and made my mind fertile to penetrate deeper."

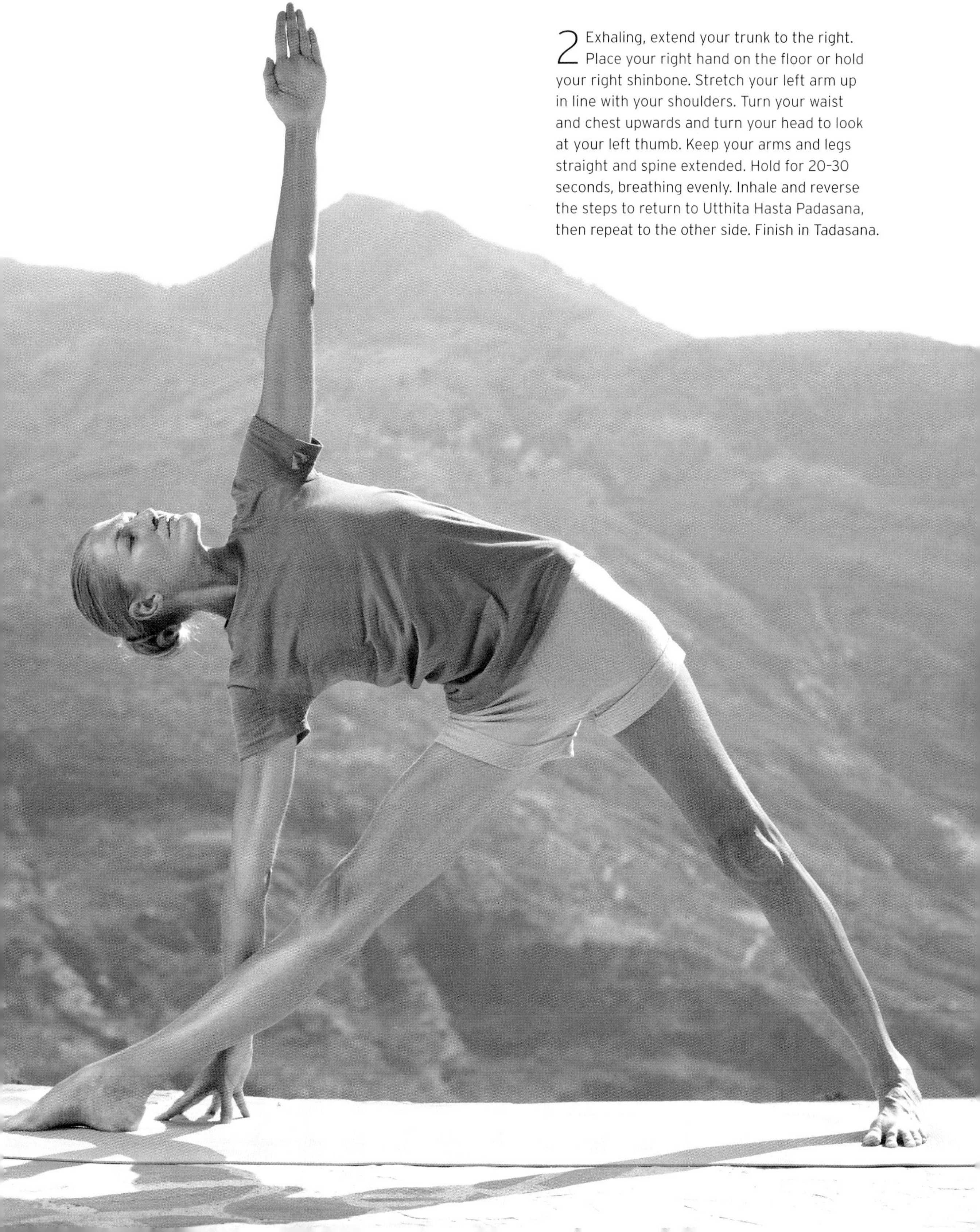

2 Exhaling, extend your trunk to the right. Place your right hand on the floor or hold your right shinbone. Stretch your left arm up in line with your shoulders. Turn your waist and chest upwards and turn your head to look at your left thumb. Keep your arms and legs straight and spine extended. Hold for 20–30 seconds, breathing evenly. Inhale and reverse the steps to return to Utthita Hasta Padasana, then repeat to the other side. Finish in Tadasana.

Virabhadrasana II

Warrior Pose II

"Equi-distribution of energy and equi-flow of intelligence within the frame of the body and the banks of the body in each *āsana* is alignment for me. The awareness has to uniformly spread all over the body through the face or the profile of the *āsana*. Alignment is to bring balance between the flow of energy and intelligence to connect the body to the mind."

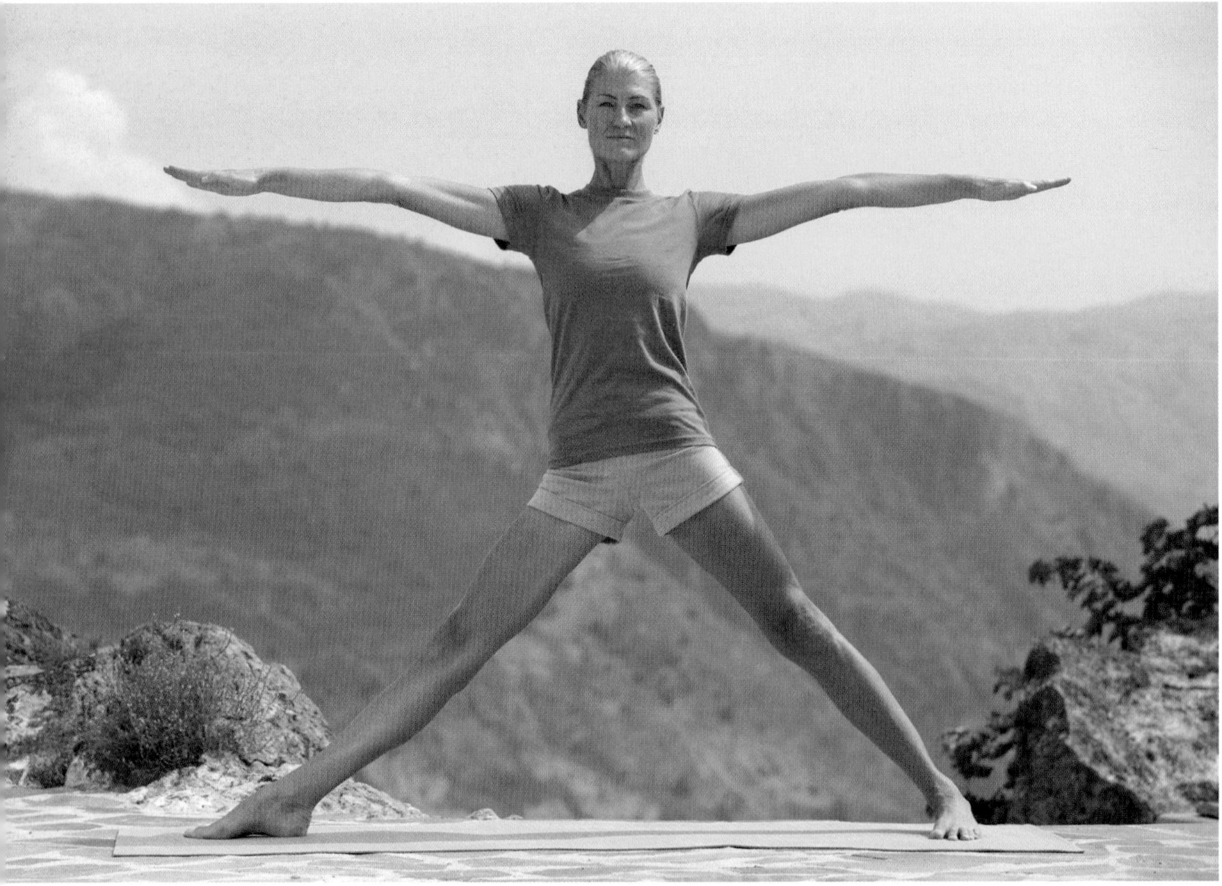

1 From Tadasana, jump into Utthita Hasta Padasana (see pages 108–109). Turn your left foot in slightly and your right leg and foot 90° to the right. Keep your arms outstretched. Look ahead and open your chest.

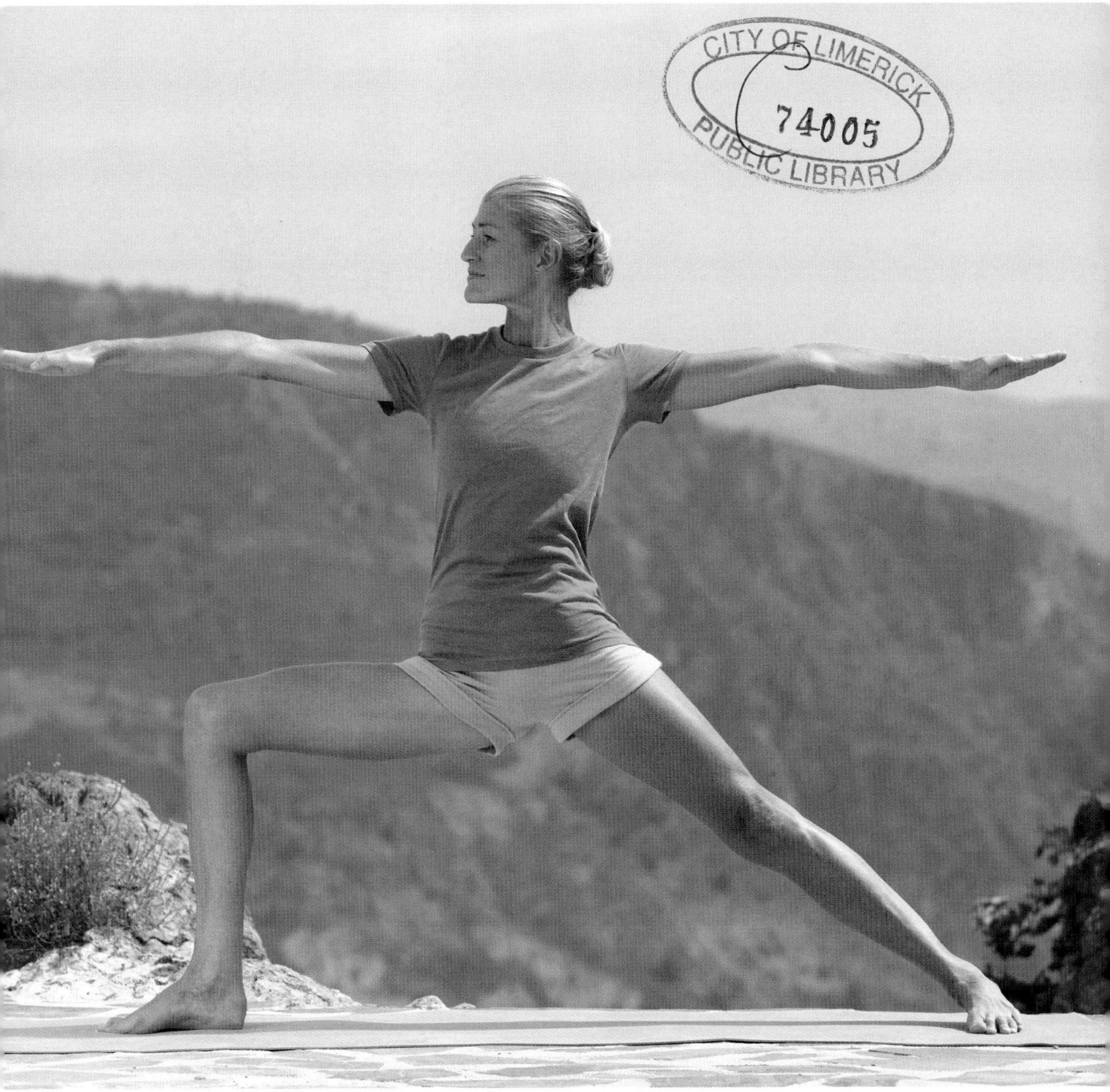

2 Exhale and bend your right knee until your shin is perpendicular and thigh parallel to the floor. Make sure the bent knee is in line with your ankle and keep your trunk lifting vertically. Turn your head to the right and gaze at your palm. Hold for 20-30 seconds, breathing evenly. Inhale and straighten your right leg, turn your head and feet forwards into Utthita Hasta Padasana, then repeat to the other side. Finish in Tadasana.

"... these props help [students of yoga] in monitoring and directing the right way to do the asana."

On Using Props

Q. *Gurujī*, the props which I've seen people using when they do their exercises - benches, blocks, and bars and other things like that - they're an innovation in yoga by you, aren't they?

"To a great extent, though my *Gurujī* started with ropes, a few *āsana,* then I built up a great deal, afterwards."

– *And did you invent these?* –

"Yes, many of the things are my own inventions."

Q. And you got local carpenters to come and make them, did you?

"Yes! I got them made by local carpenters. But it was not as simple as it looks. The guidance came from within. Realizing that the patients cannot manage to do independently to get the effect, I factualized the imagination through props. I pictured the props and gave designs to the carpenters who designed with rough wooden material. I had to practise on those shapes to try and then bring changes according to the body requirements and for the performance of various *āsana.* This way I built up and now it's easy for anybody to get and do the *āsana."*

Q. And are these props now a standard part of your yoga really?

"It's not a part of yoga. See, what happened is when Patañjali uses the word *samādhi,* he uses the word 'with seed or supported' and 'without seed or non-supported', i.e., *sabīja* and *nirbīja samādhi.* This made me think why not find ways to do *āsana* with support. Support means *ālambana.* In various *sūtra,* Patañjali refers to 'support'. I began thinking on his ideas and innovated props as 'support' for good performance of *āsana* with ease but without risk. If you read the book *Light on Yoga,* all the classical *āsana* are done without any support. No doubt it has become an authoritative book for practitioners. But I realized later that all cannot master the *āsana* easily. So I began

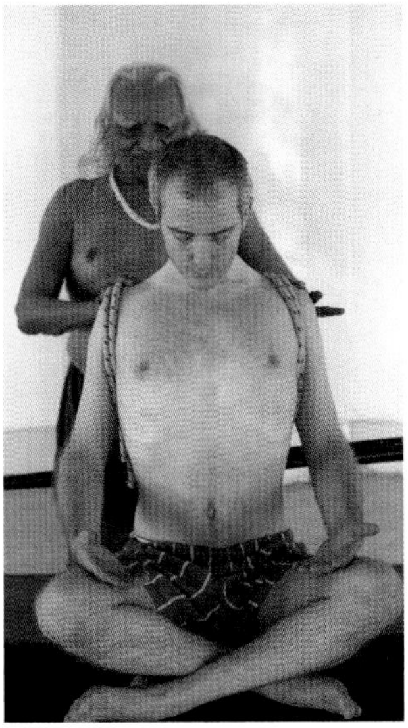

Guruji helps a student to lift and broaden his chest. He says, "As it gives a good feeling for [students] to be in a good thought by staying in those āsana *on the prop, I am happy."*

tracing supports to perfect the *āsana* without difficulties.... For years I was teaching without using any support, but realized later that these classical *āsana* cannot be done by one and all. When this Institute came into existence, people with various ailments started attending. In order to build up confidence in them, I thought that unless and until I innovate props for support to do the *āsana* with ease and also to keep their mental frame stable. I felt quick recovery from ailments may not be possible without innovating props.

In order to find props, the idea of *sabīja* and *nirbīja samādhi* came into my mind. If *samādhi* has support as well as non-support, why could not *āsana* too be *sabīja* and *nirbīja āsana?* Thus props like *sabīja* benefited in two ways; one is extension and the other is relaxation, taking place at the same time."

Q. And is the intention that eventually, like a lame person who is cured, they should throw these away as crutches?

"Yes, you can call it crutches. Once the *āsana* comes, they need not use them. These props take care of monitoring the *āsana* like intensive care units...."

From "Yoga – Head to Toe", interview for BBC Radio 4 by Mark Tully in Pune, April 1999.

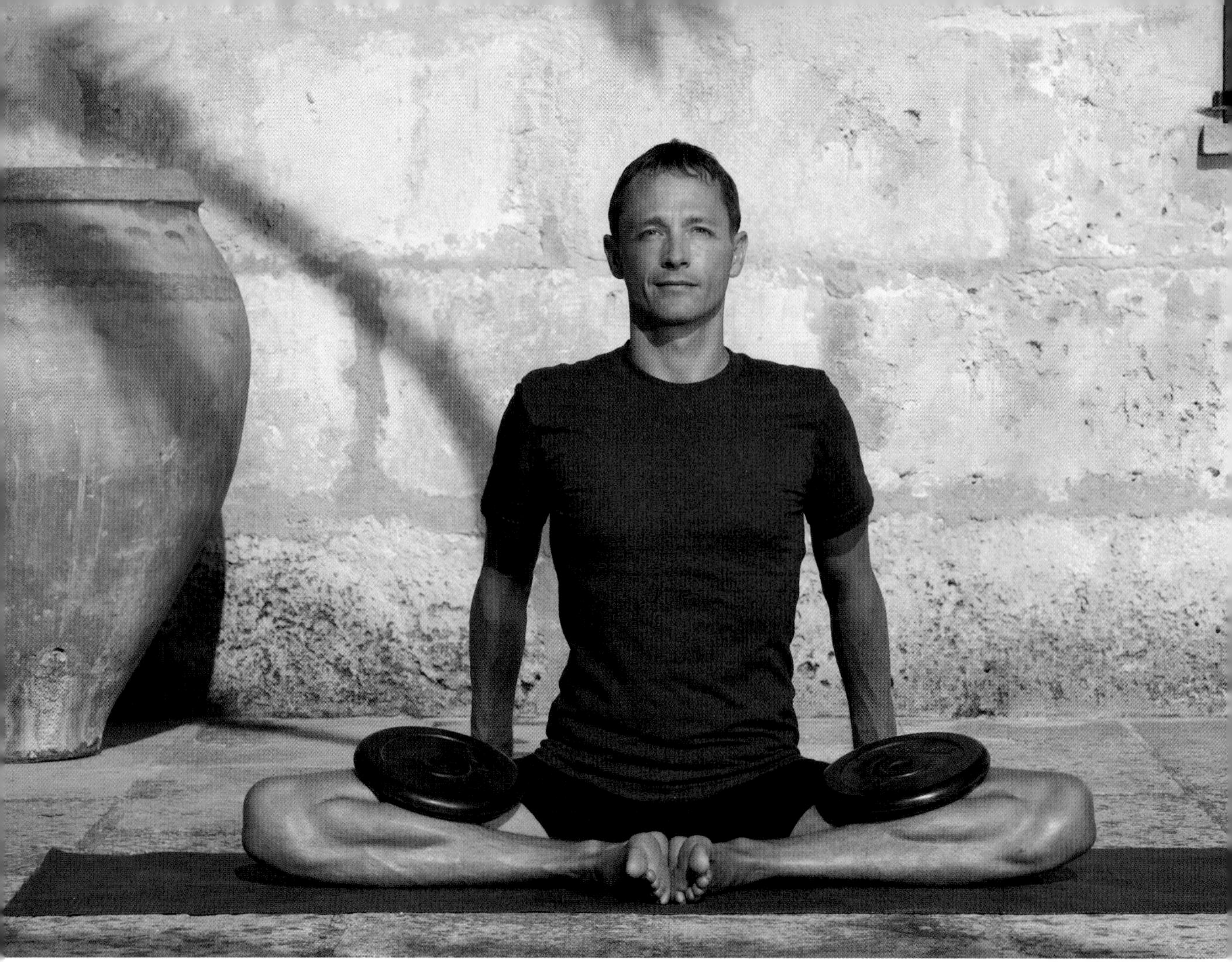

First learn Baddha Konasana (see pages 240–41). After regular practice, try the pose with weights on your thighs. Start with light weights – 5kg (10lb) – and gradually increase the pressure over a period of time.

Baddha Konasana

Fixed Angle Pose (with weights)

"In the beginning, I started using household things. For example in my early days I could not get *Baddha Koṇāsana*. So I was picking stones, cement blocks, and what are all good to learn the *āsana*, and bringing them home. People used to laugh at me.... I used to keep these stones on my thighs to get *Baddha Koṇāsana*."

Upavistha Konasana

Seated Wide-angle Pose (with a pole)

"I used to use a walking stick between my knees for *Upaviṣṭha Koṇāsana*. As I could not spread my legs apart, I used the walking stick between the knees to spread my legs sideways."

First learn Upavistha Konasana: sit in Dandasana (see pages 14-15). Take one leg at a time out to the side, then widen them. Ensure that the centre of each thigh, knee and foot faces upwards. Keep the backs of your thighs, knees, and calves pressing down. Place your hands beside your hips and lift your spine and chest, moving your shoulderblades in. Hold for 1 minute, building up to 3-5 minutes. To practise with a pole, find one that reaches from one heel to the other. Grip with your outer and inner ankles and notice the response of the head of the femurs.

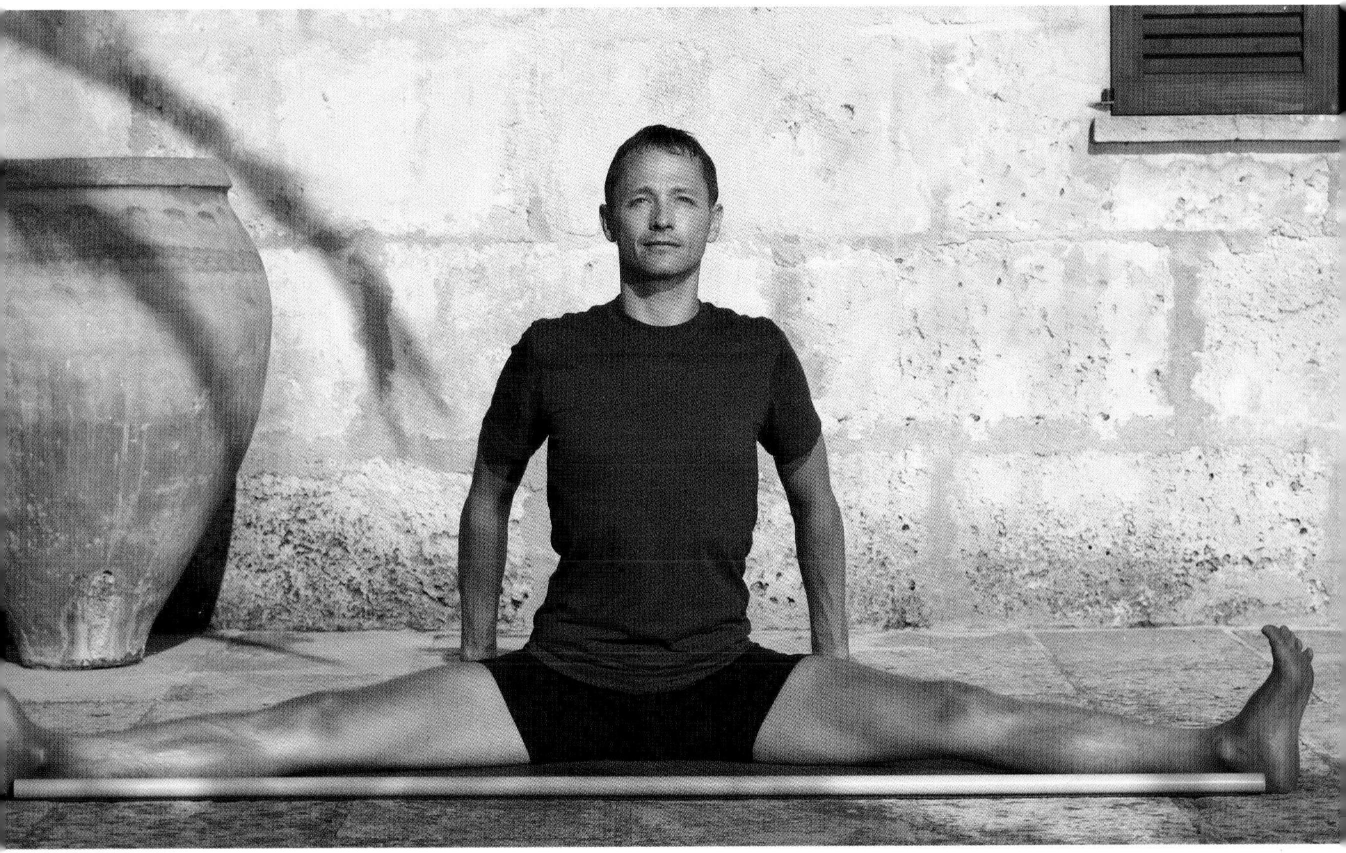

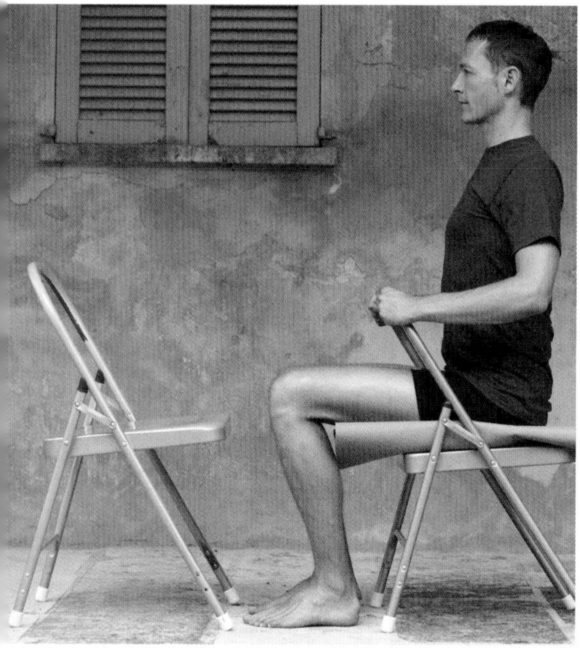

1 Place two chairs 60cm (2ft) apart and fold a mat on the front seat. Sit with your legs through the chair back, feet parallel. Hold the chair.

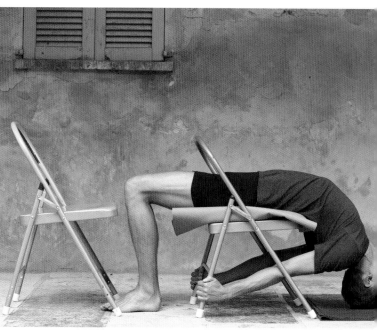

2 Lift your spine and chest, look ahead, then slide your hips to the back of the seat until your buttocks rest on the edge. Exhale, lift your chest, arch your back, and lower your torso to the floor, keeping your lumbar spine supported (place a rolled towel beneath it, if required).

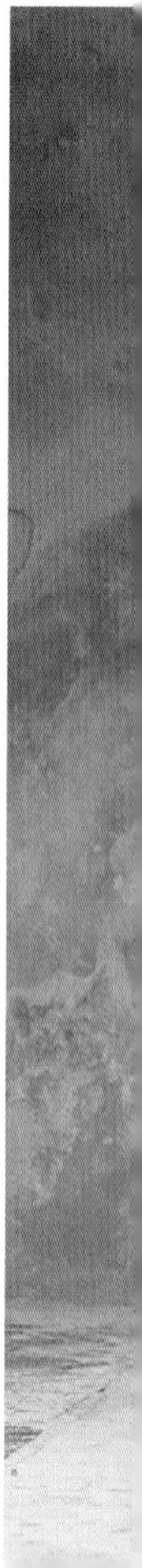

Viparita Dandasana

Inverted Staff Pose (with chairs)

"This is a very exhilarating *āsana*, but when you do it independently, it takes life out of each individual. You need to train the spine to get the correct curvature. Now everybody wants to do it, to get restfulness in their brains....on this *Viparita Daṇḍāsana* bench [or on two chairs, as shown], the head is kept down, so naturally it becomes passive on its own."

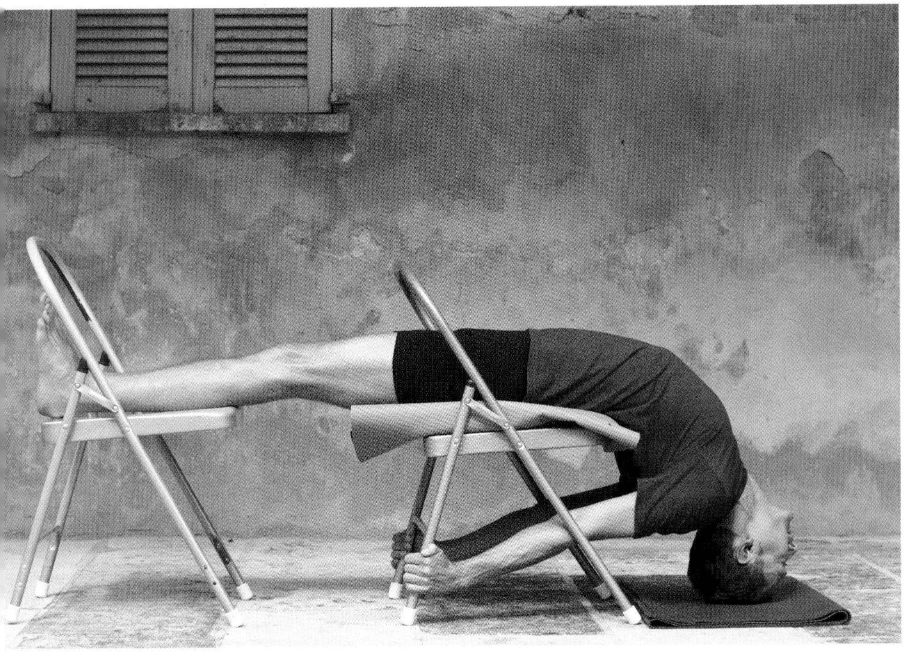

3 Rest your legs on the second chair, then arch your back further, keeping your lower spine on the front edge of the chair. Reach one arm at a time through the chair and hold its back legs. Place the crown of your head on the floor (or a bolster). If you are a beginner, hold for 30–60 seconds, then reverse the steps to sit up.

4 Now interlock your fingers behind your head (see step 2, page 73). Hold for up to 5 minutes. Release your hands and reverse the steps to sit up.

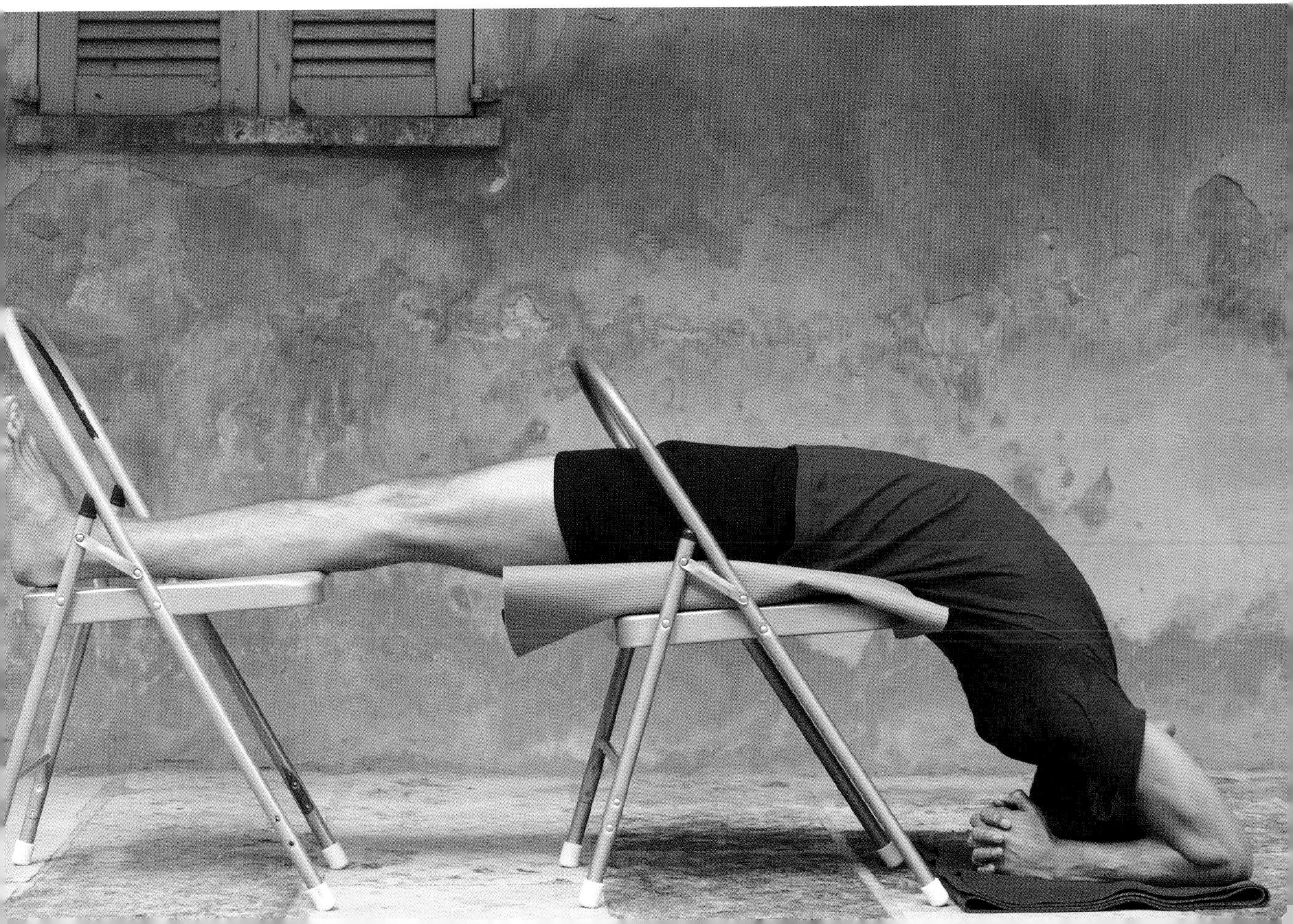

"My props became my guru and taught me how to use the body. I could sense that I did better with supports to master the asana."

A Creative Approach

Q. Another technique that sets apart your approach to yoga is your extensive use of props such as wooden blocks, sandbags, ropes, etc. How did you develop this approach?

"My *guru* was using the wall ropes, two on top, two in the middle, and two at the bottom. In those days, [people with] diseases which medicines or surgery could not handle directly were coming to *yogaśālā*, where *Śīrṣāsana*, *Sarvāṅgāsana*, *Halāsana*, *Pūrvottānāsana*, and forward bends were taught with the help of these ropes. In 1937 the principal of Ferguson College of Pune, Shri Rajawade, who was 85 years old, was suffering from dysentery. And Doctor V.B. Gokhale asked me whether I could help him as he was unable to stand or sit.

How to make him do yoga in that condition was the question I had to face. By helping him I learned the first lesson of how to teach such people. I started teaching *Trikonāsana* making him lie down. You call it *Supta Trikonāsana*. I had to lift his chest and turn it to the side so that the intestines got some movement. Since he could not spread his legs, I used to insert a walking stick between his two legs to keep the legs apart. This is how I learned to create props for getting benefits. I started treating the patients one after the other, just by instinct.

Secondly I was practising myself. I was not doing *Hanumānāsana* as I had a tear in the hamstrings. Even simple *āsana* like *Baddhakoṇāsana* was not coming. In those days, workers used to dump big stones on the roadside for road construction. Nobody would object if one picked them up. I used to bring such heavy stones to keep on my thighs to learn this *āsana*. This way I used to pick up stones, iron rods on the wayside and carry them home, which would be useful for my yoga.

You know road rollers that flatten the roads? On the front wheel I used to do backbends, because my body was not doing them on its own. So if I saw a machine on the road, I used to go to do backbends on it! Then I used drums. Because of this practice, people used to call me a mad cap. I was! Because I couldn't do the *āsana* independently, so I was always thinking of how to do so and I was finding means to learn. This way I found ways of using blocks, weights, sandbags to learn and to show the accuracy of *āsana*!"

"These supports helped in certain areas to get a better action and at the same time the sense of ease. Thus props helped me to teach well and to create a quicker healing process."

From "Iyengar Looks Back", interview by Anne Cushman, Yoga Journal*, December 1997.*

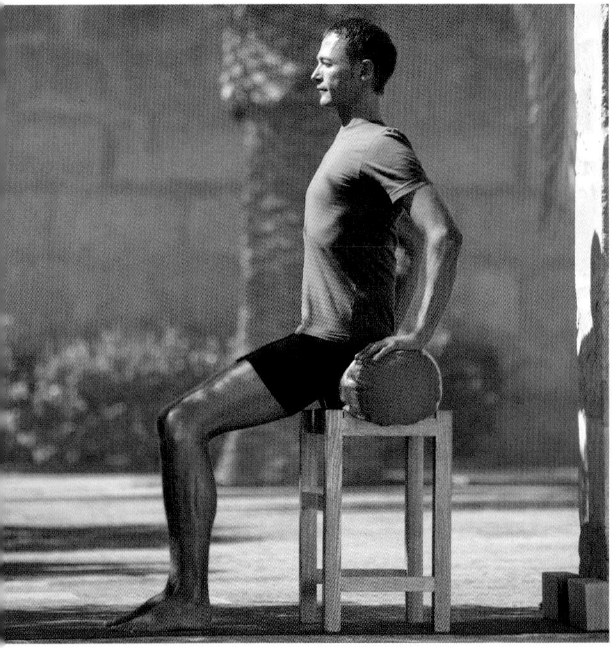

Urdhva Dhanurasana

Upward-facing Bow Pose (with props)

"Know your capacity and try to extend a little more than is possible. By this you learn the art of balancing not only the effort you put in but also the fear and courage."

1 Place a stool 46cm (18in) from a wall; further away if stiff. Place a bolster on the stool and two bricks against the wall, shoulder-width apart. Sit at the front of the bolster and lift your chest.

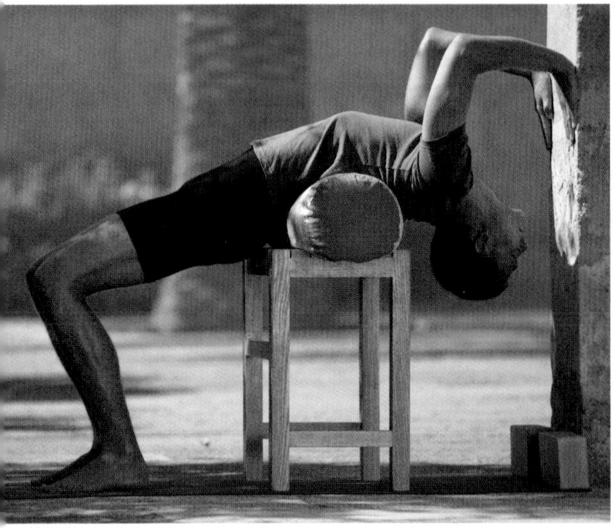

2 Slide your buttocks forwards and extend your spine over the bolster. Curve your side ribs, lift your chest, and place your hands on the wall, fingers pointing downwards.

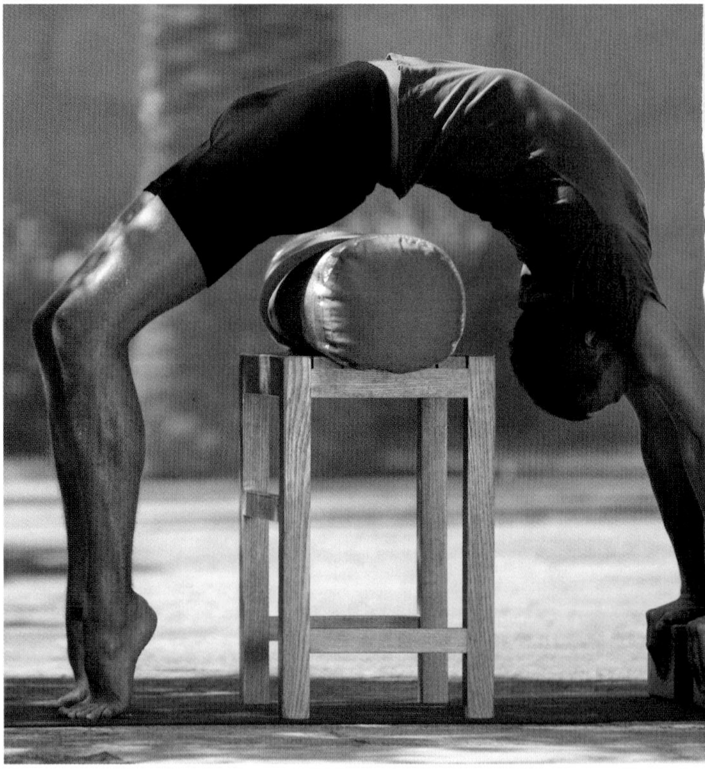

3 Curve your spine back, walking your hands down the wall until both hands are on the bricks. Press the edges of the bricks firmly and, with a lever action, raise your chest and head. Lift onto your toes and walk towards the stool. Form a good arch, then lower your heels. Hold for 20-30 seconds. Exhale and lower your trunk to the bolster, bend your legs, slide your buttocks forwards, and sit up carefully.

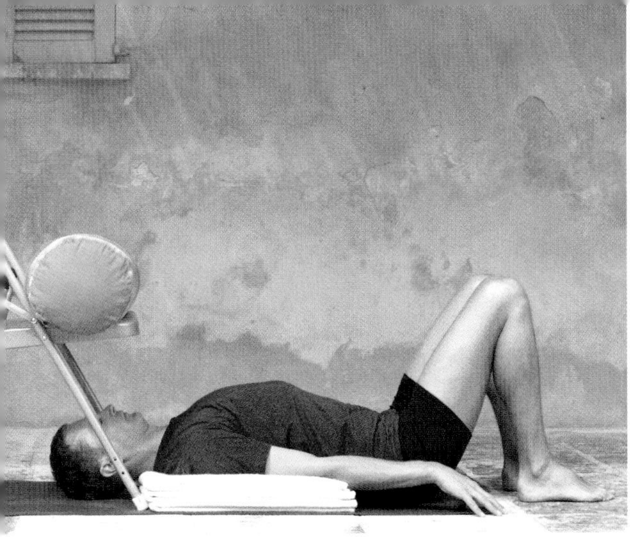

1 Place 3-5 folded blankets in front of a chair, a bolster on its seat. Recline with the tops of your shoulders at the edge of the blanket. Bend your knees, feet hip-width apart.

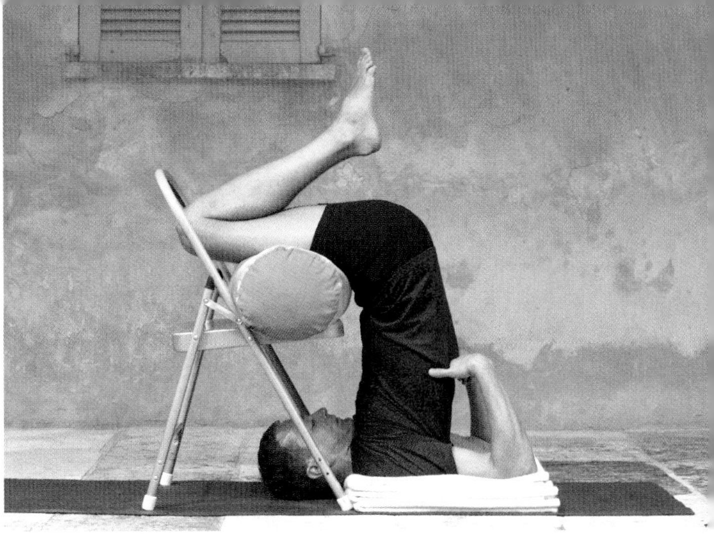

2 Exhale, lift your hips and buttocks, and place your palms on either side of your spine. Rest your thighs on the bolster.

Halasana

Plough Pose (with props)

"The most interesting observation of the usage of props is that they allow 90 per cent of the practitioners to stick to their practices. At the Institute, those who perform independently come hours before the class and practise on props and ropes. This shows that props inspire them more towards yoga."

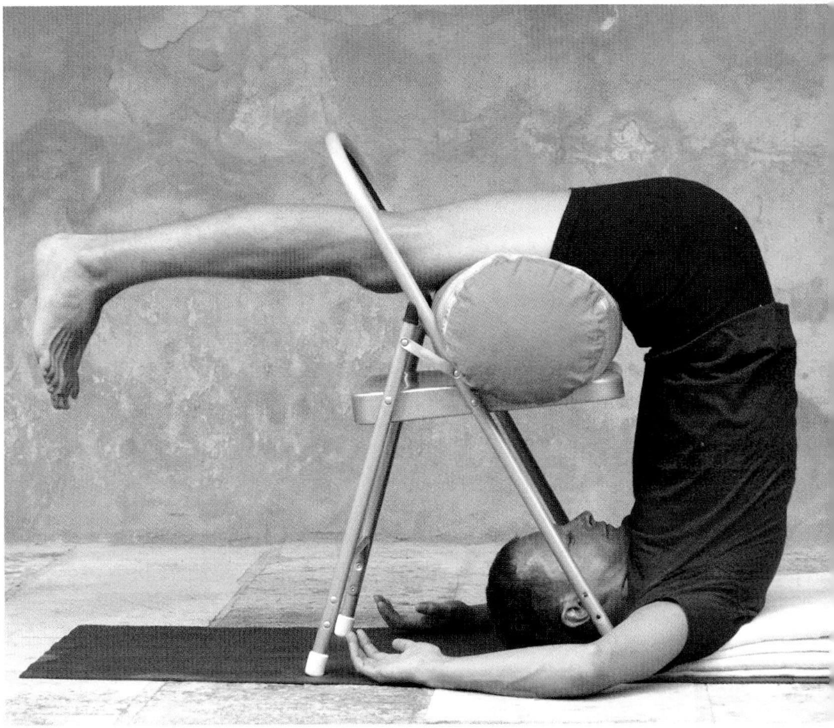

3 Lower first one leg then the other through the back of the chair. Extend your arms along the floor, parallel to each other on either side of your head, palms up. Stretch both legs from heels to thighs. Hold for 3 minutes. Reverse the steps to come out of the pose, then rest.

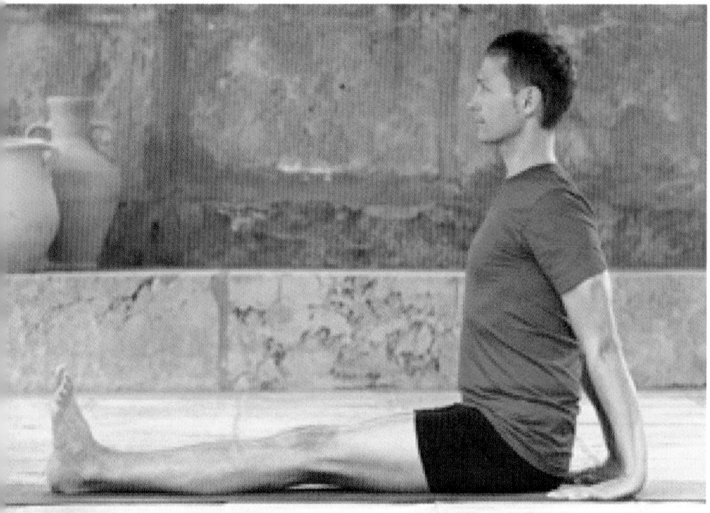

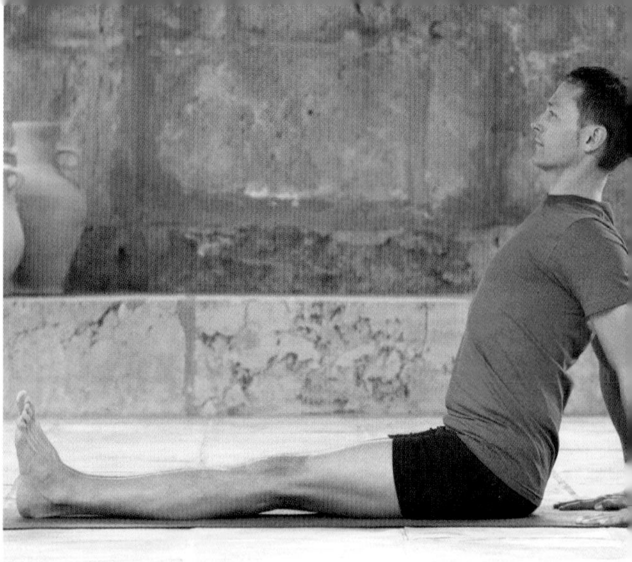

2 Take your hands back and move your dorsal spine in.

1 Sit in Dandasana (see pages 14–15).

Purvottanasana

The Stretch of the East

"The complicating and challenging *āsana* … can be learnt to perfection through props without the sense of strain or stress or fear of injury. I do not like anyone to depend on them, but use them for educating the body and mind. I continue even now, to think and develop new props. I have not yet lost my creative thinking. I am now 90 years young, and I happily use the props to retain and sustain my practices rather than escaping them on the pretext of my age. Even at this age, my body is strong, my mind is agile, and my intelligence is steady and clear."

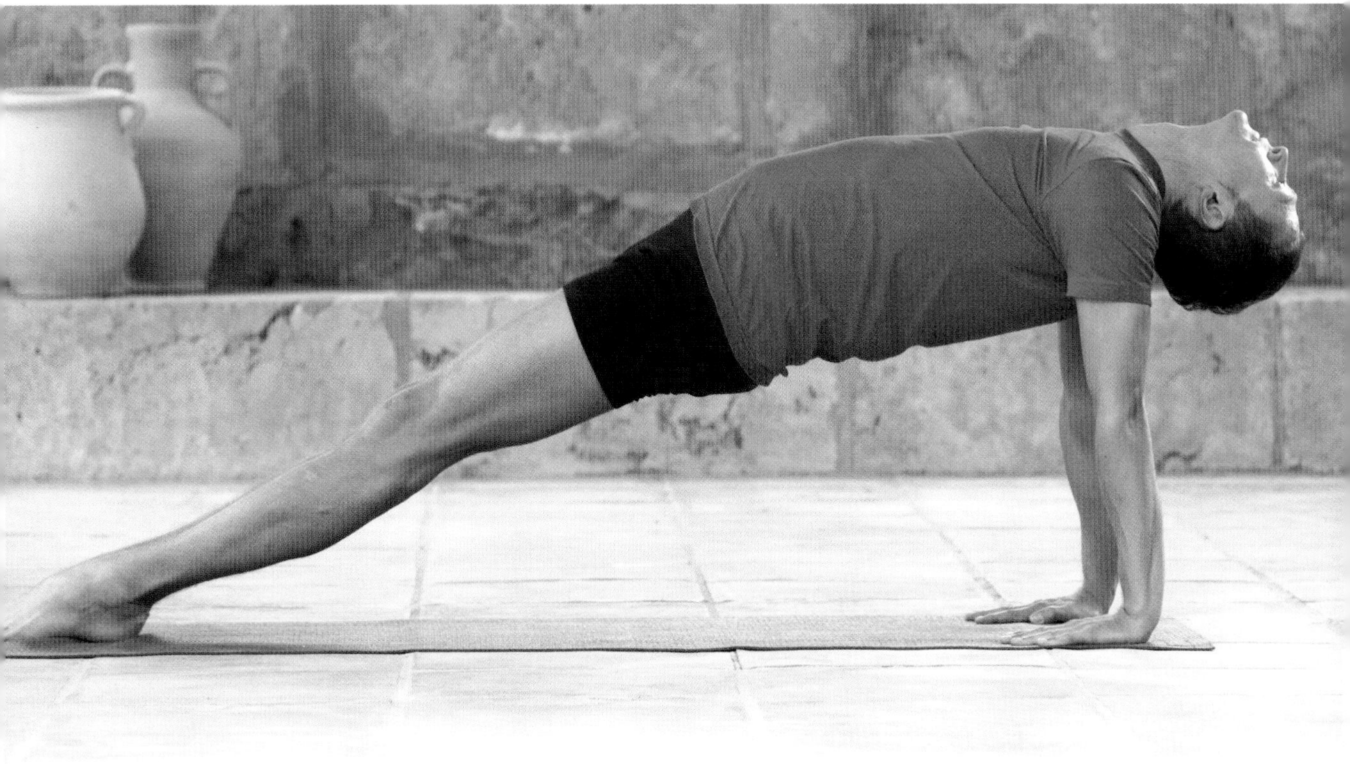

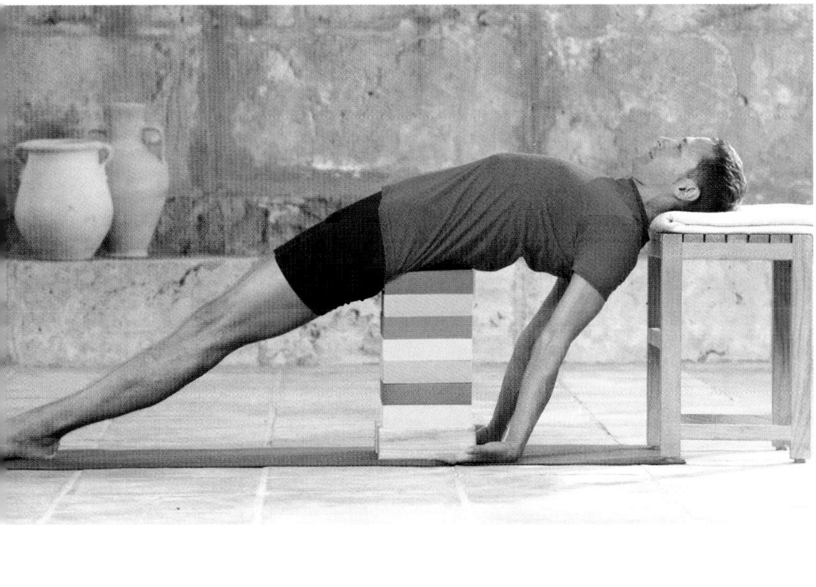

3 Exhale, press into your hands and feet, and lift your body, keeping your knees bent. Straighten your arms and legs, lift your hips, and press your toes down. Stretch your head and neck back. Hold for 1 minute. Exhale, bend your elbows and knees, and lower yourself back to Dandasana.

Pose with props: Fold a blanket on a stool. Stack enough bricks and blocks to support your tailbone when your head is on the blanket. Sit on the blocks, then lift your chest, and incline your trunk back to rest your head on the blanket. Relax your arms by your side, palms up, stretch your legs, and press your feet down. Hold for 3–5 minutes. Bend your knees, place your hands on the blocks, then sit up.

"The only thing I am doing is to bring out the in-depth, hidden qualities of yoga to the awareness of you all."

The Iyengar Legacy

Q. Not only has your name become known in the world, but also your yoga, so people speak of "Iyengar Yoga". I believe you don't accept this distinction.

"How can I give my name to a universal art? Because they learnt from me, the pupils began to identify my teaching compared to others and started naming my work as 'Iyengar yoga'. As yoga has spread like wildfire, my students shortened the terminology by calling my work as 'Iyengar yoga'. But how can an individual name prefix this great art which is existing since time immemorial? Only I must have revitalized this art by new adaptations and made it palatable, attractive, and educative by linking up what was missing in the progressive sequential practice in this chain of yoga. I was blessed by the grace of God, as well as by my *guru,* to find out the various missing links in each movement of motion and action in the body and the flow of the breath. With my *sādhanā,* whether it is *āsana* or *prāṇāyāma,* I not only observed the movements but the moments also while I practised which gave the depth of understanding of the *āsana* and *prāṇāyāma.*

God and my *guru* graced me to look, think with understanding, and feel while in the *āsana* and *prāṇāyāma,* about the state of the body, mind, breath awareness, intelligence, existence of consciousness, and presence of the self.

First I started learning the physical aspect due to my ill health, but the tremendous inner urge inside me made me feel that energy flowing along with the consciousness. I started uniting that infinite flow within the finite body, which is the frame for the flow of life's elixir. This new method of uniting the energy with the consciousness, which I gave to people, brought a new awareness on yoga and for convenience sake they call it as Iyengar Yoga. Unfortunately, it shouldn't be called that way at all. I cannot stop people, though I have shown my uneasiness by protesting against it."

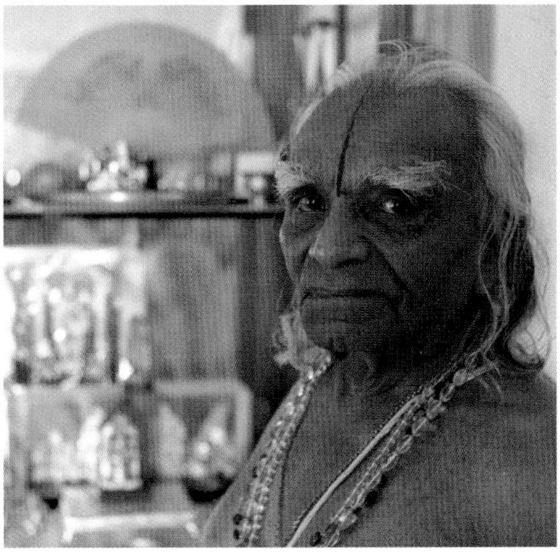

A lifetime of achievement: Guruji beside one of the numerous display cabinets at the Institute filled with awards from statesmen, universities and medical bodies across the globe.

"It is wrong to differentiate traditional yoga from Iyengar yoga...there is no distinction between one yoga and another; they all have the same root and the same purpose."

Question from "Meeting B.K.S. Iyengar", interview in London May 1984, published in Yoga Today *(now* Yoga and Health, *UK) July 1984 and August 1984.*

"If the slightest idea comes to me that my body cannot take it, I am lost.... So I practise with more zeal than before."

A Continuing Practice

Q. Have you felt your own practice changing as the years go on?
"I won't say changing – no. My practice is not changing. It is transforming. It is becoming subtler and finer. The change is impermanent. There can be constant changes occurring, and one may progress or regress in those changes. In me, only progressive transformation is taking place."

Q. What sort of transformations are you finding now?
"Clarity, precision, the feel of the inside body. Even my toe – if it's slightly wrong, I know my toe has gone wrong. Can you know that in your practice? Tell me."
– *Not usually.* –

"You can see me when I am practising, I will tell you which knee is out, which calf muscle is in, which toe, nail is stretching straight and so forth, as my presentation appears perfect. You cannot perceive these defects, until I say and you look. This I consider transformation. The light is coming from within to those areas. In the early days there was no light, it was all darkness.

All these years I practised yoga to get maturity in my body and mind. Now I am practising yoga after maturity. Then I was seeking. Now, I am seeing. Even if it is a small or petty mistake, it reflects on me at once. Being a raw student, you may not understand. As you go on practising, one day this illuminative light also may dawn on you. For me, previously it was all crude, now the subtle things surface. In the earlier days I used to think like you, 'This muscle is not working, that one is not working.' Today my cells speak to me. My mind speaks to me at once. I perceive the movement of my energy, of my mind, of my intelligence. Not only do I observe, but I am with myself – I am there. This is concentration and meditation. A hunter hunts in the jungle, I hunt within me. A searcher wanders in a wonderland; I wander within myself....

When people see me doing the most difficult *āsana,* they say, 'He just does *āsana.*' But what am I seeing inside is unknown to them. They cannot see that. A saint may meditate. Can you see his meditation? Do you know what he does? He says that he is seeing God, then do you see what he sees? How do you know what I see when I do *āsana*? Do you know how I penetrate within myself? Do you know how I penetrate the opaque body so that it becomes transparent? Not only each and every part of my body, but my mind, intelligence, and consciousness become transparent to me. This transparency reflects the very being. That is the transformation."

Q. Do you still find challenges in your practice?

"Yes, the challenges have to be there, but these challenges today are quite different. Previously I used to challenge the body, now the body challenges me. Nature plays its own role. The body hasn't got that strength which it had years ago. So I have to fight. Earlier my mind was demanding the body to do in certain way. Now the body says what the mind has to see and feel in the *āsana.*

At this stage I am a bit at the precipice. The body is giving way. If I surrender to this weakness, I am lost."

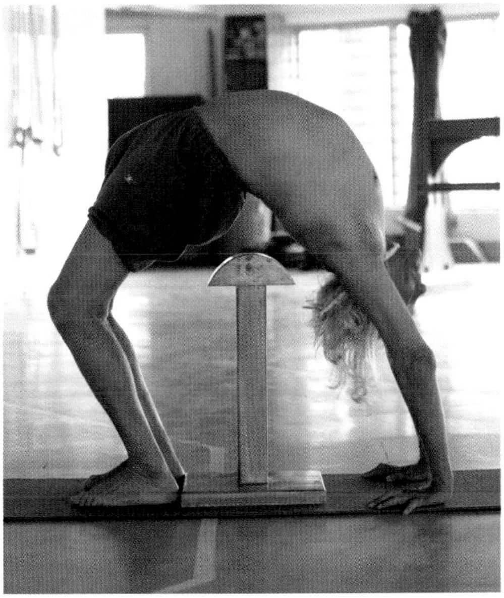

Guruji spends 2–3 hours each morning on personal practice in the main hall at RIMYI, beginning with supported and then unsupported backbends, such as Urdhva Dhanurasana.

From "Iyengar Looks Back", interview by Anne Cushman, Yoga Journal, *December 1997.*

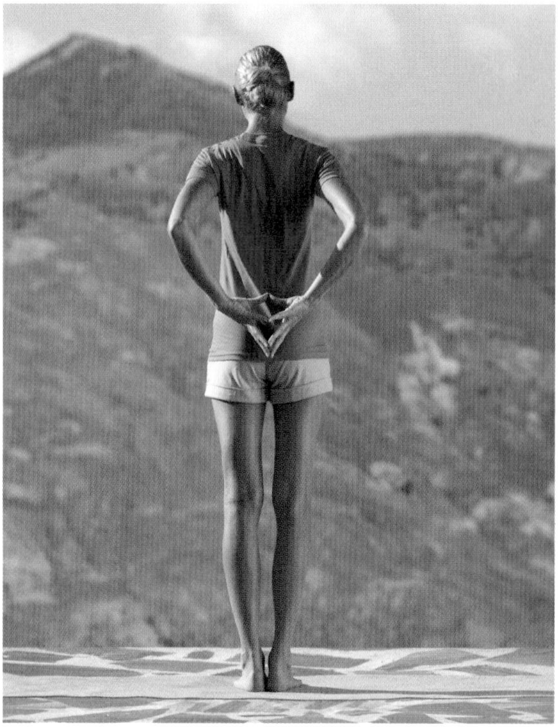

1 Stand in Tadasana (see pages 26-27). Stretch out your arms, then take them behind your back. Join the tips of the fingers of both hands, with your fingers pointing down.

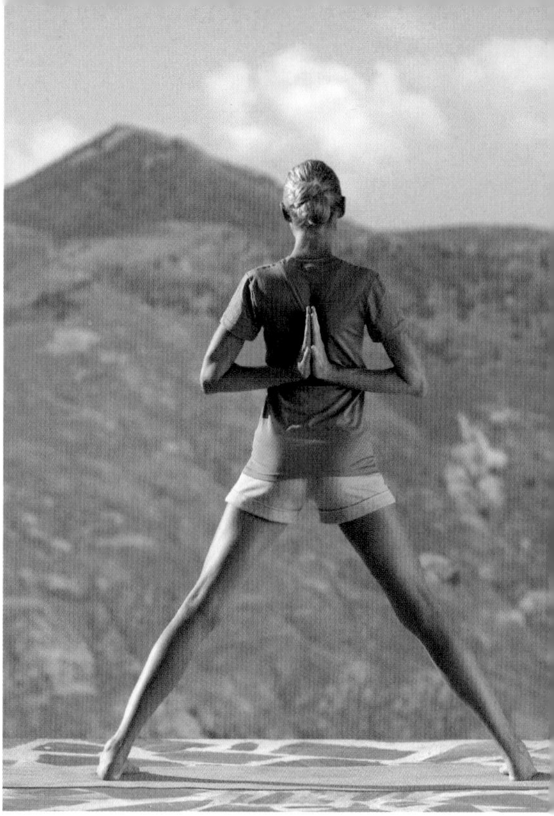

2 Rotate your wrists so your fingers point inwards, then move your spine forwards and up. Press your palms together and slide them up between your shoulder-blades. Draw your shoulders and elbows down and back, and press your fingers and palms together. Exhale and jump your feet 90cm (3ft) apart.

Parsvottanasana

Intense Torso Stretch

"If *āsana* has to be complete you cannot forget any part. You cannot remain absent anywhere. The body and mind both have to be free from pleasure and pain to experience fullness in the practice of an *āsana*. The completeness brings contentment. Contentment leads towards quietude."

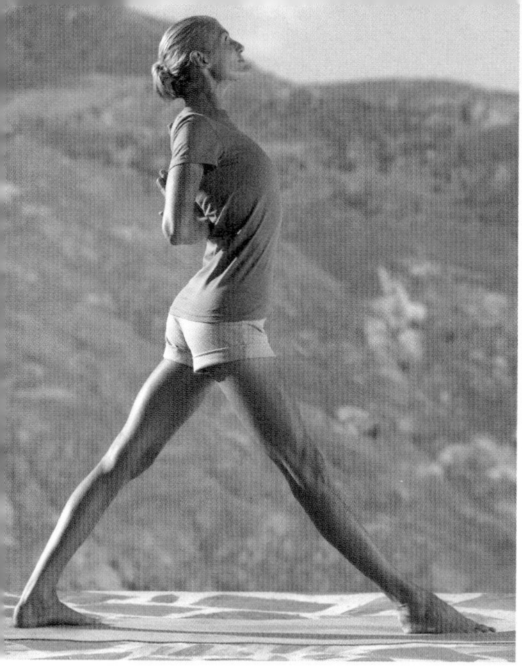

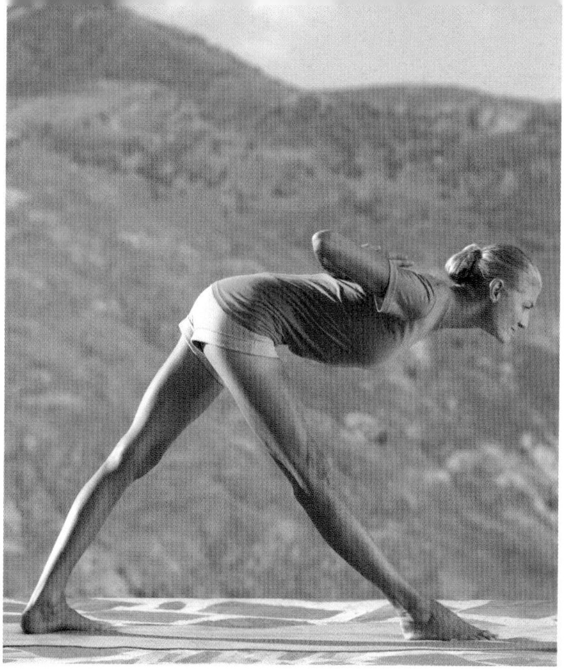

3 Turn your left foot in by 60', your right leg and foot 90° to the right. Rotate your torso 90° forwards. Inhale, lift your abdomen and chest and look up. Curve back over your fingers.

4 Straighten your head and, on an exhalation, extend forwards from the tops of your thighs. Press your palms together to open your chest and extend your spine until your trunk is parallel to the floor.

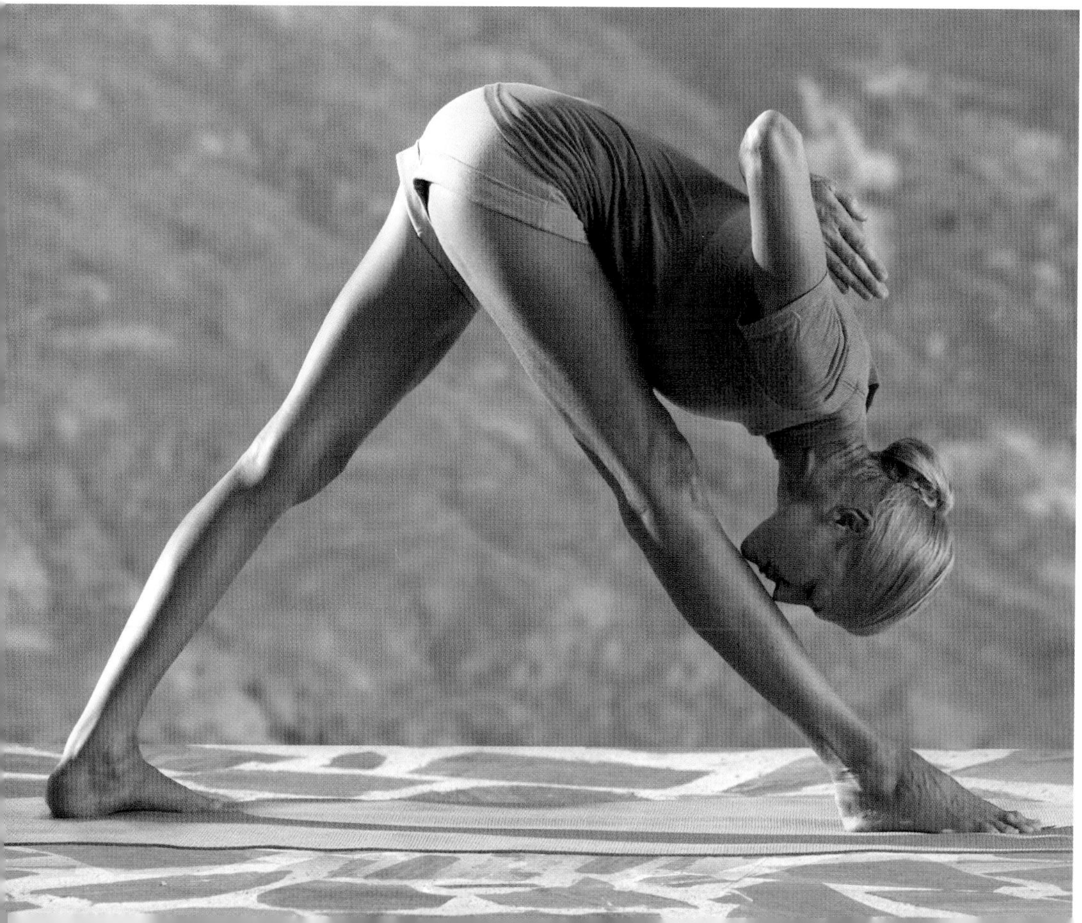

5 Continue to extend your trunk evenly to bring your chest towards your right thigh and your head towards your shinbone, until your nose, lips, and chin rest beyond your knee. Hold for 20-30 seconds, breathing evenly. Inhale, lift your trunk to return to step 2, then repeat to the other side. Finish in Tadasana.

"In the mornings I do advanced asana and in the evenings recuperative asana so that I am fit for the next morning."

A Day in the Life

Q. Could you run through your day for us..., what time do you get up in the morning?
"Previously, I used to get up at three-thirty or four in the morning for years.... I used to practise like a fanatic sometimes even at three o'clock in the mornings. But now as I am semi-retired, I take it easy... I'm semi-retired and in a semi-retirement I just want to remain in studentship. Now I get up at five-thirty or so. Though I am awake I may only be tossing on my bed, as I do not like to disturb others. I have a cup of coffee, finish my morning chores and do *prāṇāyāma* for one hour. After doing *prāṇāyāma* for one hour, I glance through the morning papers."
– I can't imagine you being very interested in newspapers. –
"Well, one should be in contact with the world at the same time in order to know what is happening around the world."

Q. Do you take any interest in India's favourite subject, politics?
"I'm interested in politics but I don't get involved in politics. I see the right and the wrong of the politicians and society. In politics, power has become important and not the humility to serve the poor in helping them in education, health, and to meet their daily needs. That is a pity, for me."

Q. When you finish your newspaper reading, what time of day is it?
"After *prāṇāyāma,* I glance through, but I read the editorials.... I get three or four newspapers. *(Laughs.)* After reading the papers, I have another cup of coffee..."
– Haven't we got to about nine o'clock then... –
"Yes, the classes end at nine. So, I adjust the timings for my practice after the class and not earlier.... So I am there at nine-fifteen to eleven-fifteen or eleven-thirty and I'll be practising. Sometimes students who come to practice ask me questions and I answer them as I practise. Then I go home, take bath, pray and have a little food and then relax for half an hour."

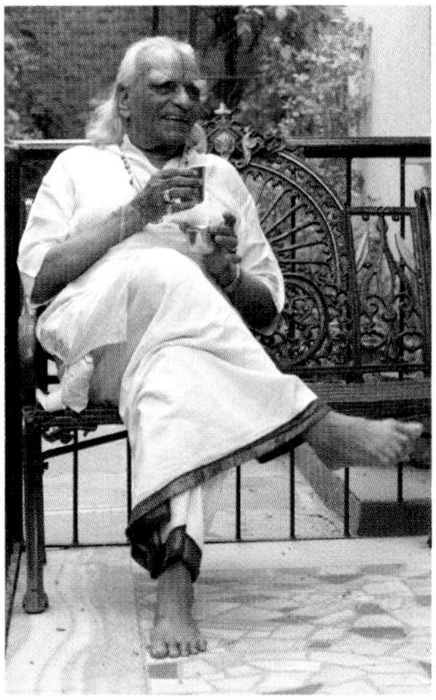

The guru's daily schedule is as regular as sunrise and sunset seven days a week. He regards it as reverence to the "Universal spirit".

Q. How long do you pray for?

"... About fifteen, twenty minutes."

– Do you have a little pūja... –

"Yes, I've got in my room...my family deity.... I've installed it in my room and I sit there...."

– Then after that, that takes... –

"I relax for about half an hour or so, and I come to the library, reply to letters, read some books, write on the subject, up to six in the evening...."

Q. By this time, you have only had one very light snack in the whole day?

"Yes." *– And aren't you hungry? –*

"No, I'm not. It was built up from the childhood and now it has become a natural thing for me...."

Q. So when is your main meal of the day?

"Only in the night, at about eight-thirty or nine."

– And what would that meal consist of, vegetables? –

"Vegetables, rice, curds and sometimes *rasam*. That's all. Very mild, light food. I can take food with anyone, in any party, anywhere though I'm a practitioner of yoga."

Q. And television?

"Yes! I see. There is a news item at nine o'clock and if there are good things, I see. Sports, because I'm fond of all sports. Then there are serials, dramas, which I see, and then I go to bed...it would be about ten-thirty or eleven o'clock. And sometimes I play with my grandchildren in the evening, have fun with them...."

From "Yoga – Head to Toe", interview for BBC Radio 4 by Mark Tully in Pune April 1999.

"People remind me of my age, but while practising I am beyond my body and its age."

Yoga and Ageing

"Ageing is a natural phenomenon. It is growth from childhood to adolescence, to middle age and to old age. It is a change from one phase of life to another phase although the owner remains the same.

The fragrance of life in each of us begins to dry out as we age, similar to a sapling which grows into a healthy, gigantic tree bearing tasty fruits each year and then withers away.

I am also ageing but my yogic practice, for hours together, is very regular like the rising and the setting of the sun. I began yoga when I was sixteen to free myself from my sickly existence. I gained good health after four years of regular practice and this encouraged me to share my knowledge of yoga with people who are suffering – as I did. I have relentlessly worked to make yoga attractive and appealing and have carried the message of 'yoga for health in body and peace in mind' throughout the world and am glad that now yoga is considered as a form of alternative medicine.

I have gained sixty years of bonus life because of my regular practice, therefore I am not afraid of death. I am ready to embrace death with ease because through yoga I made life worthy for myself and for others. I still continue with my early practices so that I can have a natural, majestic, and noble death. I have given my own example to encourage people of my age group to take to yoga.

I feel that old age is a blessing which brings with it a great deal of respect from the youth, provided one pays attention to keep oneself healthy and is not dependent upon others like a parasite. At this age, one should reflect on one's thoughts and one's

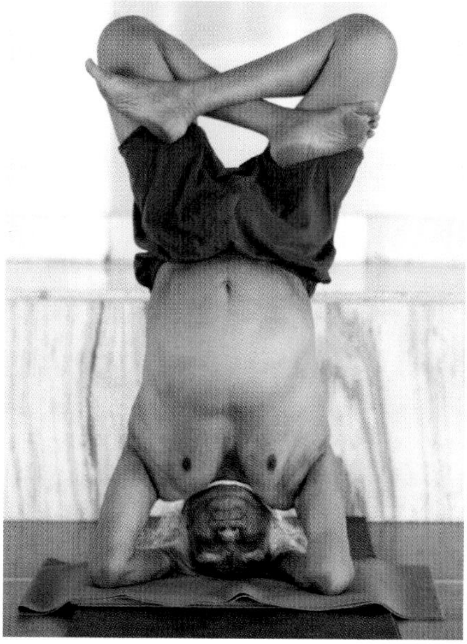

"Even though age is telling upon me," says Guruji, "I am still experiencing new feelings" in daily practice, which includes inversions such as Padmasana in Sirsasana. He shares this insight with his pupils.

actions. One should guide one's family and friends so that they do not commit the same mistakes as oneself, which acted as a stumbling block in one's progress through life.

God has given us this body to evolve in the spiritual world and it is meant to serve one's self as well as one's surroundings.

The body ages but the soul does not. When one is aged, the mind fuels a negative attitude towards life. By the power of will over mind, old age can be lived benevolently through yogic practices. ”

From "Yoga and Old Age", a talk for senior citizens, published in Yoga Rahasya *Volume 3, number 1.*

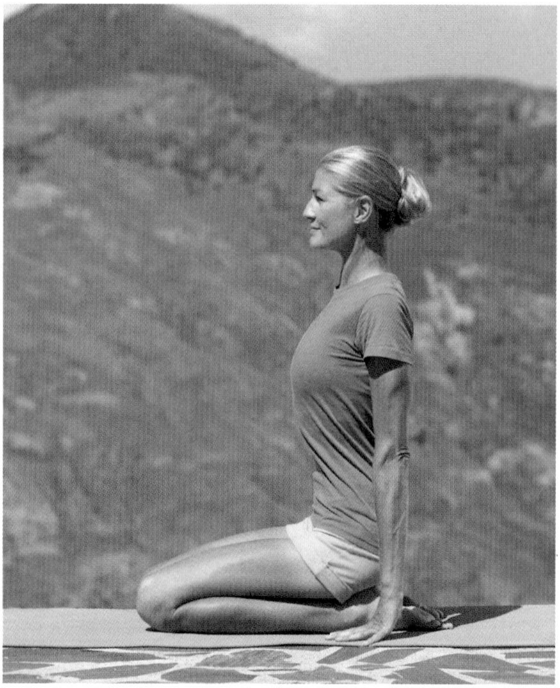

1 Sit in Virasana (see pages 138–39). Place your hands on the floor beside your hips. Align your spine and stretch upwards. Lift your sternum and open your chest.

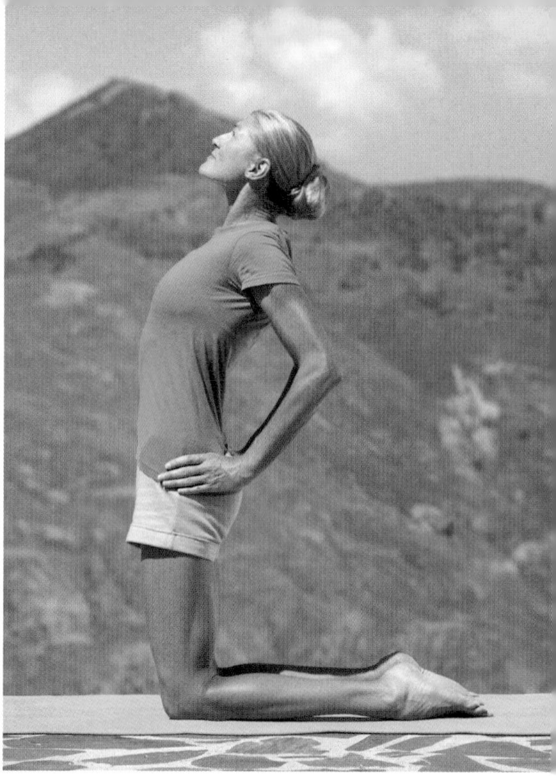

2 Kneel with your knees and feet hip-width apart and your thighs perpendicular to the floor. Place your hands on your hips. Tuck in your buttocks, extend your spine, and open the chest.

Ustrasana

Camel Pose

"I do not get pains or aches like you, but I feel dryness and shrinking sensation in the sternum while doing backbends. This is how I have learned how old age sets in. The sternum is known as a dry area, where energy recedes. Even a doctor will tell you that this area is a bony structure and movement is very little....and again with my determinative practice, I eradicated this dryness and shrinkage."

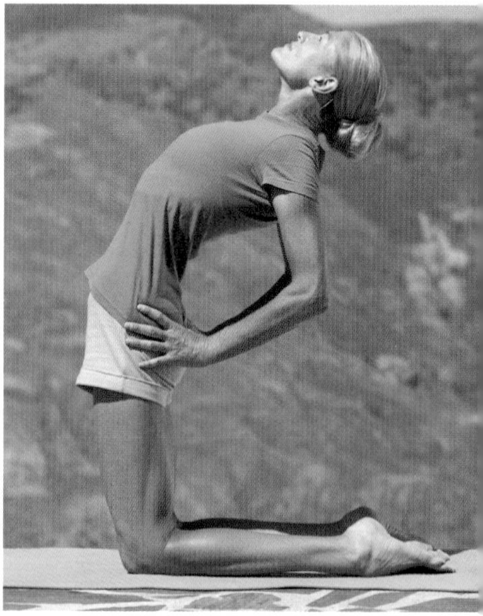

3 Exhale and curve your trunk backwards. Keep your thighs perpendicular to the floor and your chest well lifted.

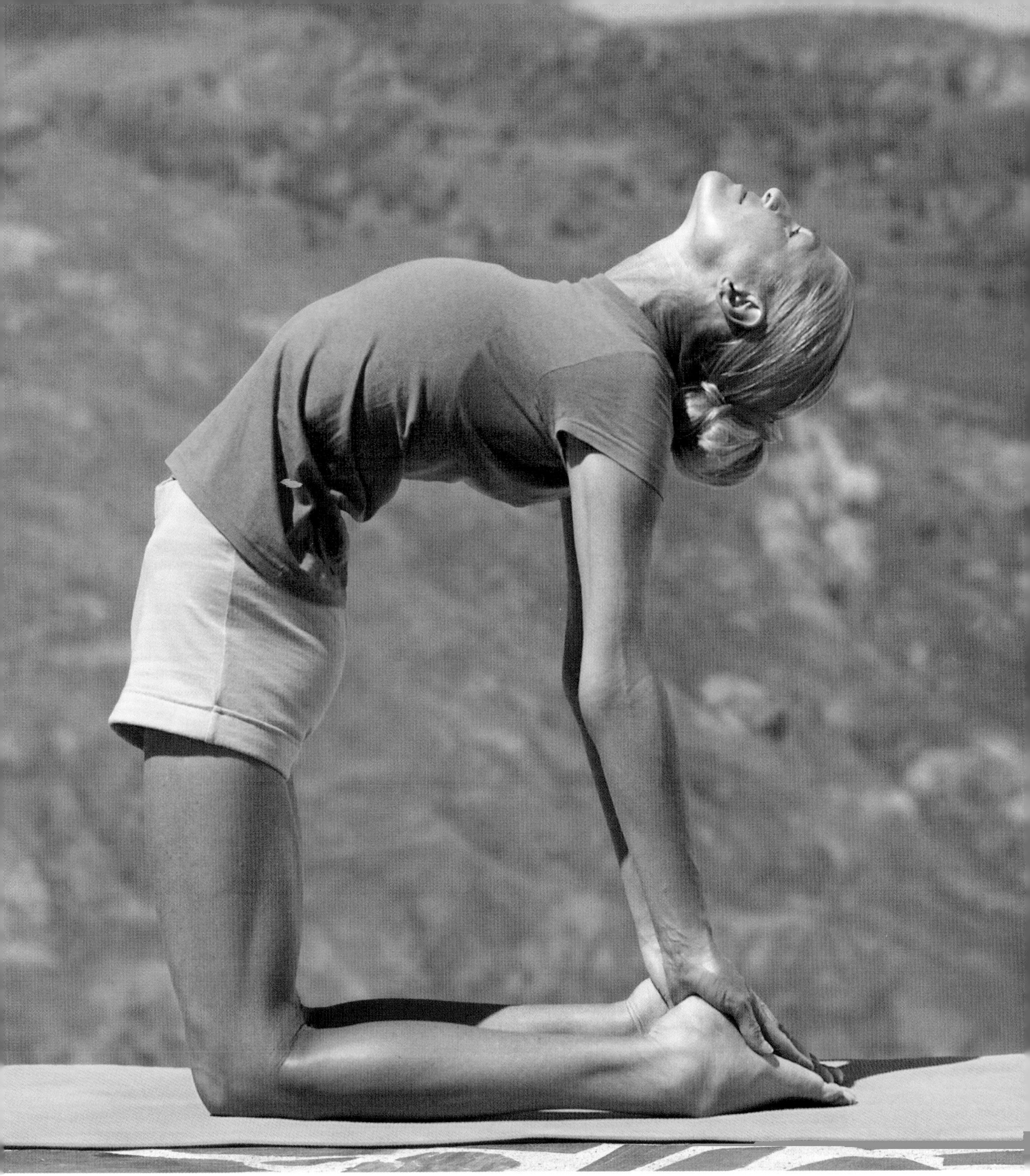

4 Take your arms towards your feet, reaching back towards your toes. Press your hands onto your heels, or the soles of your feet, to move your shoulderblades deeper inside. Keep your neck long, take your head back, and look back. Hold for 20–30 seconds, breathing evenly. Release your hands, lift your head and trunk, then sit in Virasana.

1 Lie face-down with your legs extended and arms by your sides, palms facing upwards. Keep your feet together, knees tight, and toes pointing backwards.

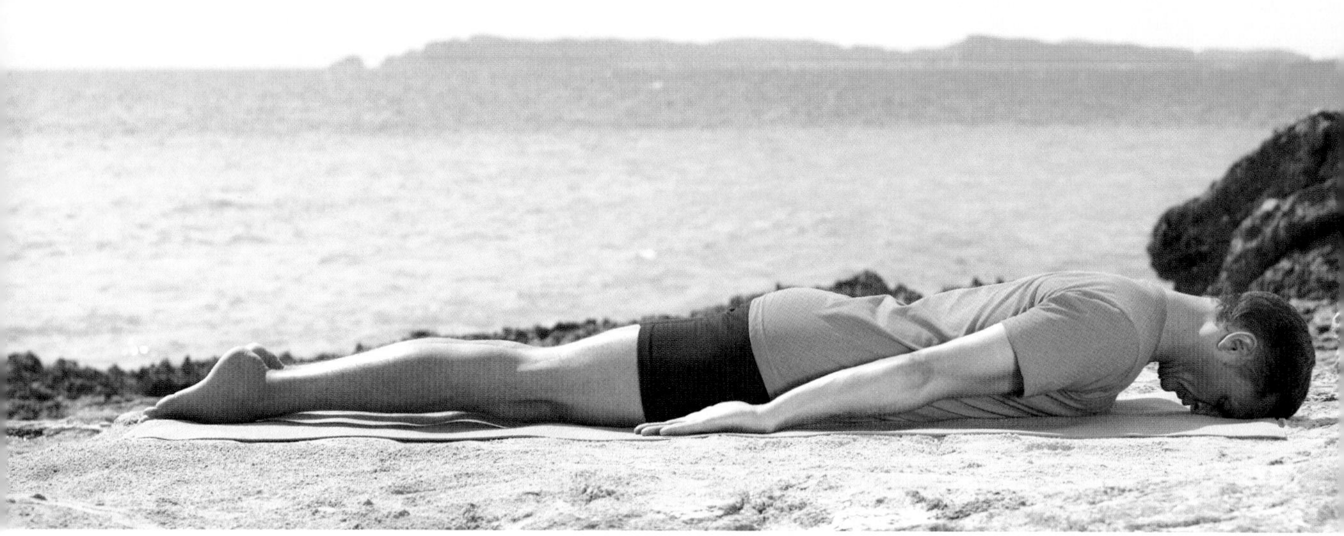

2 Place your palms by your ribs. Inhale, press down firmly on your palms and lift your trunk. Take two breaths.

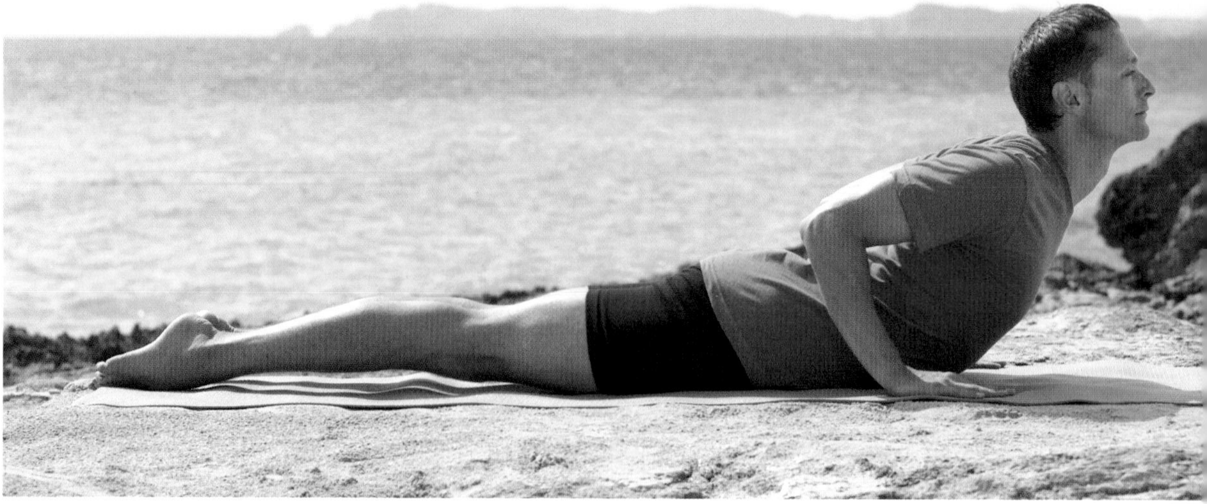

Bhujangasana I

Serpent Pose I

"If one wants a good garden, he needs to tend it each day. The moment he stops taking care of it, it dries up. If one does not use a blade, it rusts. If one needs to play a violin each day, he needs to tune it as well. It is the same with the body, breath, and mind. They need to be tuned each day. Otherwise they become insensitive."

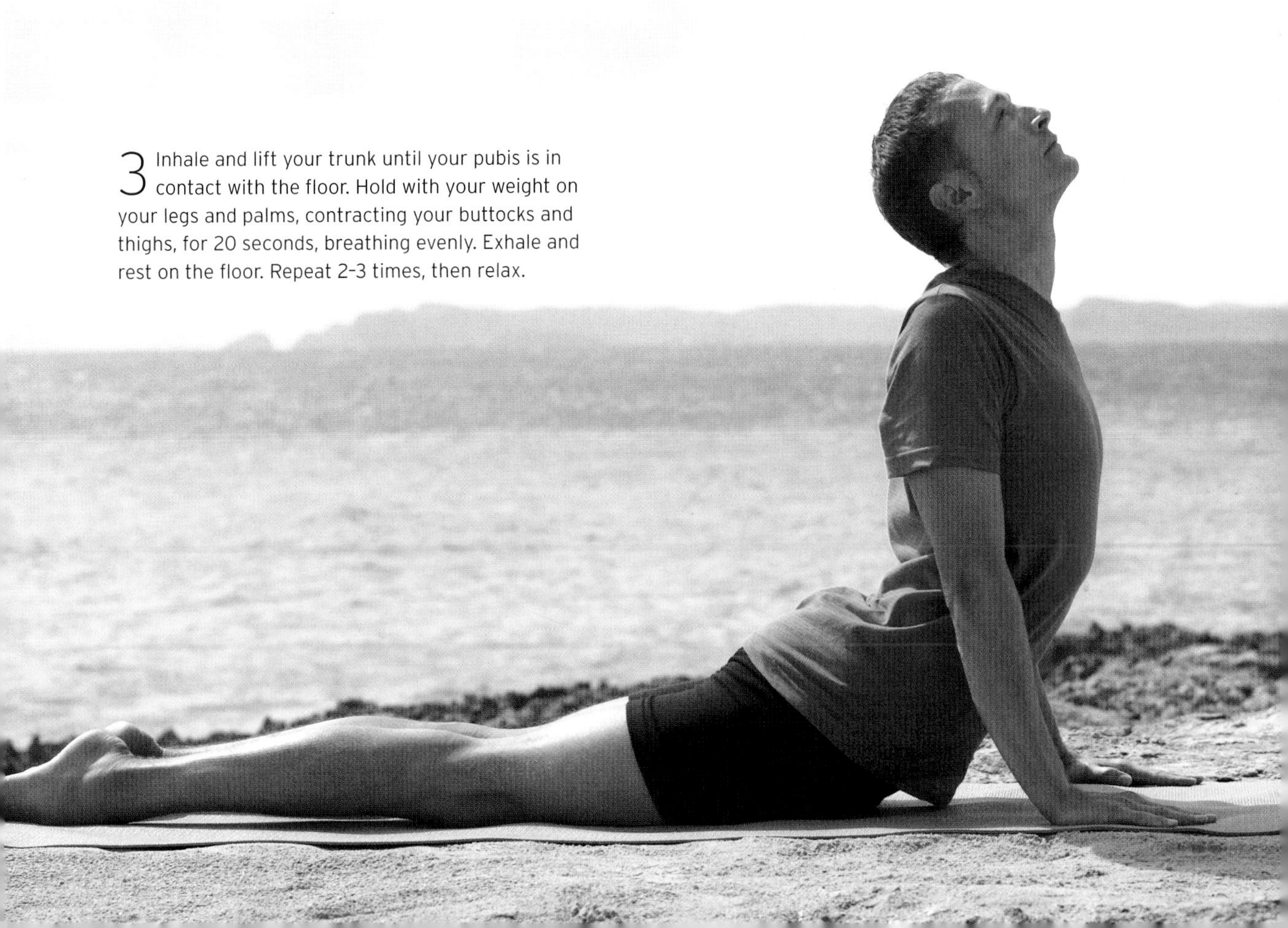

3 Inhale and lift your trunk until your pubis is in contact with the floor. Hold with your weight on your legs and palms, contracting your buttocks and thighs, for 20 seconds, breathing evenly. Exhale and rest on the floor. Repeat 2–3 times, then relax.

On Death and Dying

“Birth and death are beyond man's control. They don't belong to our domain. Life departs when the time comes. According to our scriptures, death is a natural phenomenon of *prakṛti* (nature) while life is *vikṛti* [see glossary], as *Kālidāsa* puts beautifully in *Raghuvaṇśa.* Birth and death are not in our hand. But life in between birth and death needs to be shaped, baked, and cultured. Lord Krishna says that life is in unmanifested form before birth, it becomes manifest after birth, and goes back to its unmanifest form in death (*Bhagavad Gita,* II.28).

Death and dying are two different things. Death is full stop to the present life, but dying is a process. By the word death one should not get frightened by the dying process. It is told that: 'Every form of meditation is in essence a rehearsal of death.' But I do not think so. For me meditation is a new life. It is a death from worldly pleasures and enlivenment towards spiritual light. A Zen adage says, 'If you die before you die, then when you die, you won't die.' This means that one has to live positively until death. This is what *abhiniveśa* means. We die due to the fear of death rather than actual death.

I am neither concerned about death nor dying. But I would say this much. If my body becomes fully non-functional though living, I would consider it as my death. So, I do not waste my time on thinking of death but do yoga to live holistically every moment. Face the fear of dying courageously; then death becomes glorious and majestic.”

"I would like to practise yoga till my last breath, as a humble service to yoga. My only wish is to prostrate before God, surrendering my last breath in a yogic posture."

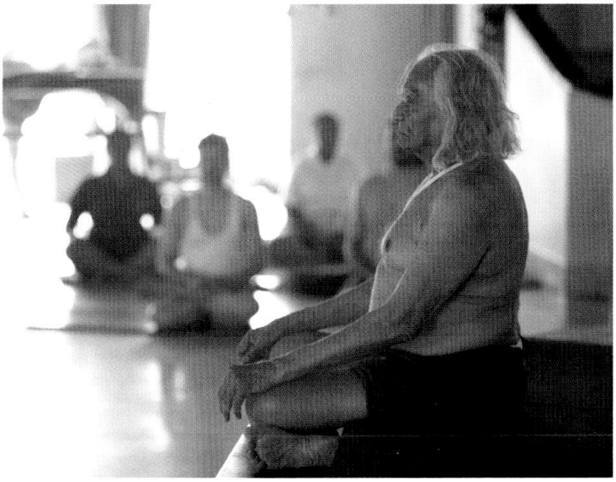

Guruji shares his morning practice space with his pupils, who come from every corner of the globe. "I was supposed to have only lived for twenty years or so, but the practice of yoga has not only made me live a full life of satisfaction and joy, but it has made me its messenger all over the world."

From "The Practical Psychology of Yoga", Aṣṭadaḷa Yogamālā *Volume 7, pp279–80.*

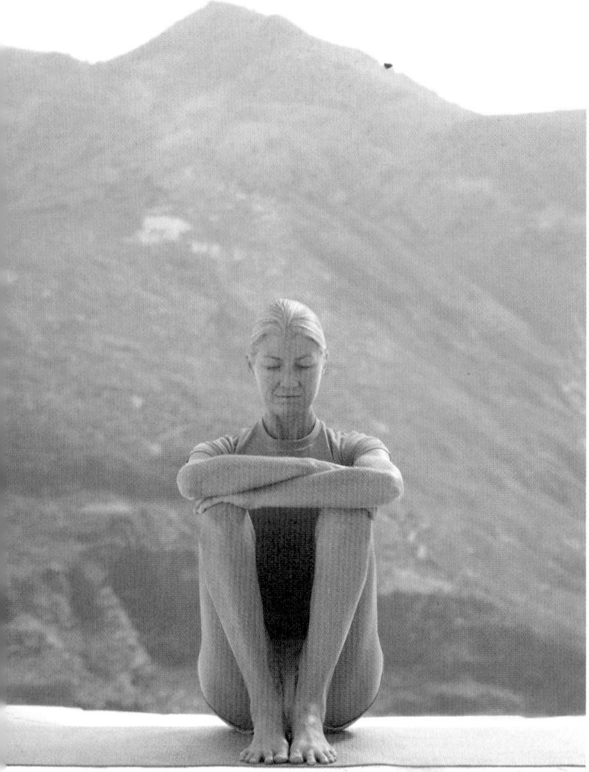

1 Sit in Dandasana (see pages 14–15). Draw your legs in, feet together, to make a straight line from big toes and heels to the centre of your forehead. Rest your buttocks evenly on the floor.

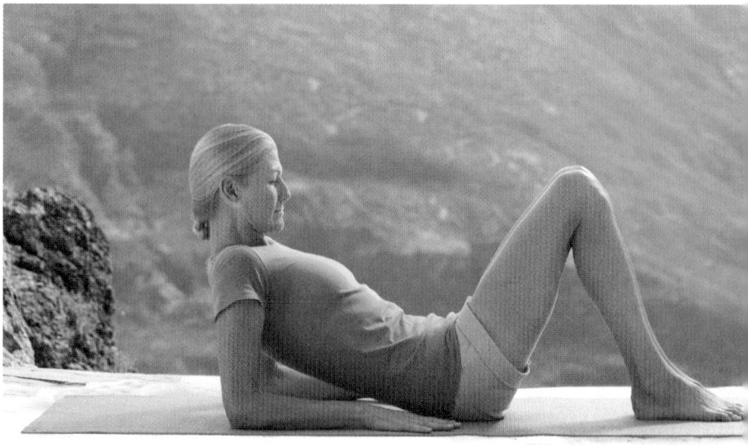

2 Place your palms beside your hips and lean back onto your elbows. Do not move your legs or feet.

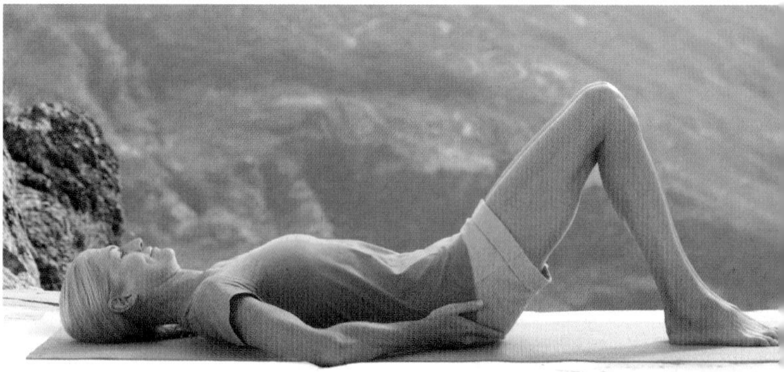

3 Lower your trunk, vertebra by vertebra, until your spine and head rest on the floor without tilting to one side or the other. Check that the backs of your shoulders, buttocks, and hips rest evenly on either side of your spine.

Savasana

Corpse Pose

"By *āsana* practice we can know how to face the ultimate relinquishing of all our attachments and addictions. In *Śavāsana* we begin to train and educate ourselves for surrender.... Learn how to do *Śavāsana* well, that simulates death and brings silence and non-movement. After all, what is death? It is a non-existing and a non-feeling state that one experiences often in *Śavāsana*."

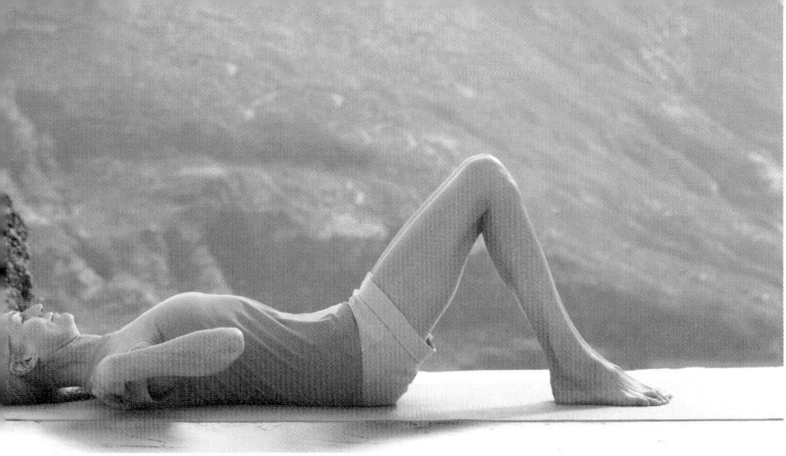

4 Bend your arms and touch your shoulders. Gently elongate the backs of your arms towards your elbows to position your shoulders and shoulderblades evenly. Rest your arms 15° from your sides, palms up. Keep your chin perpendicular and the bridge of your nose parallel to the floor.

5 Close your eyes. Then stretch one leg forwards, keeping it straight, and rest the heel on the floor. Stretch the other leg forwards so that both legs are together and aligned along a straight line. Check that both halves of your body lie evenly on either side of your spine. If you tilt to your stronger side, adjust the weaker side. Keep your head straight.

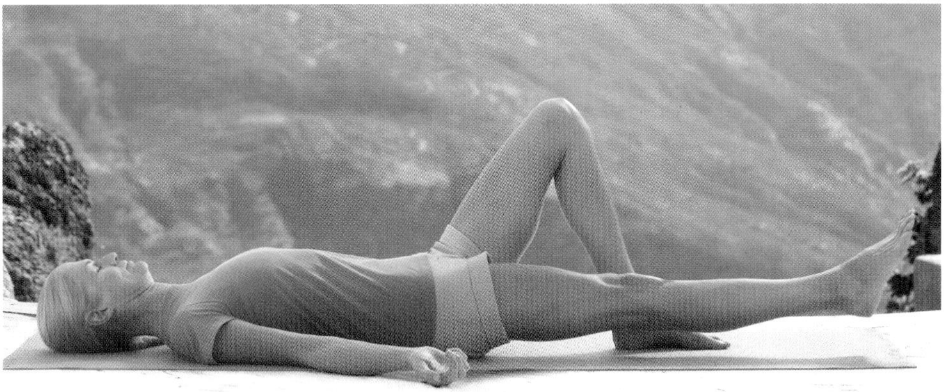

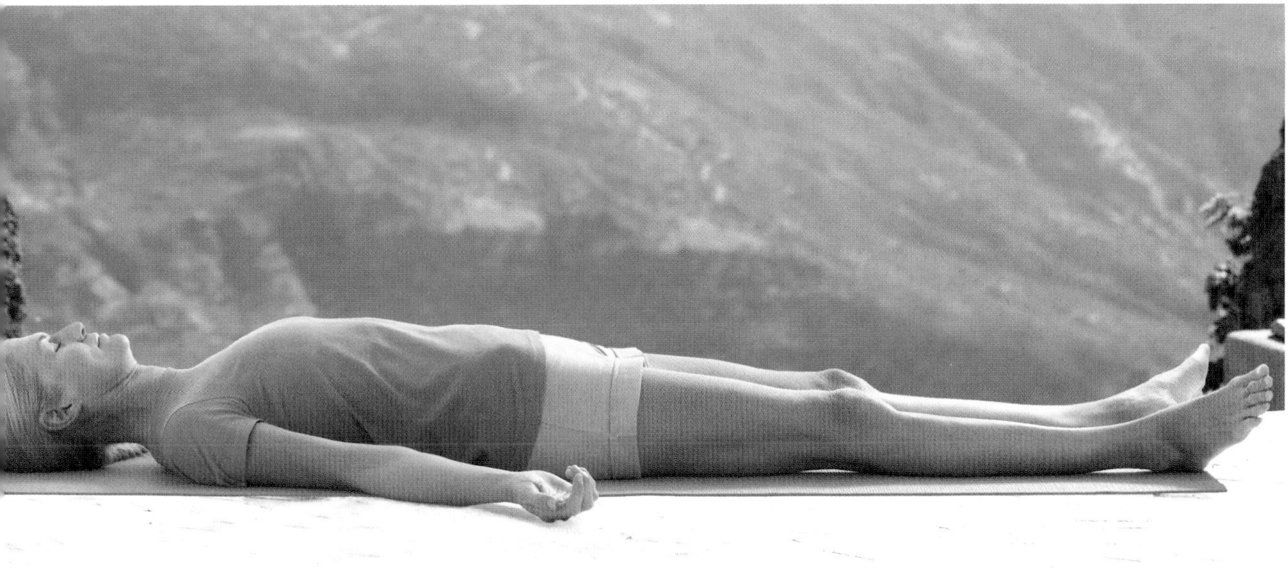

6 Relax your feet away from each other. Roll your shoulders down and relax your arms and palms. Release all expression and let go everywhere. Relax for 10 minutes or more. Open your eyes, lift one arm, then the other to your body and bend your legs, bringing your feet towards your buttocks. Turn to your right to rest before sitting up.

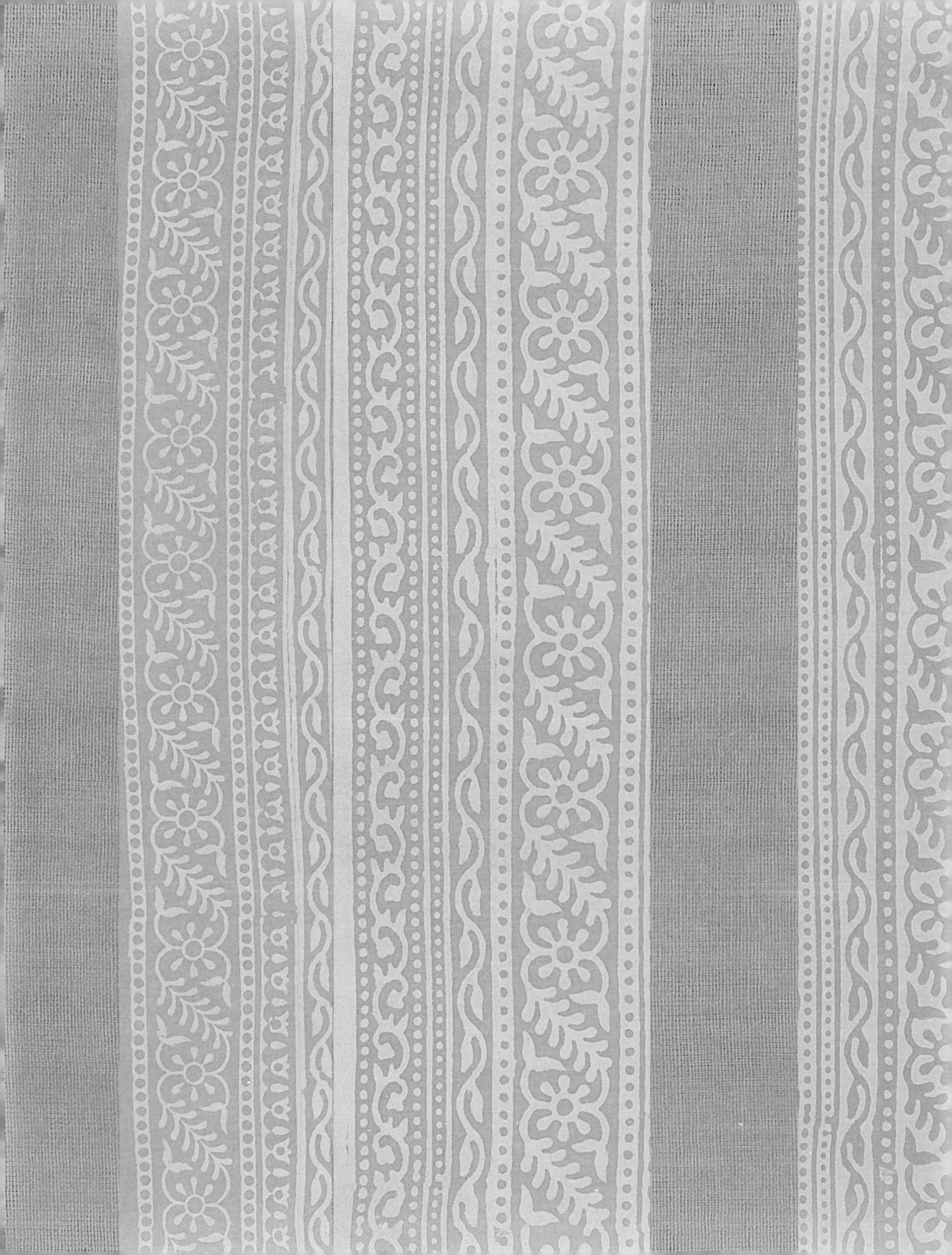

Light on Daily Practice

Yoga Defined

"Our sages enumerated four paths for the evolution of man: *jñāna* (knowledge), *bhakti* (love or devotion), *karma* (action), and *yoga* (control of the consciousness). The trouble and confusion arose with these names when each path began to be called 'yoga', *jñāna yoga*, *bhakti yoga,* and *karma yoga*. As the last path could not be called *yoga yoga*, the subject was sub-divided, bearing different names.

Thus, we have *mantra yoga* (the yoga of thoughtful prayer), *laya yoga* (the yoga of love and dissolution in the object of devotion), *haṭha yoga* (the yoga of firmness and determined discipline), and *rāja yoga* (the royal path of yoga). If one carefully examines these so-called divisions of yoga, one finds that those ways explained are almost identical, with emphasis on one or the other facet of the subject, depending upon the favourite field chosen by the author.

Man is a product of intellect (*vidyā*), intelligence (*buddhi*), emotion, action, and determined will. While the seat of the intellect is the head, the seat of the emotion is the mind. The hands and feet are meant to be the limbs for action. If one is to be pure in action, in love (lust-free emotional life) or in intellectual pursuits, the foundation is the path of yoga. Patañjali, the codifier of yoga, has not called his treatise '*rāja yoga*', but has enumerated it as *aṣṭāṅga yoga* (eight-petalled yoga). The first of these petals is *yama* (social discipline) – the great commandments transcending creed, geographical origin, age, and time, namely, *ahiṁsā* (non-violence), *satya* (truth), *asteya* (non-stealing), *brahmacarya* (continence), and *aparigraha* (non-coveting). The second petal is *niyama* (individual discipline), encompassing *śauca* (purity), *santoṣa* (contentment), *tapas* (ardour or austerity), *svādhyāya* (study of the Self), and *Īśvara praṇidhāna* (devotion to the Lord). The third petal is *āsana* (posture), which brings physical health as well as mental steadiness and lightness. The fourth petal is *prāṇāyāma* (control on breathing), which makes the body and mind fit instruments for the purpose of concentration. The senses are brought under control directly by the mind in the fifth petal, *pratyāhāra*. Then comes the sixth petal, *dhāraṇā* (complete attention of the consciousness on a single point or task). The seventh petal, *dhyāna* or meditation, is an uninterrupted flow of concentration. *Samādhi* is the eighth petal, where the body and senses are at rest as if in sleep, but the mind and reason are alert as if one is awake, beyond the pale of consciousness. ”

"These aspects of yoga are like a gigantic mango tree which starts from the seed to the root, root to the trunk, trunk to the branches, branches sprouting into leaves, leaves aerating the entire tree supplying energy in the form of sap through the bark, and later blossom into flowers, culminating with tasty fruit."

From "Yoga Defined", Bhavan's Journal, *September 1977.*

"I have not called this Iyengar yoga, but others call it so, maybe for the sake of convenience."

Methods of Yoga

Q. There is a difference between yoga practised by others and Iyengar yoga?

"Yes, that is because of the inner sight of Patañjali's, which I brought out not merely in expression but in experiences of the body, mind, and self. The important point in my practice and teaching is the guidance given by Patañjali regarding the interpenetration of attention and touch of awareness of intelligence from the skin to the self and from the self to the skin. The second point is the conscious interweaving together of the physical, physiological, mental, intellectual and spiritual levels of the practitioner. This interweaving and interpenetrating attention that I built up gained ground as time moved on.

I think that many people do not know how to connect the body, the mind, and the soul in their practices. They consider *āsana* as a conative action and say that it is good for the body like any other physical exercise. But they cannot explain how the same can be done connecting the intelligence to ignite and discipline the consciousness to reach the soul. The *āsana* are not mainly the conative actions, but consist of cognitive, mental, intellectual, and spiritual aspects. Therefore, the practitioner has to connect and coordinate all the five sheaths [*see glossary*] of the body while practising *āsana* and *prāṇāyāma*. This I consider as true yoga. On account of my precise presentation and explanation of the yogic philosophy in *āsana* as well as in *prāṇāyāma*, people named it as Iyengar yoga. I never claimed yoga by my name.

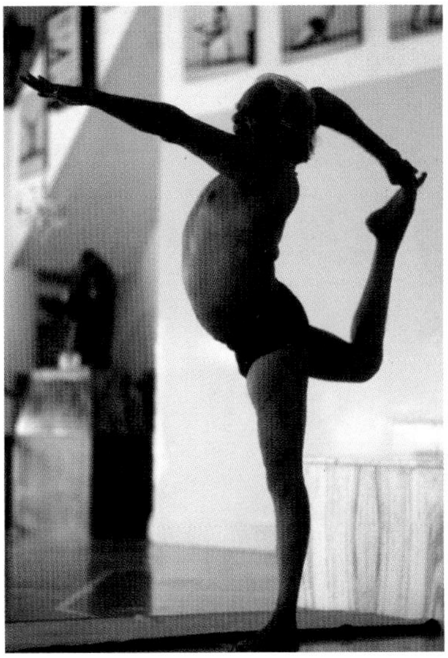

Guruji in Natarajasana demonstrating the importance of keeping the intelligence alert, active and sharp in yoga practice.

We need to train the I-ness through the consciousness – *citta*. The small self or I-ness is the needle and the intelligence is the eye of the needle. The mind is the head of the thread. In order to insert the thread into the eye of the needle, you sharpen the thread with the hand. If the thread is loose or thick it doesn't pass through the eye of the needle. So you sharpen it by wetting it with water or saliva before inserting it into the eye of the needle. In our body, the nervous system, the cellular system, the fibres, the tendons are like threads. The skin fibres, muscle fibres, bone fibres, nerve fibres are threads. The moment the thread is inserted, the mind pierces the eye of the needle, the intelligence, and it disappears. Similarly, in the practice of *āsana*, the mind acts like the sharp edge of the thread, which passes through the intelligence and leads the fibres to sew the body in the right direction.

Then the intelligence takes the lead, the mind disappears or rather it follows the intelligence. The intelligence is the eye of the needle. The intelligence makes the needle to weave the entire body into a perfect cloth. A weaver through his skill weaves the cloth. Similarly, the consciousness, as weaver, skilfully weaves the fabric of our existence. I do this in all the *āsana* and *prāṇāyāma* as well as in *dhyāna*."

From "Yoga – A Divine Embroidery", interview by Zippy Wiener in the Library at RIMYI, August 1997.

"The credit of collating, systematizing and codifying the entire philosophy of yoga goes to Patanjali."

Patanjali and his Yoga Sutra

" Let me tell you a little about the background of Patañjali. He is said to have been born some time between 500 and 200 BC. Nobody can give the exact date because in India the dates of the lives of the great sages were measured according to the grammar that was in vogue during their time.... He had no parents, and according to Indian mythology, was the incarnation of Lord Ādiśeṣa.

Ādiśeṣa is a great King Cobra whose body is the seat of Lord Vishnu. It is said that once Lord Shiva, the king of dance, invited Lord Vishnu and other deities to see his famous dance, *tāṇḍava nṛtya*. As Lord Shiva danced, Lord Vishnu became absorbed in it. He began to vibrate with the rhythm of the graceful movements of Lord Shiva. Lord Vishnu was seated on Ādiśeṣa, the great cobra. The great King Cobra became breathless under the weight of the Lord, which was increasing, and began gasping for air. When the dance came to an end, Ādiśeṣa felt the lightness in the Lord's body. Amazed by this change of weight, he asked the Lord, 'How is it that you were so heavy when Lord Shiva was dancing and as soon as the dance finished you became light?' Lord Vishnu replied, 'I was so fully engrossed in His movements that my nerves and body vibrated as if I myself were dancing. That is why you felt it'. Seeing how impressed Lord Vishnu was with the dance, Ādiśeṣa decided to learn the dance himself.... He began looking for a mother who was both a

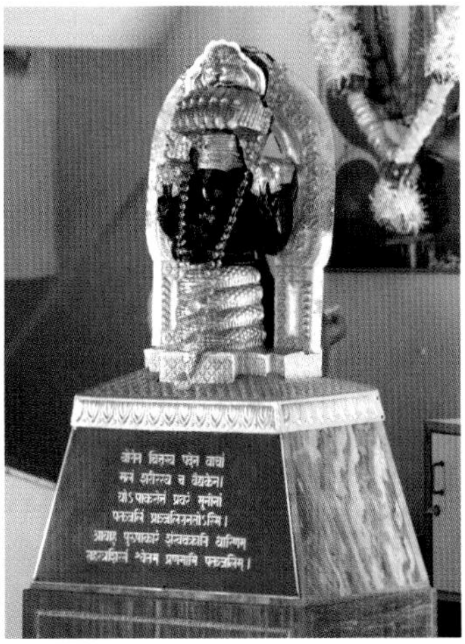

Students pay their respects to the Patanjali statue in the main hall at RIMYI before class.

yogini and a *tapasvini* (a woman who had done much yoga and fervent penance).... After some time he found Gauṇika, who had no children and who had done penance for several years. She was praying to the rising sun.... She took some water to offer as oblation, closed her eyes, and prayed. As she opened her eyes to offer the water to the Sun God, she saw a very tiny snake moving in the water that she was holding in her palms. At first she was terrified and said, 'What polluted water I have taken!' As she was saying this, the tiny snake at once assumed human form, prostrated and begged her to accept him as her son. She accepted him as her son and named him Patañjali – *pata* means fall and *anjali* means the folding of the hands during prayer. He is also known as Gauṇika *putra* (son of Gauṇika). Thus, Patañjali means 'fallen into the palms at the time of prayer'.... Eventually Patañjali completed his first duty, the commentary on grammar. Then he decided to learn dance. As he was learning dance the idea struck him that the various movements of the body could be used for understanding the functions of the body. He studied the system of the body, using the knowledge of matter, the elements, and their qualities. Through the study of the outer and inner body he brought out the system called *Āyurveda*. *Āyuḥ* means life and *veda* means knowledge, so *āyurveda* is the knowledge of life.... Finally, he composed the aphorisms on yoga, known as the *Yoga Sūtra*. ”

From "Essence of the Yoga Sūtra of Patañjali", Aṣṭadaḷa Yogamālā *Volume 1, pp200–202.*

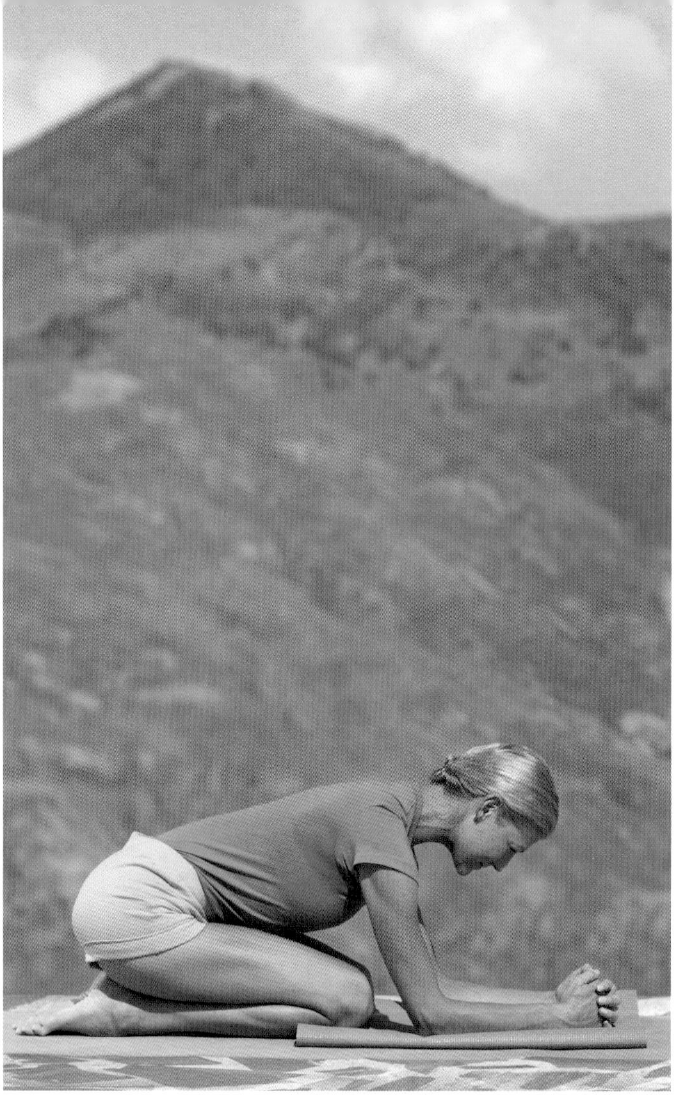

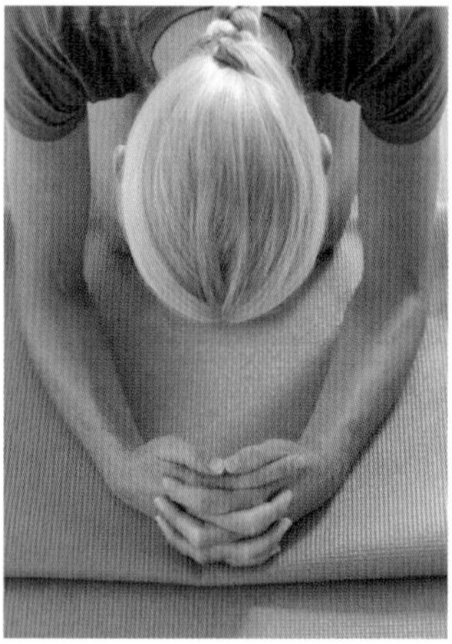

Arm position viewed from above.

1 *Caution: It is best to learn this pose with an experienced Iyengar yoga teacher.*
Fold your mat in four and kneel in front of it. Place your elbows on the mat, shoulder-width apart, with the tips of your elbows facing your knees. Interlock your fingers so that your palms form a cup, then place your forearms and wrists on the mat as shown (see above).

Salamba Sirsasana

Headstand

"If a line is drawn from the centre of the head to the centre of the foot, these two points should be in a single thread from the head to the arches of the feet. This single connecting thread from the head to the arches of the feet is the intelligence. The two heads – the crown of the head and the middle of the arches of the feet – are like the South pole and the North pole. They have to be evenly balanced in *Śīrṣāsana*. This is the spiritual or mystical root of *Śīrṣāsana*."

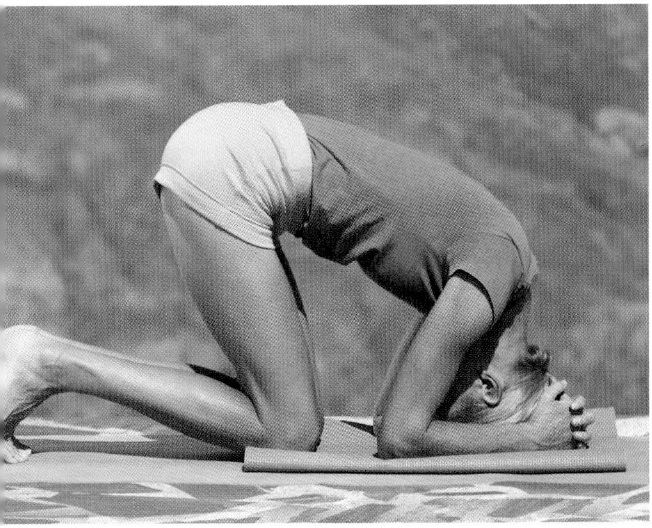

2 Place the crown of your head on the mat with the back of your head touching your cupped palms. Only the crown of your head should be on the mat.

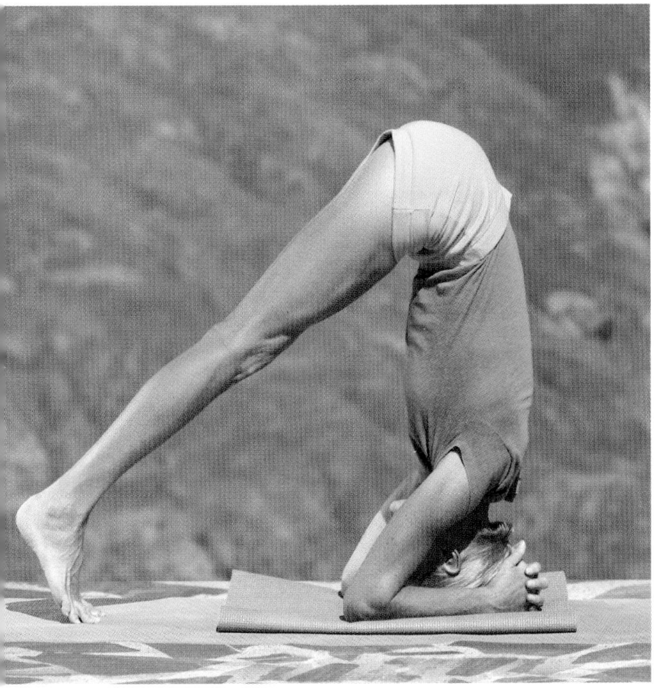

3 Press your arms down, lift your shoulders, raise your knees, and straighten your legs, stretching your spine upwards. Lift onto tiptoes, then walk your feet towards your head until the back of your body is vertical, from head to back of the waist. Keep lifting your shoulders so that your dorsal spine does not drop.

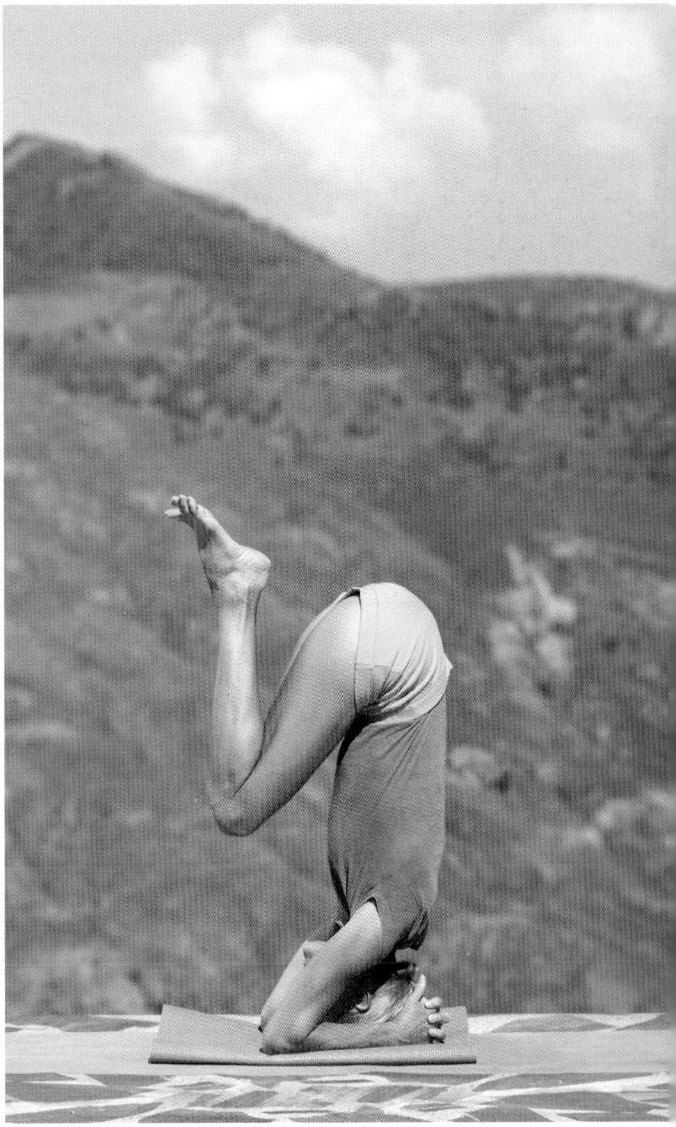

4 Exhale and, bending your knees, lift both feet off the floor simultaneously in a smooth arching movement.

→ continued

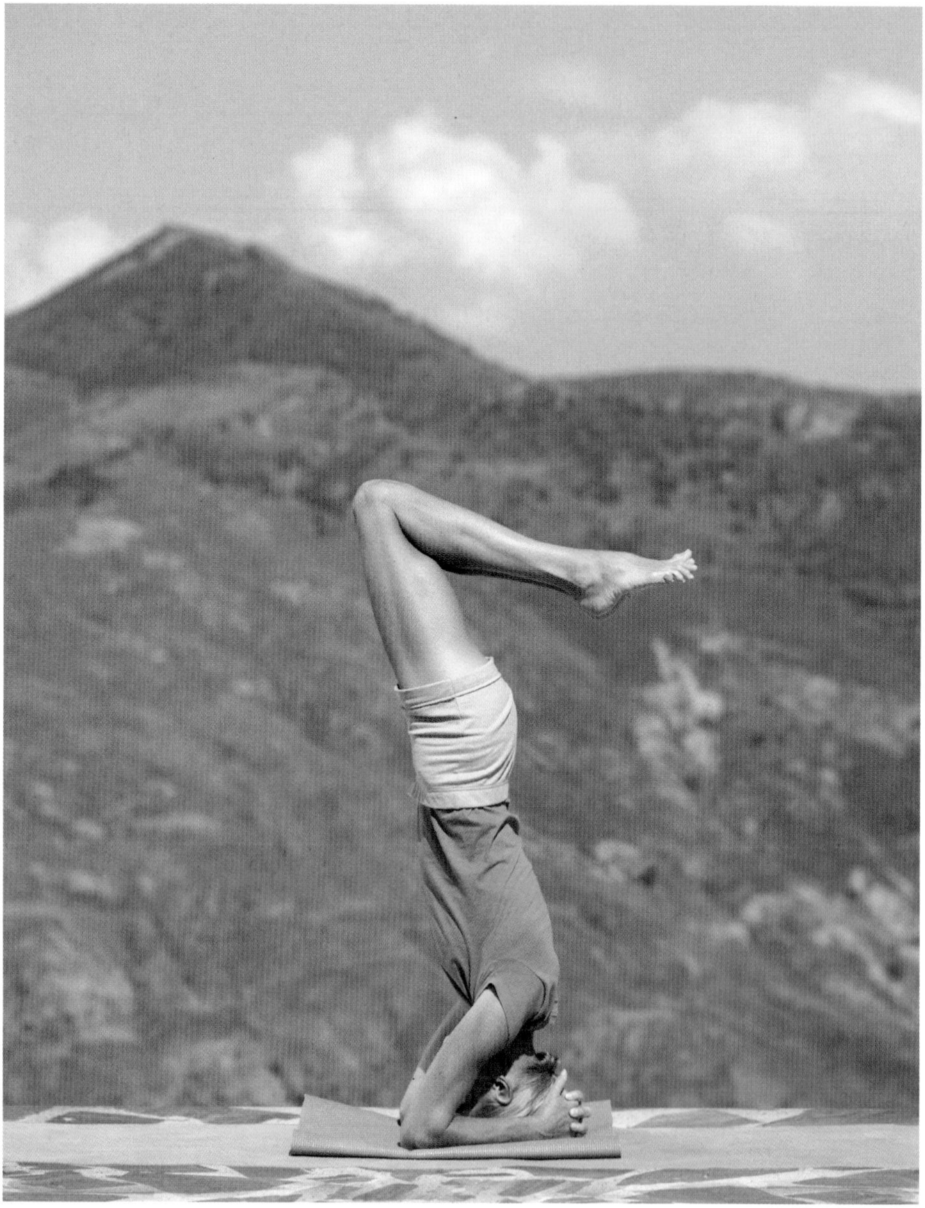

5 Slowly lift your knees until they point directly upwards. Try to keep your heels close to your buttocks. Once your thighs are vertical, hold the position for a few breaths.

6 Extend your legs, stretching your toes and heels up so you form a vertical line from ears to ankles. Keep lifting as you hold for 1–5 minutes. Reverse the steps to come down. Sit on your calves and rest your forehead on the floor, arms forwards, for a few seconds before sitting up.

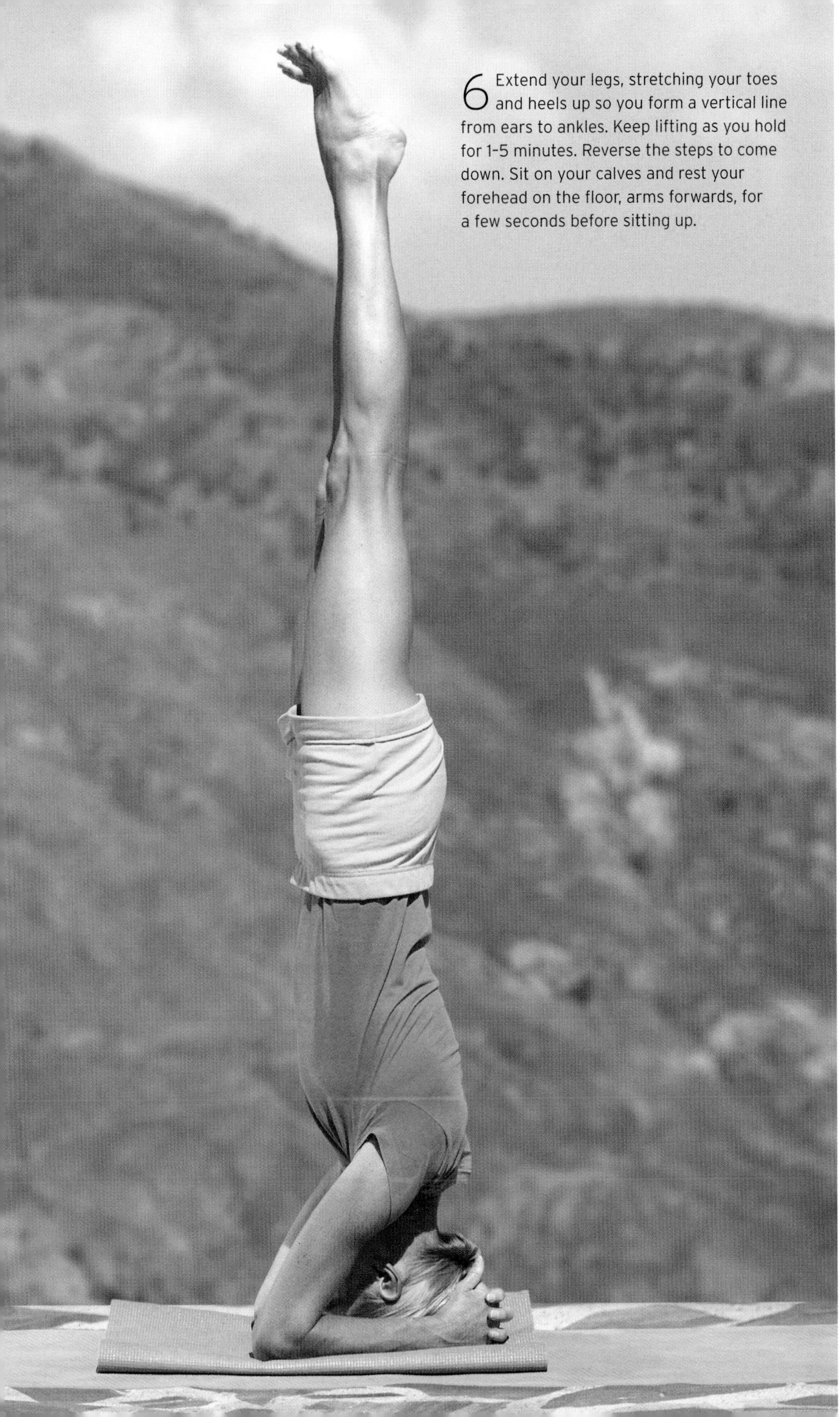

"There is no age limit and no geographical restriction. Differences of sex and health too are no drawback."

Yoga is for All

"All that is required for success in yoga is cheerfulness, perseverance, courage, correct knowledge of the techniques to be followed, moderation in one's habits, and faith in the practice of yoga. Then the effects of yogic practice as enumerated by the sages follow. These are beauty and strength, clarity of speech and expression, calmness of the nerves, an increase of one's digestive power, and a happy disposition that is revealed in a face full of smiles."

Q. How would you advise a follower of your method to plan his regular practice of *āsana*?

"In the sixties, when I wrote my book *Light on Yoga*, I outlined a course of 300 weeks (more than five years). I had in my mind my own practice and measured, according to my dedication, the possible time it would take to learn, but I never thought of practitioners at large. I didn't think that people who follow my method could dedicate ten hours a day that took me to come to that level. Now, as a mature man, I realize I should have divided the course into 900 weeks. At least that much is required to this measured control of *āsana*.

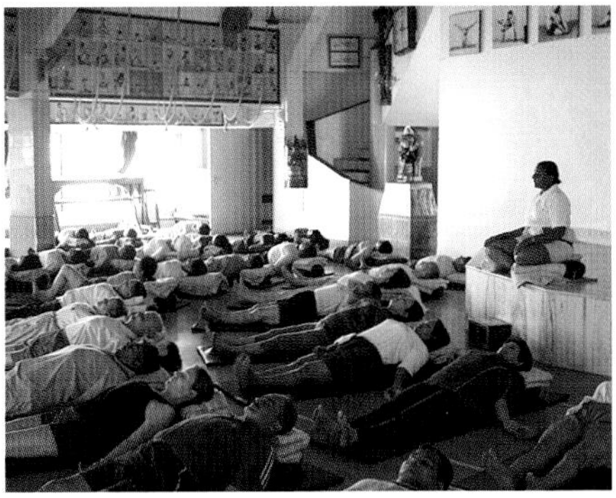

Geeta Iyengar leads a class at the main practice hall at RIMYI. Students are of all ages and backgrounds, from both sexes and in various states of health.

Actually there are no prescribed rules. Only one who practises has to establish his own sequential series of *āsana* to maintain rhythm and exhilarative feelings. There are many yoga books without a healthy sequential practice. The sequential series given in my book offer protection in their practices.... As I tried to give a sequential method in *āsana* practice in *Light on Yoga*, I also gave a sequential progressive method of practice of *prāṇāyāma* in my book *Light on Prāṇāyāma*."

Q. The majority of people do yoga on a "once a week" basis. What would you say is the value of yoga done this way?

"Something is better than nothing. Today people cannot find sufficient time to practise. Under the guidance of a teacher, if they work once a week, the right thought will be imprinted on their minds and it will have a good effect. And this effect will last for about two or three days on the entire human system. Then it starts deteriorating. If people go to a teacher once a week to learn correct presentations and practise at home twice or thrice a week, retardation will not take place. The functioning of the human system, and the clarity in the brain, and maintenance of equilibrium in body and mind will increase if one practises daily."

Extract opposite from "Pathway to Salvation", Bhavan's Journal, *December 9, 1973.*

Question 1 from "The Yoga of Intelligence", interview by Conchita Labarta in Madrid, October 1997, Mas Alla de la Ciencia, *January 1998.*

Question 2 from "The Guru Who is Just a Family Man", interview by Pauline Dowling, Here's Health, *November 1981.*

"If the body is supple, the mind should resist and make itself hard for the body to perform the asana."

The Supple and the Stiff Body

Q. And could you discuss the difference between a supple body and a stiff one?

"Many people see the photographs of *āsana* and think that the supple body alone can perform such *āsana*. But one should know that often the supple body, too, cannot give any feedback to the brain or mind, as the body lacks sensitivity. Though supple bodies do not experience pain, these tax the nerves, causing fatigue, restlessness, and headache or heaviness. They run out of energy. Instead of receiving the energy, the cells get squeezed and this may introduce hoards of diseases. A supple body does not trigger the intelligence to think what is wrong and what is right in performing an *āsana*. On the contrary, a rigid body has resistance, action, and counter-action, which triggers the intelligence to study the *āsana* in the right perspective. There is no action, counter-action, or resistance from the supple body to give clues to intellectual thinking and emotional stability. They get the *āsana* easily without inner resistance or response. If one is pregnant and there is no response, then the fear surfaces that the child is still with no life. Similarly, the *āsana* done without resistance is an *āsana* without life, like a stillborn child."

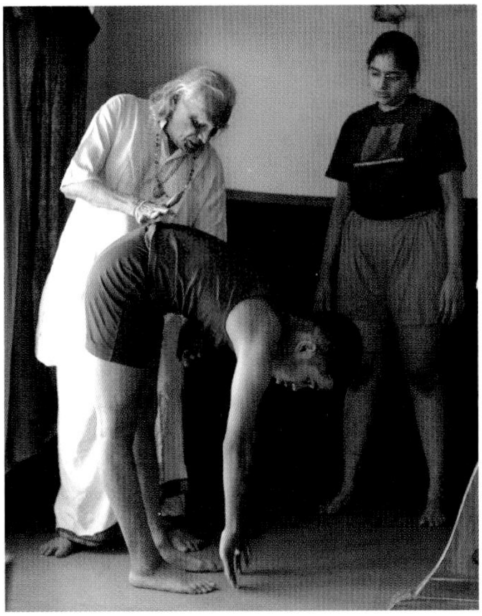

Guruji adjusts a less supple student in a medical class at RIMYI observed by his granddaughter Abhijata Sridhar.

Refining your Experience

"Suppose you remember a poem word by word without knowing its meaning, does it make any sense to you? The moment you begin to know the depth of the poem's meaning, you begin to appreciate the poem. This appreciation is interaction. You begin to reflect on the poem and this reflection reflects with new thoughts on you.

Similarly, while doing or being in *āsana* there has to be the interaction between the body and mind as well as mind and intelligence. The body may act but the mind has to react. The intelligence has to reflect on the interaction between the body and mind.... Otherwise, the body does on its own accord without giving any message to the mind or intelligence. This does not open the gates of intelligence to interpenetrate or outerpenetrate the fullness of the *āsana.*"

From "Seed of Practical Yoga Sown in America", interview by Laurie Blakeney, Rose Richardson, Sue Salaniuk and Toni Fuhrman, July 1992, published in Yoga 93, *American Yoga Convention, Ann Arbor, Michigan, 1993.*

Ardha Chandrasana

Half-moon Pose

"One benefits from yoga in terms of physical balance (*śārīrika santulana*), physiological balance (*aindriyika santulana*), mental balance (*mānasika santulana*), intellectual balance (*bauddhika santulana*), and the balance of the soul (*ātmika santulana*)...."

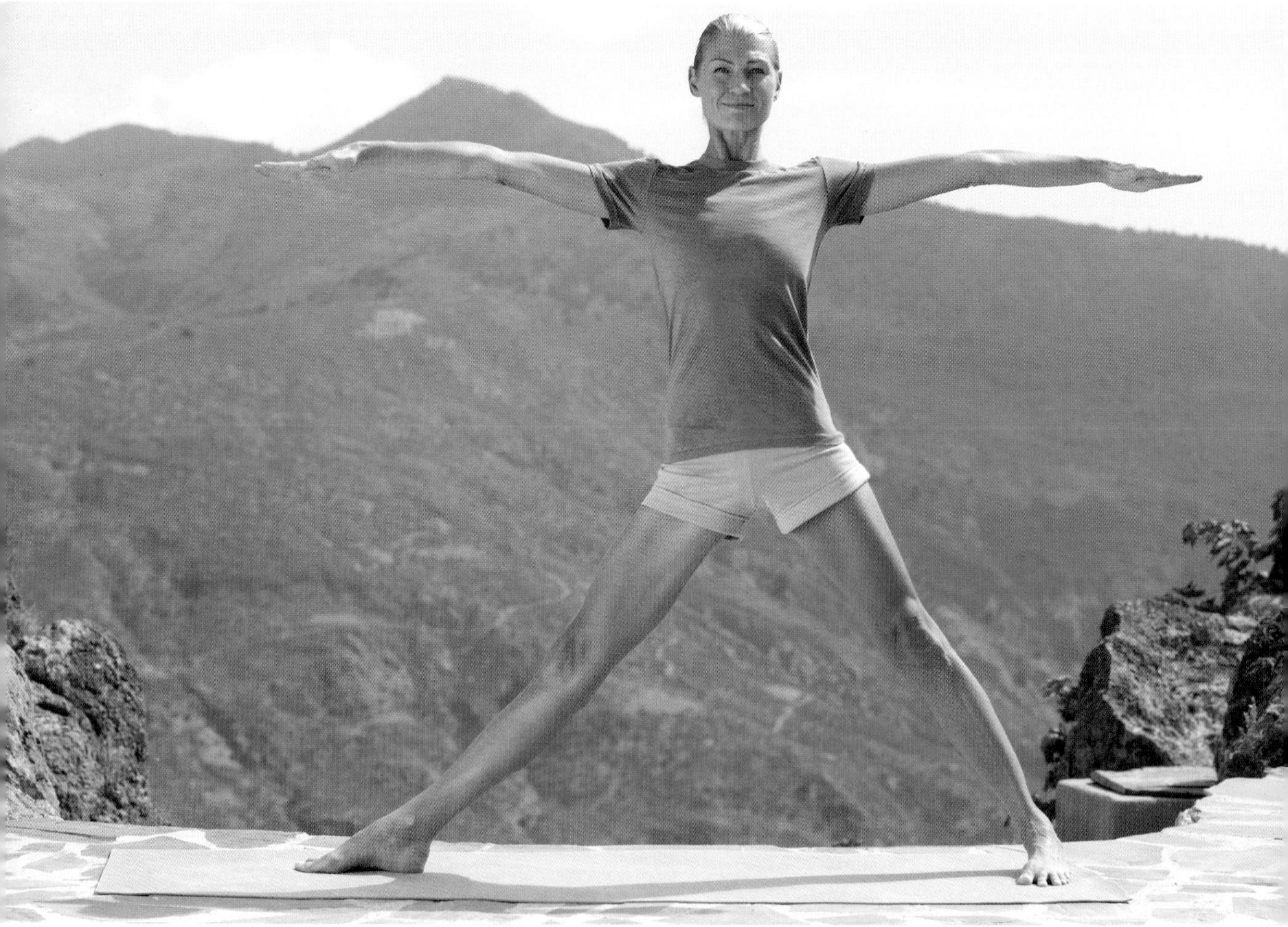

1 From Tadasana, jump into Utthita Hasta Padasana (see pages 108-109). Then turn your left foot in slightly and your right leg and foot 90° to the right. Keep your arms outstretched. Look ahead and open your chest.

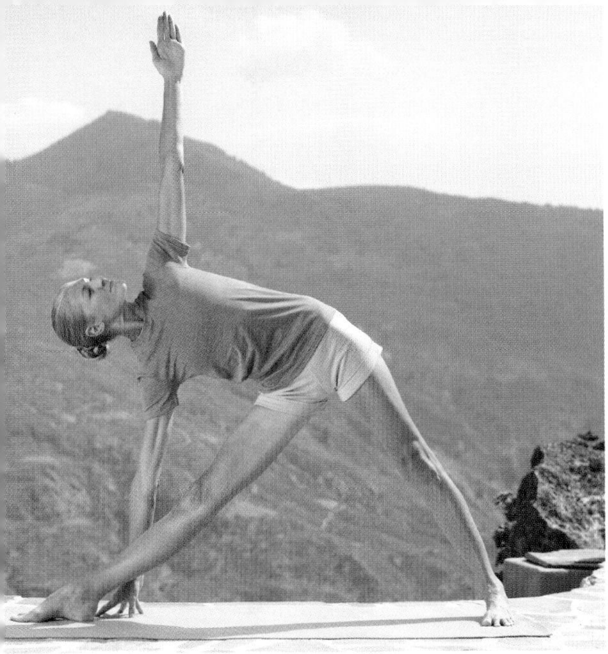

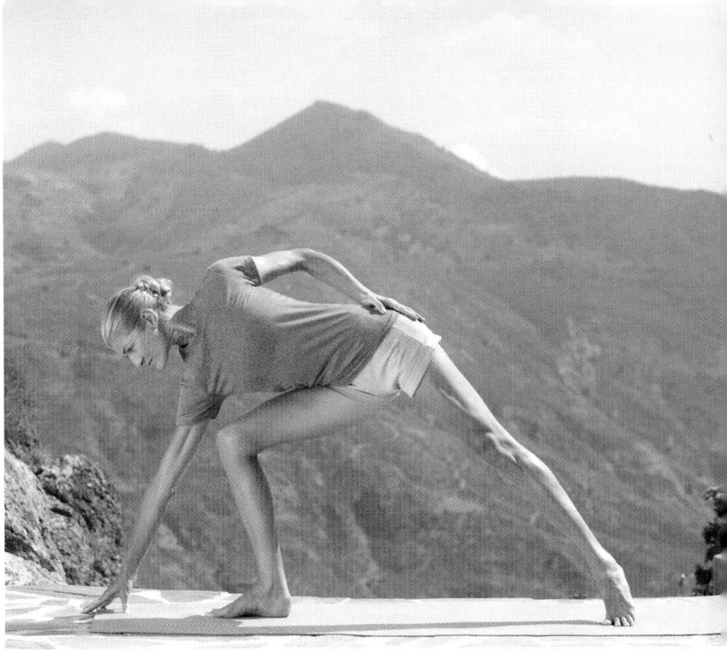

2 Exhale and extend your trunk sideways to the right, moving into Utthita Trikonasana (see pages 30–31).

3 Exhale, bend your right knee, step your left foot in a little and place your right hand about 30cm (1ft) in front of and in line with your right foot. Rest your left palm on your left hip. Look in front of your hand.

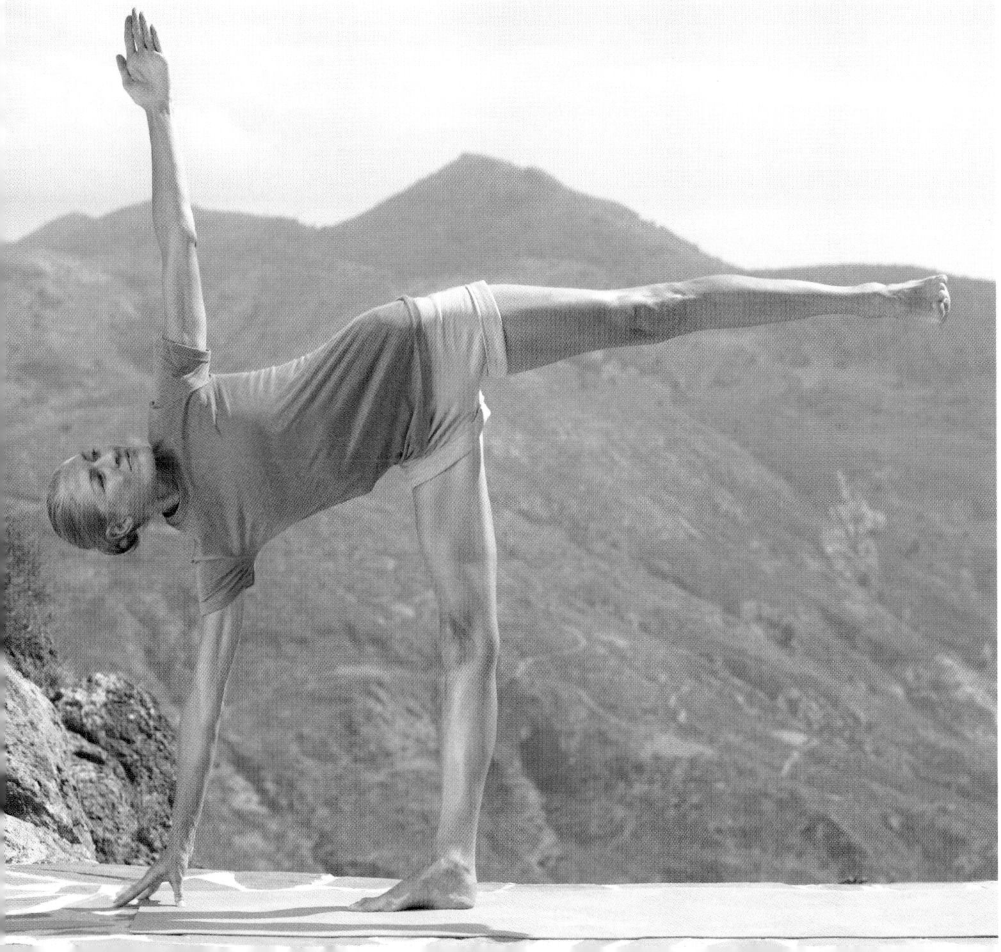

4 On an exhalation, raise your left leg, keeping it straight, and straighten your right leg. Extend your left arm in line with your shoulders. Look ahead or turn your head to look up. Hold for 20–30 seconds, breathing evenly. Inhale, bend your right leg and step your left foot back to the floor. Reverse the steps to return to Utthita Hasta Padasana, then repeat to the other side. Finish in Tadasana.

Yoga for Women

“ God created men and women equal. Yoga too was created by Him. Yoga too does not differentiate or shun or exclude anyone by gender, colour or class.... In the early days women had all the rights and opportunities to practise for the realization of the soul. They were recognized as having every right to practise the four paths of *karma*, *jñāna*, *bhakti*, and *yoga* in order to experience the establishment of the soul. The names of such *yogini* may be found in the *Upaniṣad* and the *Purāṇa* or the stories of past legendary figures....

Men and women have the same fluctuations in thoughts and reflections, diseases, sorrows, and obstacles. Only their approaches differ from each other because of their inherent natural disposition (*svabhāva*). Though both are endowed with intellect and emotions, man's intellect grows vertically filled with pride and ego, whereas woman's intelligence develops horizontally with compassion and sympathy. If women are gifted with instinctive and intuitive feelings, men work with their analytical head. If women are endowed with emotional intelligence and devotional qualities, men are endowed with intellectual deliberation. Man disregards his emotional feelings and tries to resolve the emotional weather by means of his intellect, which is usually founded in the pride of 'I' ('I' decide, 'I' know) rather than the reason and logic (*tarka*) of an objective mind. Women, however, instinctively bring to bear their emotional intelligence to solve emotional upheavals.

Yoga helps both men and women to develop intellect in the head and intelligence in the heart to lead a balanced life maintaining harmony, balance and concord not only at home but in the community and society as well....

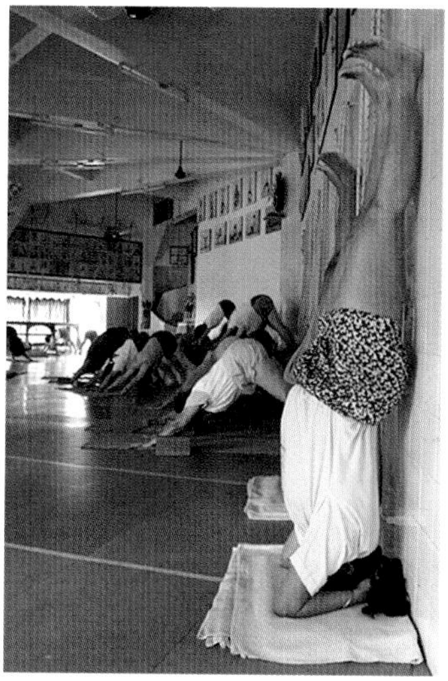

In a dedicated class for pregnant women at RIMYI, students practise the helpful poses Salamba Sirsasana (foreground) and Adho Mukha Svanasana (background).

Yoga in pregnancy

During pregnancy women normally are afraid or nervous to practise yoga. They cannot imagine standing on their heads during pregnancy. Let me assure them that these *āsana* are a boon for them. Daily practice of *āsana* and *prāṇāyāma,* which are essential during pregnancy, has to be done regularly. Then they maintain physical and mental health and also create good and auspicious *saṅskāra* in the baby while carrying.... Practice at the time of pregnancy establishes the 'feel of contact' with the baby inside the body and showers good and auspicious thoughts with peaceful and untainted mind as its mother keeps her body healthy with relaxed nerves. Her digestive, circulatory, excretory systems function well and the glandular system undergoes a sea change in its hormonal functions. Besides these benefits, its practice will take care of keeping away diseases and infections and help in maintaining a good hygienic health with perfect immune system, preparing her mind for an easy delivery without stress, tension, agitation, fear, or anxiety. ”

From "Yoga A Saviour in Women's Life", Aṣṭadaḷa Yogamālā *Volume 8, pp354–82.*

Paripurna Navasana

Boat Pose

"Inevitably as beginners we want to generate energy and momentum, or speed through the water, so we pull nearer to *abhyāsa*...where the current races fast. Seeing where that might lead we edge over towards *vairāgya*...where the current is slacker but treacherous rocks are concealed, so we must redouble our watchfulness. This corresponds to Patañjali's II.47, exalted effort is cessation of effort. At this moment, the helmsman's hand rests lightly on the tiller but his eyes remain sharp."

1 Sit in Dandasana (see pages 14-15), fingers pointing at your feet.

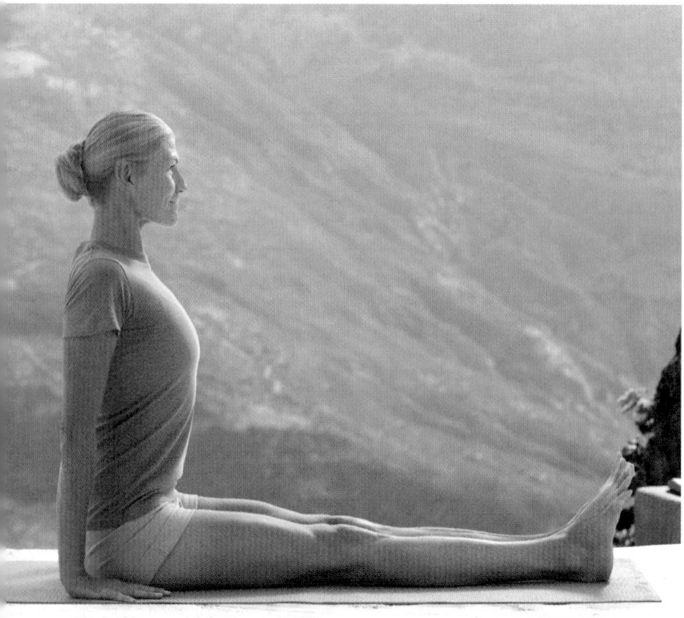

2 Exhale, recline your trunk slightly and raise your legs by 60° (keep them straight, with knees tight). Press your palms down, lift your spine from the base, and keep your chest up.

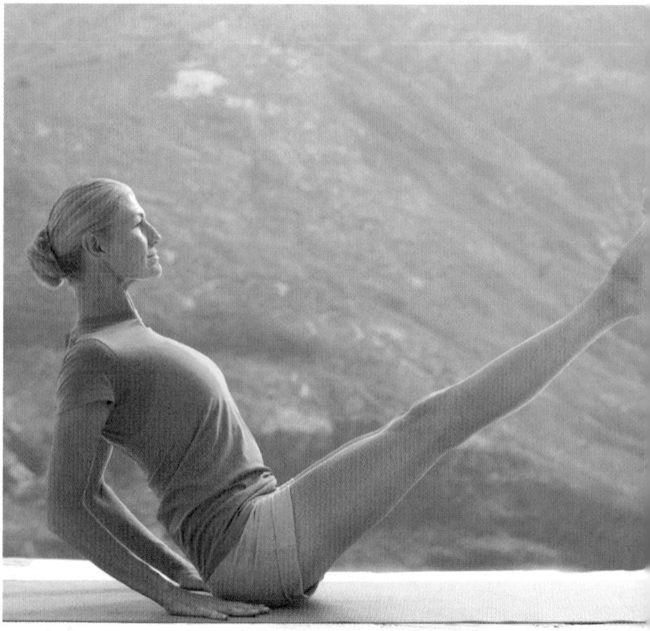

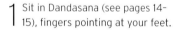

3 Raise your arms to shoulder-level and stretch them forwards, parallel to the floor, palms facing each other. Extend your legs, stretch your spine, lift your chest, and look at your feet. Hold for 20–30 seconds (do not hold your breath). Exhale, and lower your legs and hands back to Dandasana. Rest by lying on your back.

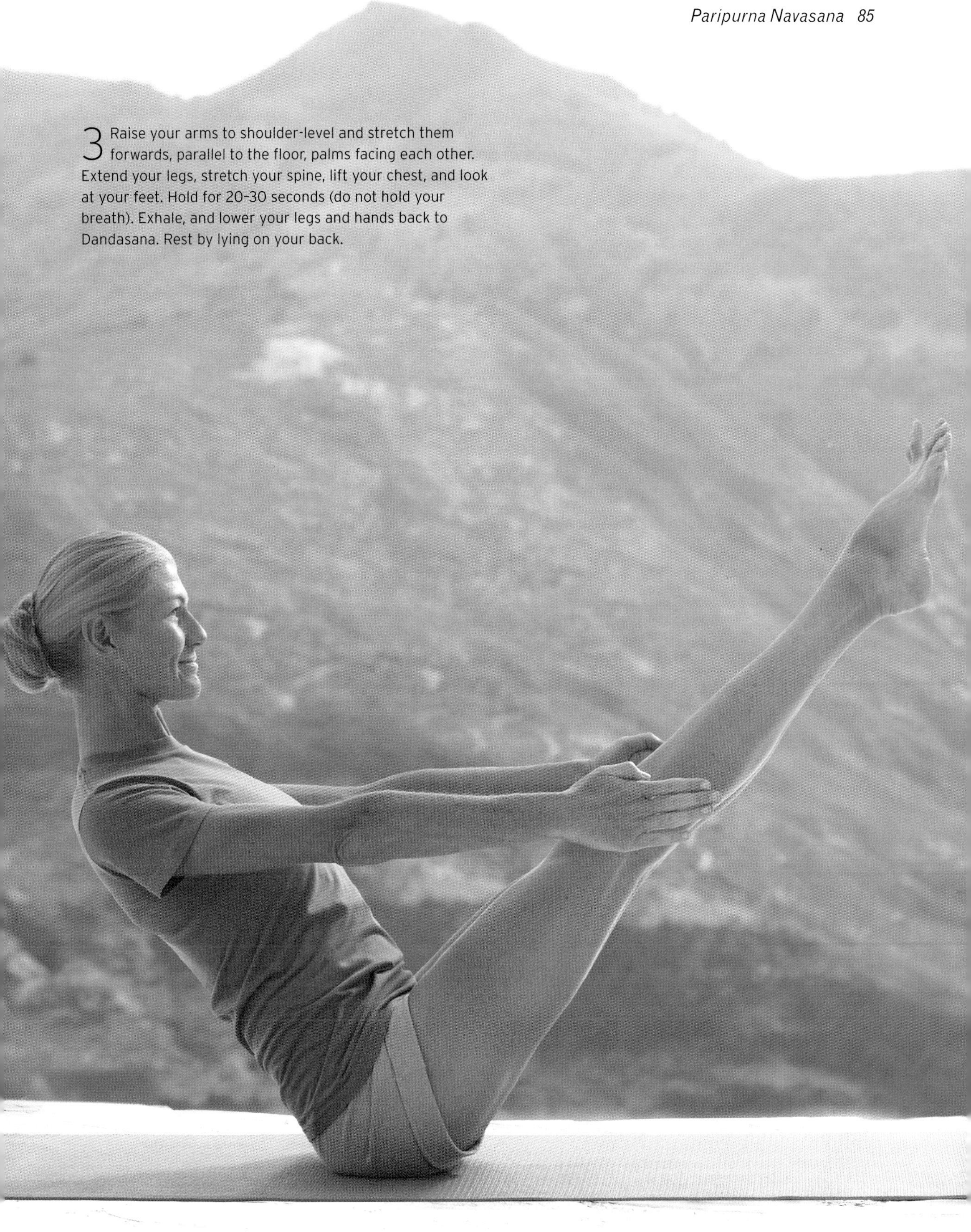

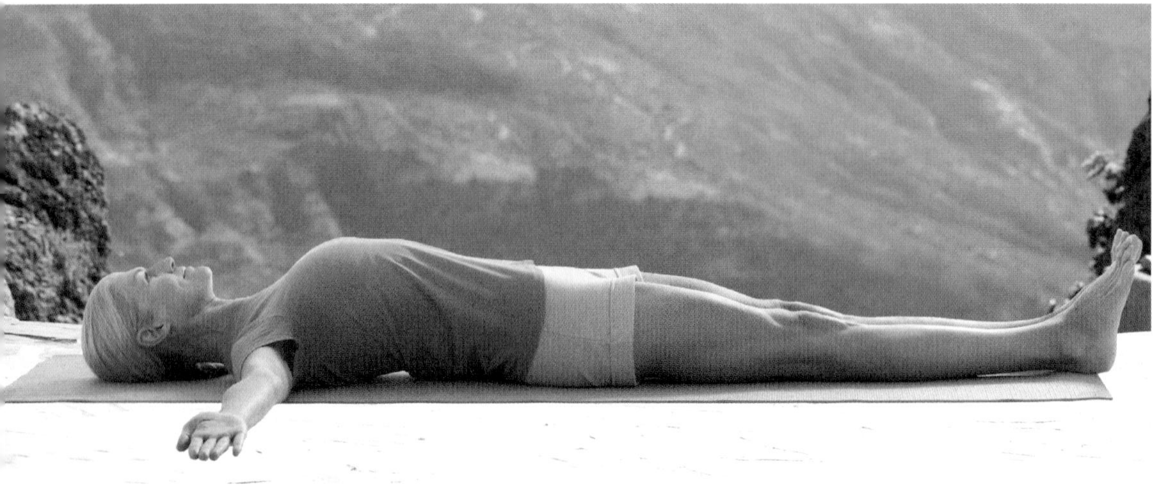

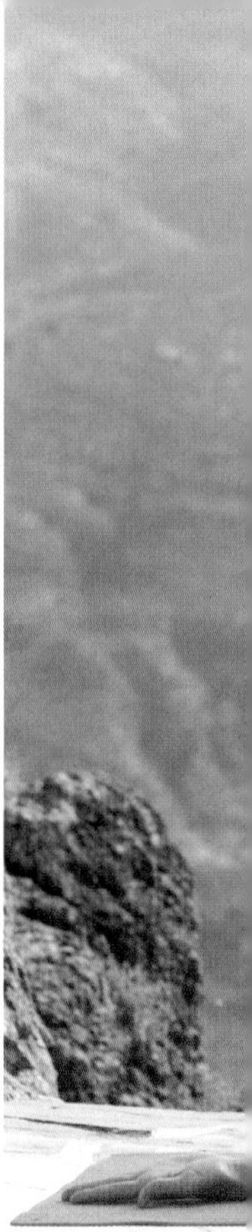

1 Lie on your back with your legs outstretched and together. Stretch your arms to the sides, in line with your shoulders, palms facing upwards. Make sure that the centre line of your body is straight and forms a cross with your arms.

Jathara Parivartanasana

Turning the Belly Pose

"Yoga is an inner bath. Blood gives us a bath inside the body. To do this, the blood has to circulate extremely well, and with a constant, even power or force. Think of a waterfall, how much energy it generates. By the practice of yoga, we have to generate energy in our blood to nourish every part. Then the cells sense comfort and freedom, and send the message: 'I am happy'."

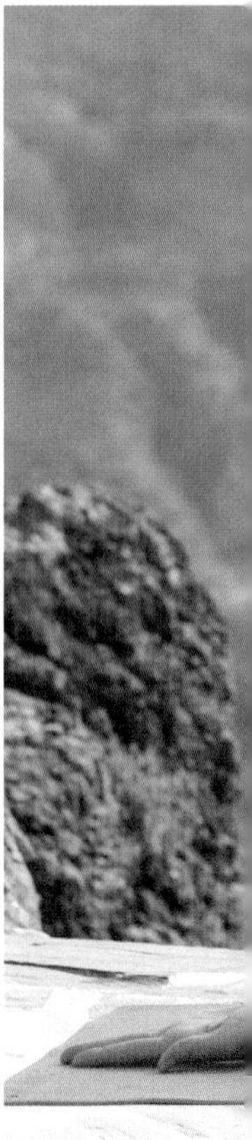

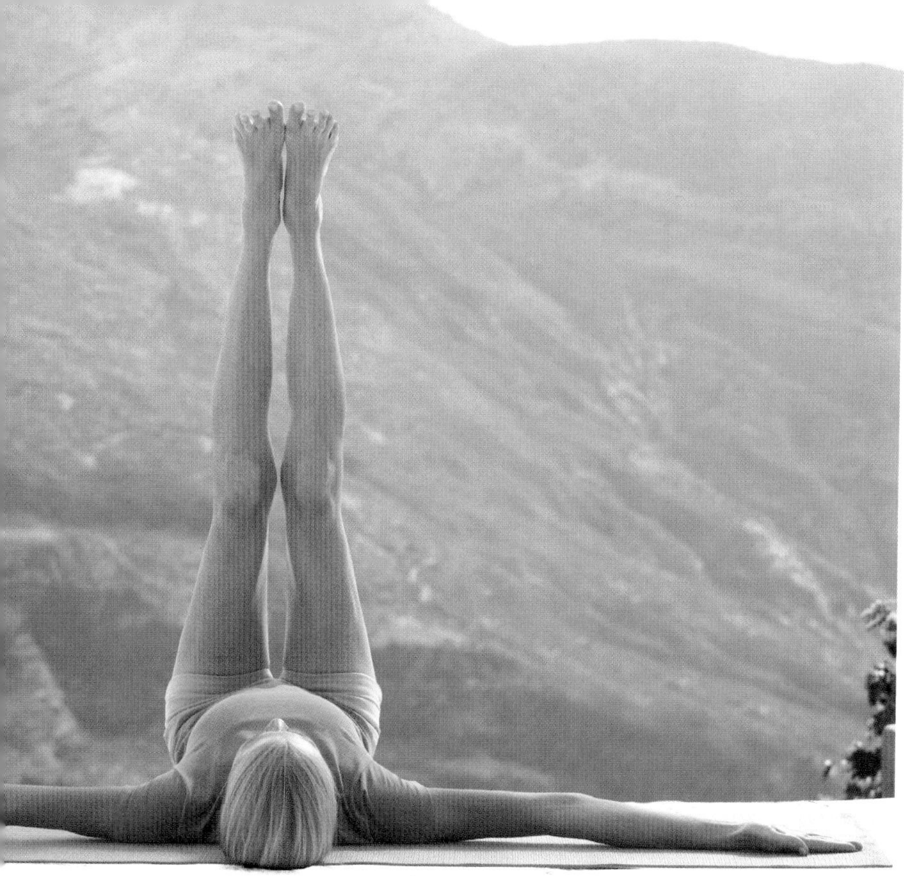

2 Exhale and raise your legs together, keeping your knees firm, until they are perpendicular to the floor. Turn your big toes a little towards your right side.

3 Exhale and lower the legs towards your right hand. Keep your feet together and knees tight. Press your left shoulder down and keep your lumbar area close to the floor. Roll your belly to the left to keep your navel centred. Hold for 20 seconds (do not hold your breath). Inhale and raise the legs back to centre. Turn your big toes left and repeat to the left. Lower your limbs and relax.

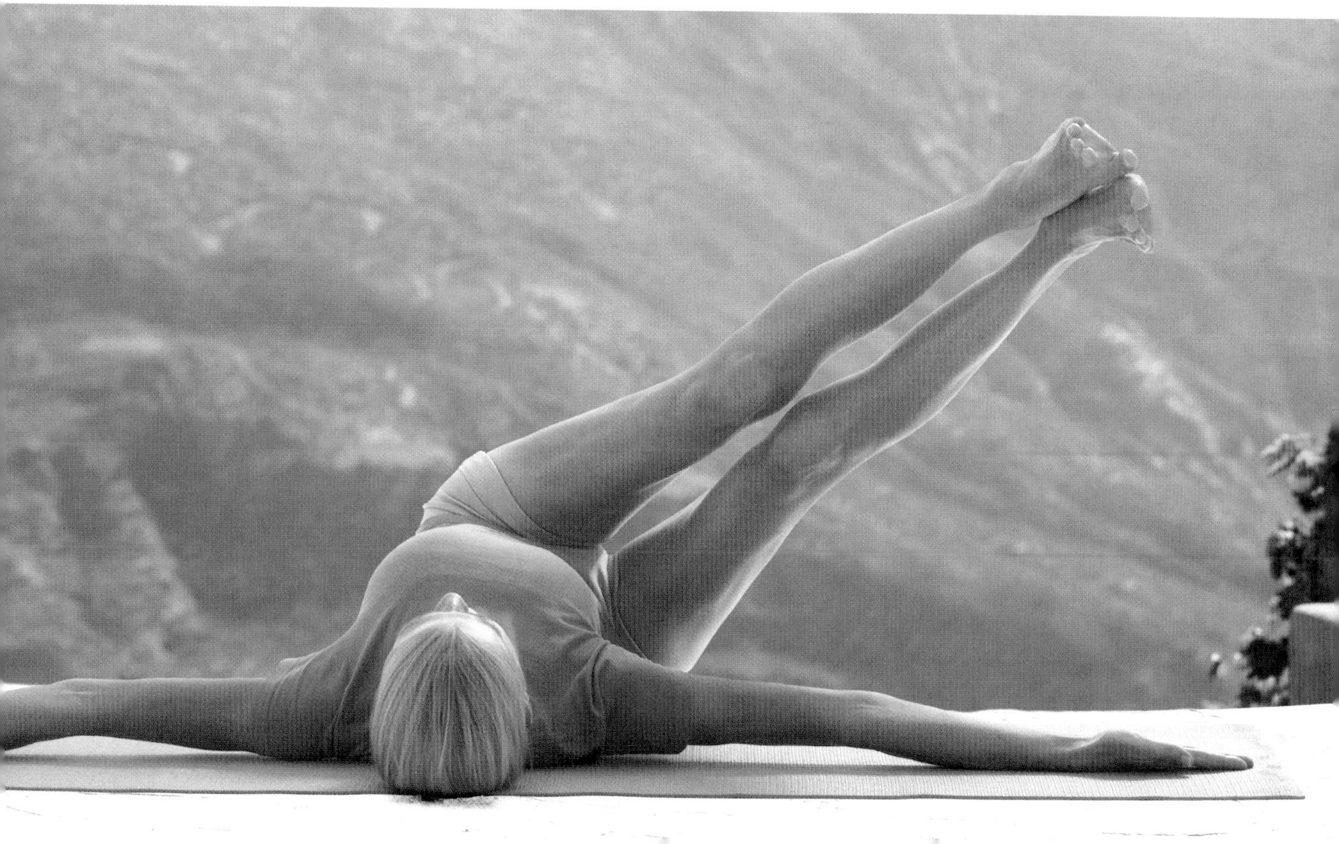

Invocatory Prayers

“I request all of you to recite the invocation on Patañjali when you start your classes. If you cannot recite it in Sanskrit, you may recite the translation. In this way, we may invoke his presence at the time of our practices. We recite this invocation for the simple reason that we consider him as our *Guru* in yoga. This great sage gave us grammar for right speech, medicine for health, and yoga for mind culture. When we are in our yoga *sādhanā*, we should think of him and pay our reverential respects to him so that our minds may be tuned to the good thoughts of his works.”

Invocation on Patañjali

“Yogena cittasya padena vācām
Malaṁ Śarīrasya ca vaidyakena
Yopākarottaṁ pravaraṁ munīnāṁ
Patañjaliṁ prāñjalirānatósmi
Ābāhu puruṣākāraṁ
Śaṅkha cakrāsi dhāriṇam
Sahasra śirasaṁ śvetaṁ
praṇamāmi Patañjalim.”

“To the noblest of sages, Patañjali,
Who gave yoga for serenity of mind,
Grammar for purity of speech,
And medicine for the health of the body, I bow.
I prostrate before Patañjali,
Whose upper body has a human form,
Whose arms hold a conch and disc,
Who is crowned by a thousand-headed cobra,
O incarnation of Ādiśeṣa, my
salutations to Thee.”

Q. Could you elaborate a little bit on the meaning of each of the symbols: the conch, the disc, the cobra, and the human torso?

"As the conch can be blown, it represents a kind of alarm if any danger such as evil spirits or diseases interferes, and the disc indicates that one can destroy, the evil thoughts, evil spirits or diseases. *Asī* means a sword. On one hand, he holds the sword of knowledge to destroy nescience. On the other hand he blesses those who practice yoga. In another aspect, he folds his palms and salutes the seat of the *antarātman* – the God, symbolically showing that through yoga, one reaches God."

Q. And then the cobra.

"You know the cobra is the one which is holding the Earth. It is the protector of the universe. In the *Haṭhayoga Pradīpikā,* the first stanza of the third chapter says: 'Ananta, the Lord of Serpents, supports the Earth with its mountains and forests, similarly *kuṇḍalinī* – serpent energy – is the main support of all yoga practices'.... From early civilization almost all the religions have worshiped the Snake God. Every mythology had some sort of serpent worship. It was a belief that snakes do not die but they shed their skins and emerge as new. This eternity of snakes became symbolic. This ageless quality of the serpent is known as *ananta* – never ending. The snake is a symbol of eternity, fertility, and regeneration. It is a symbol of wisdom too. The snake is depicted with the good and bad deeds of man. Is it not? All religions say that we have to conquer emotional upheavals like lust, greed, anger, malice, and so on. The snake is poisonous but its venom is medicinal too. Similarly, anger, lust, etc. are poisonous. We have to convert our nature and develop the opposite qualities such as quietness, control or continence, love, contentment, and so on."

Q. And then the fourth is the human torso.

"You must have heard the story of Patañjali's birth. He was like a worm which took human form, and his mother, Gauṇika, was a virgin, just like Mary. This indicates the process of evolution, how one can progress from small creature to human being. It is the growth and expanse of intelligence. This head in the human form is to explain the essence of Yoga."

Extract opposite from "Pearls of Yogic Wisdom", Aṣṭadaḷa Yogamālā *Volume 1, pp234–35.*

Questions from "Invoking Patanjali", interview by Bonnie Anthony, first published in Newsletter of the B.K.S. Iyengar Yoga Association of Southern California, *Spring/Summer 1991.*

"Each asana has a beautiful shape, grace and elegance that bestows power and makes the practitioner as strong as a diamond and at the same time as soft as a flower."

On Asana

" *Āsana* means a seat as well as a posture. The word *āsana* comes from the root *āsa*, which means to sit or to lay down. It means to assume and assert a particular position bringing both description and definition in the position. It also means to exist, to present, to dwell-in, to abide.

Āsana is a state where one arranges and assumes a particular position or form and re-forms it for a right configuration with study (*svādhyāya*). Positioning the body for posing means action. Re-posing means reflective action. So after action one has to observe, re-think, and re-reflect on parts of the body that work and parts of the body that are not working. Similarly, one has to observe which part of the body the mind is penetrating, and which part is not penetrating. Again, one has to look and see along with the body's extension, expansion, and contraction, whether the mind and intelligence concurrently and evenly occupies the entire body in its extension, expansion, and contraction. This is reflective re-posing. While performing the *āsana,* this action, reflection, and

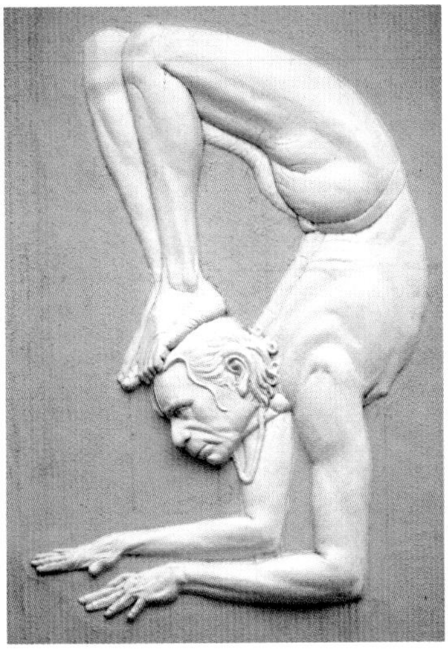

Frieze from the outer walls of RIMYI. Guruji counsels that, "These pictures are meant to be looked at and observed by you. They are meant to make you understand their depth. They are archetypal icons using architectural elements within the frame of the human body."

"Constant study and trial is needed to educate and mould the limbs of the body to fit into the right frame of each posture."

reaction makes the practitioner to re-adjust his intelligence sensitively and accurately to cover each limb from end to end. If one learns to extend equally this intellectual sensitivity to all parts of the body along with the self, the *āsana* transforms into contemplative or meditative *āsana*. This must be the aim of each *sādhaka*, to reach the ultimate descriptive and definitive condition in all the *āsana*. Then his practice turns divine. ”

From "On Aṣṭāṅga Yoga – Asana", Aṣṭadaḷa Yogamālā *Volume 7, pp101–102.*

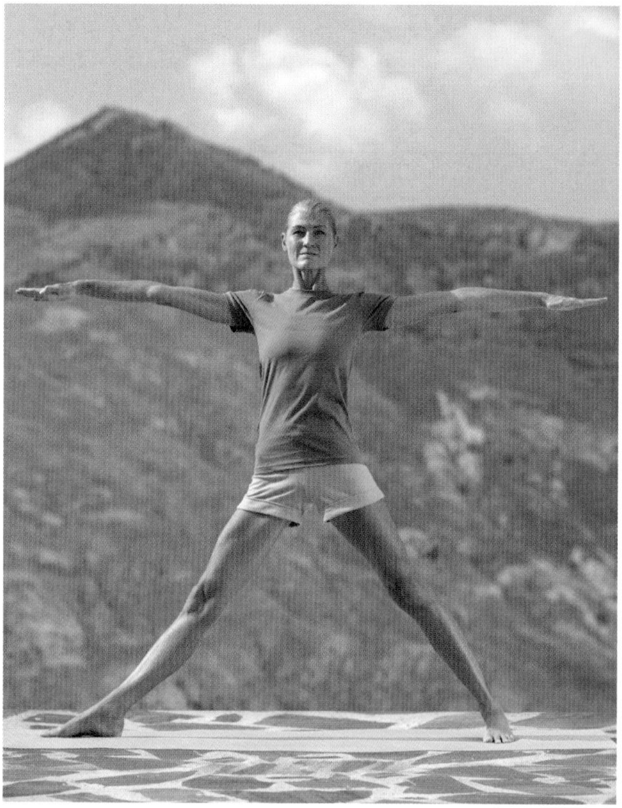

1 From Tadasana, jump into Utthita Hasta Padasana (see pages 108–109). Turn your left leg and foot in by 60° and your right leg and foot 90° to the right. Keep your arms outstretched. Look ahead and open your chest.

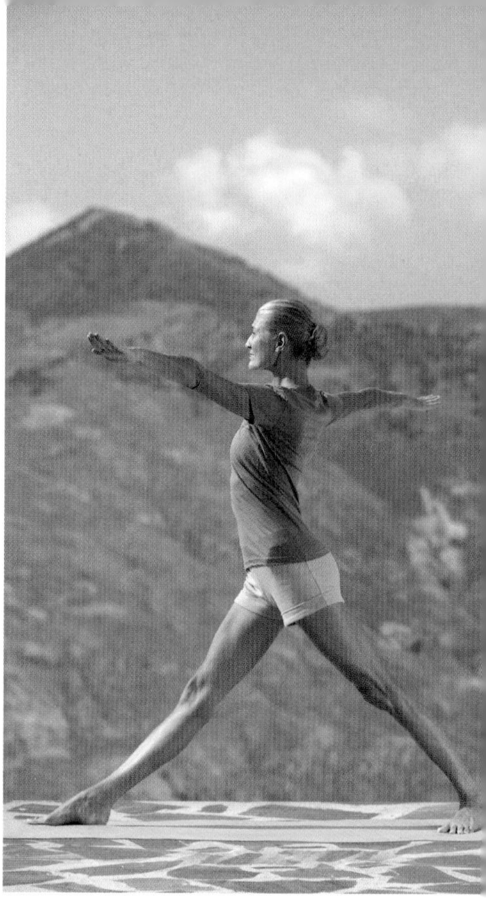

2 Exhale and rotate your entire trunk to the right, bringing your left side forwards and right side back. Keep both your arms and your legs straight and extended.

Parivrtta Trikonasana

Revolved Triangle Pose

"Trim the jewel of the body like a well-cut diamond by creating space in joints, muscles, and skin so that the fine network of the body fits into the *āsana*. This helps the senses of perception to cognize the conative action. This conjunction between organs of action and senses of perception brings about reflection in thought and subjective understanding begins to prompt re-adjustment. Then one begins to act, react, reflect, readjust, correct, and perform the best..."

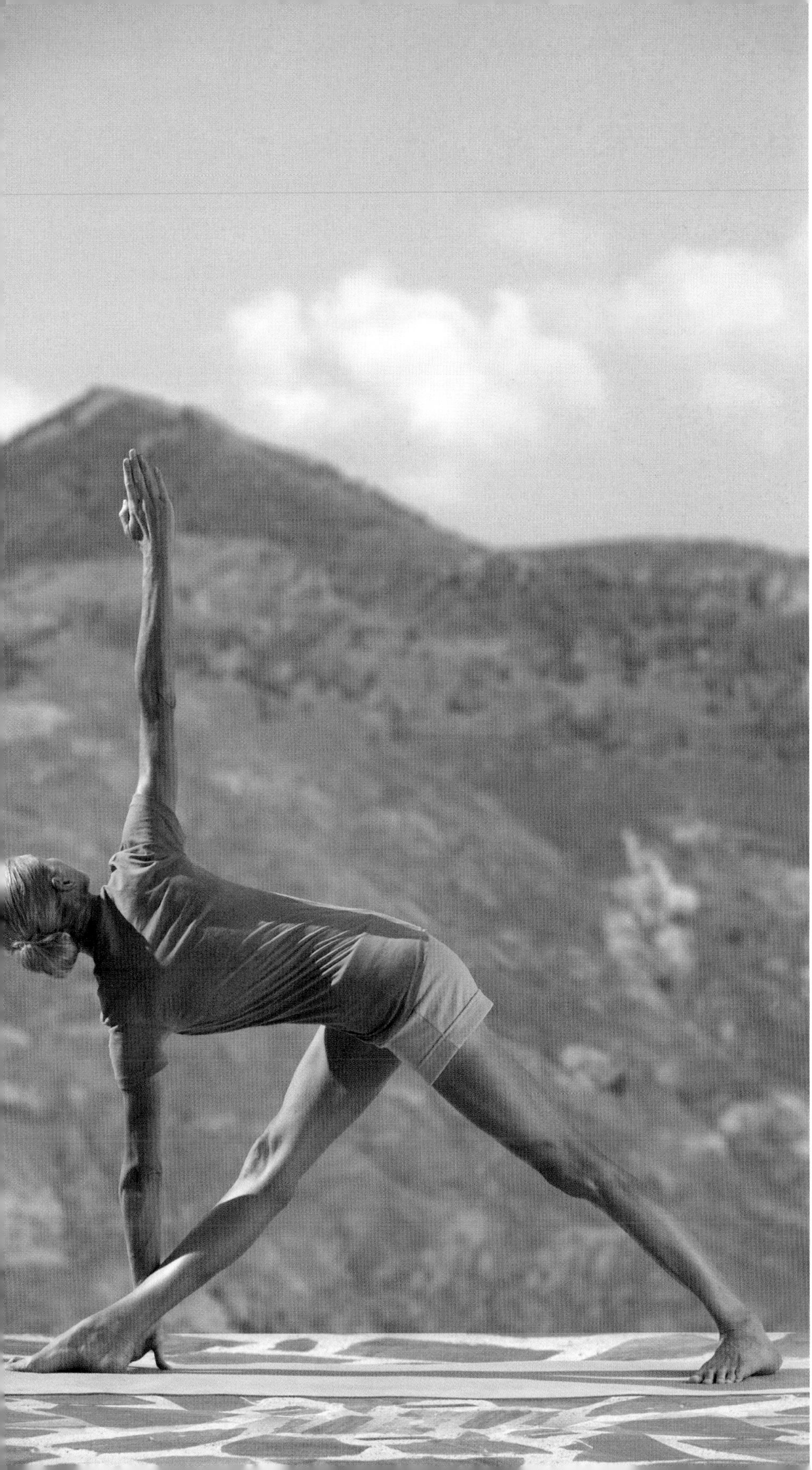

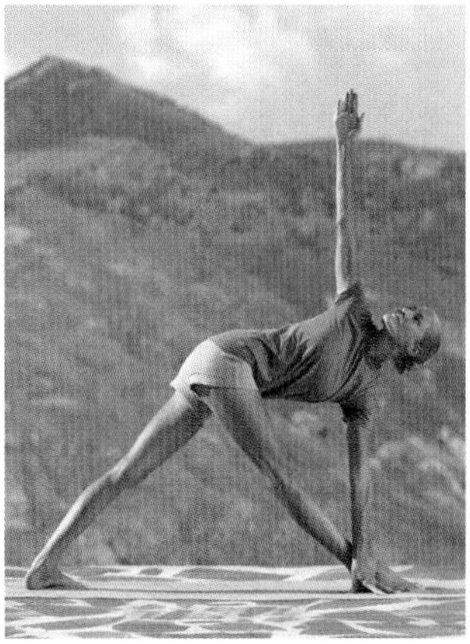

Parivrtta Trikonasana viewed from the back.

3 Exhale and bring the left side of your trunk towards your right foot, placing your left hand on the floor beside the outer edge of your right foot. Stretch your right arm up in line with your shoulders. Open your chest and look up at your right thumb. Hold for 20–30 seconds, breathing evenly. Inhale and reverse the steps to return to Utthita Hasta Padasana, then repeat to the other side. Finish in Tadasana.

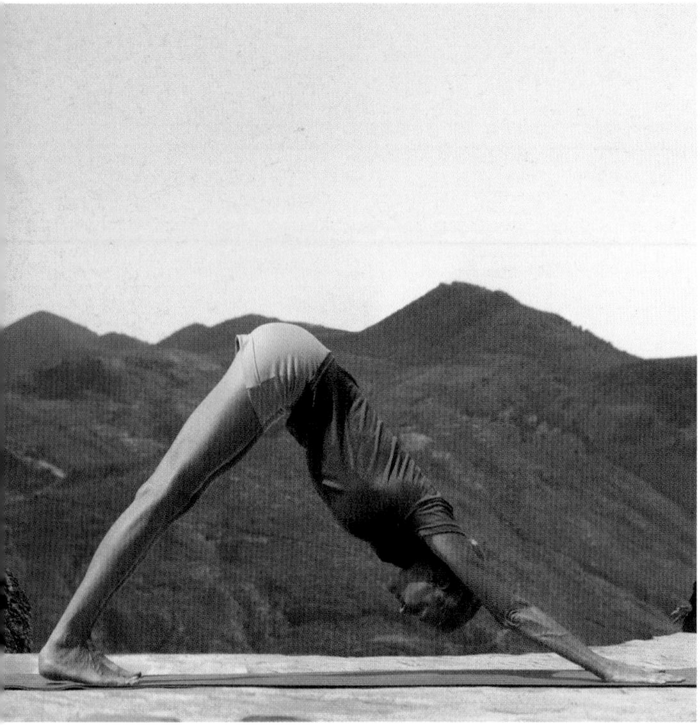

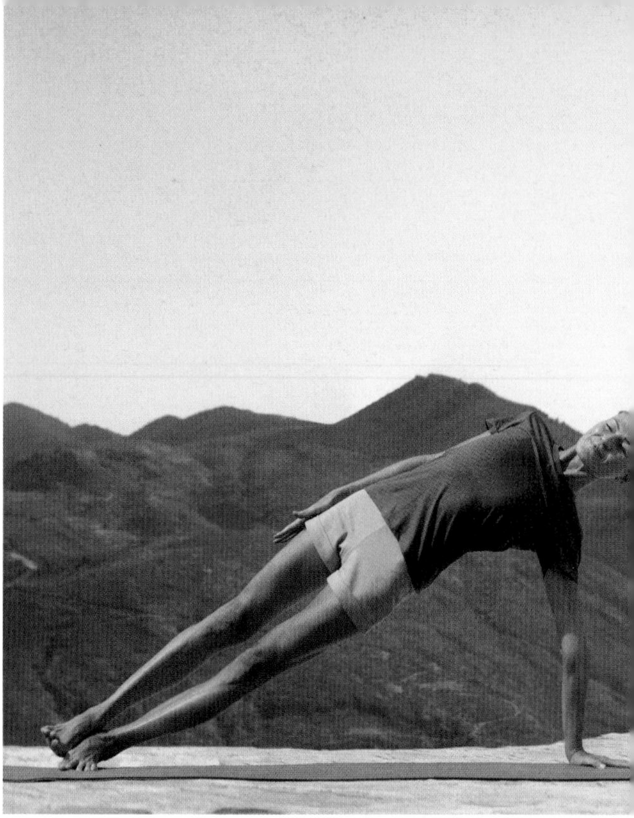

1 *Caution: This is not a pose for beginners.* Begin in Adho Mukha Svanasana (see pages 104-105).

2 Turn your whole body and left foot sideways to the left, stretching your big toe down. Balance your right foot over your left. Rest your upper arm along your right side and keep your head in line with your spine.

Vasisthasana

Asana Dedicated to the Sage Vasistha

"Conscious and regular practice not only cultures and keeps the cells of the body healthy but develops clear and pure intelligence and memory in them, creating purity of thought for one to move closer towards the *ātman*. The practice of *āsana* with reflective and meditative attention leads the *sādhaka* to move with the right attitude, right poise, and stability, bringing about loveliness, liveliness, and dynamism."

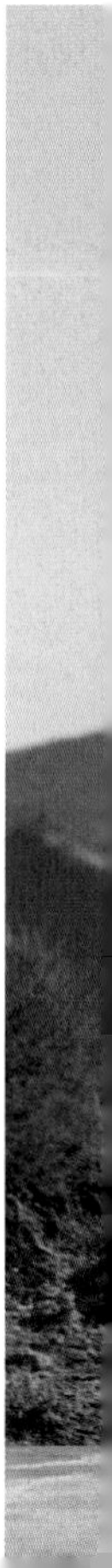

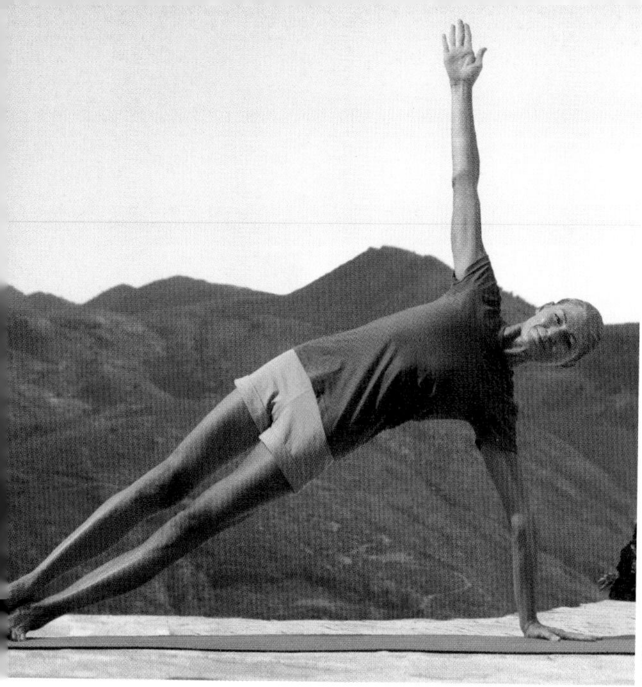

3 Lift up through your lower arm and stretch your top arm upwards. Keep your legs and arms straight and lift your chest.

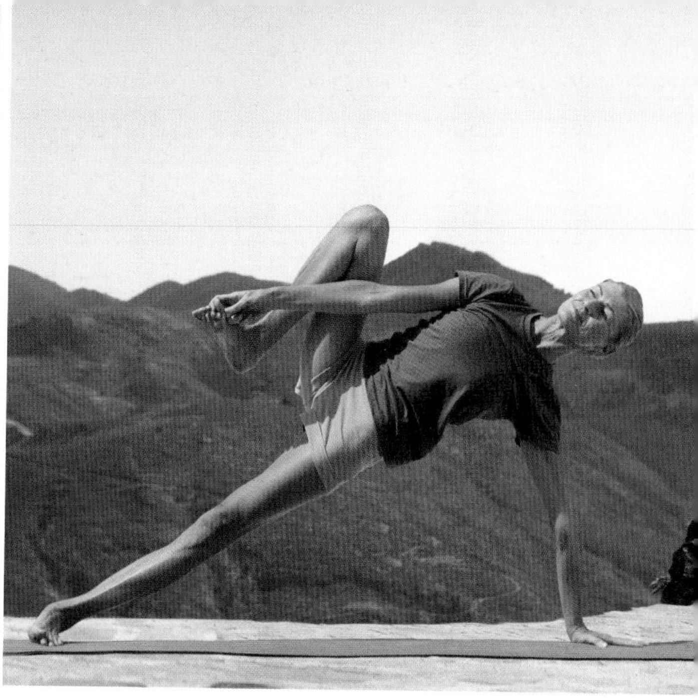

4 Exhale, bend your right leg, and grip the big toe firmly between the thumb and the index and middle fingers of your right hand.

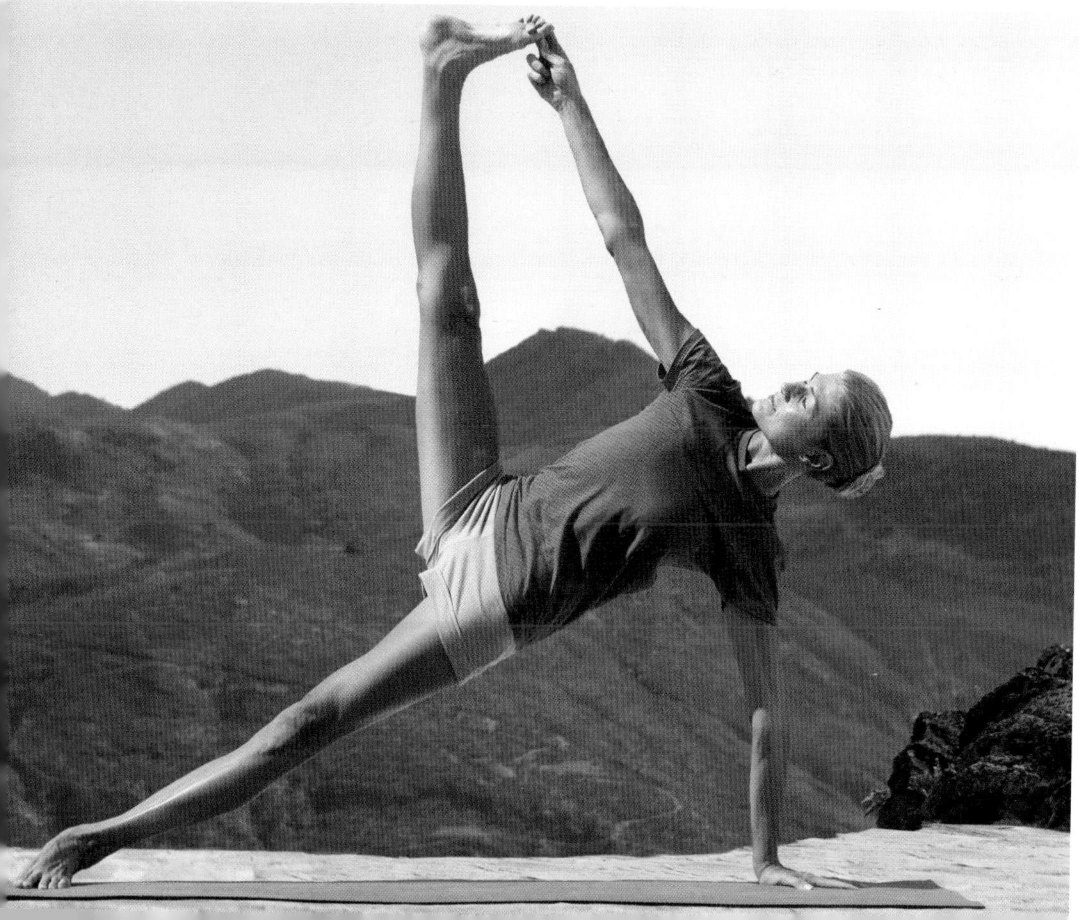

5 Lift your arm and leg and look towards your foot. Hold for 20-30 seconds, breathing evenly. Release your toe, lower your arm and leg, then turn back to Adho Mukha Svanasana. Repeat to the other side. Finish in Adho Mukha Svanasana.

"Wrong presentation of asana dislodges the position of intelligence, consciousness, and the core."

Alignment in Asana

Q. What is the theory of alignment that you teach?

"Perfect alignment of body, mind, and self. If I am intelligent here in the head, then I should be intelligent at the other places too. Say in my toe also.... Let me explain to you about my way of practice. I practise yoga in such a way that my intelligence stretches and spreads everywhere instantaneously. If my intelligence sticks at one place, I immediately work to see that it spreads equally everywhere. This means that when I do *āsana* or *prāṇāyāma*, I allow the intelligence to flow to each and every part of my body, so that I know and I understand what practice conveys to one for re-study and adjustment of *prāṇa* or energy to flow evenly. This is how I learnt, with attention and study, and I developed a progressive sequential method. If my intelligence is stretching here in one finger, if it is not stretching in the fingers of the other hand, I have to think and work out for the intelligence to flow in the same area of the other hand. Years of practice developed in me the instant feel to observe at once even the subtlest of the subtle disparities in my practice of *āsana*, *prāṇāyāma*, and *dhyāna*."

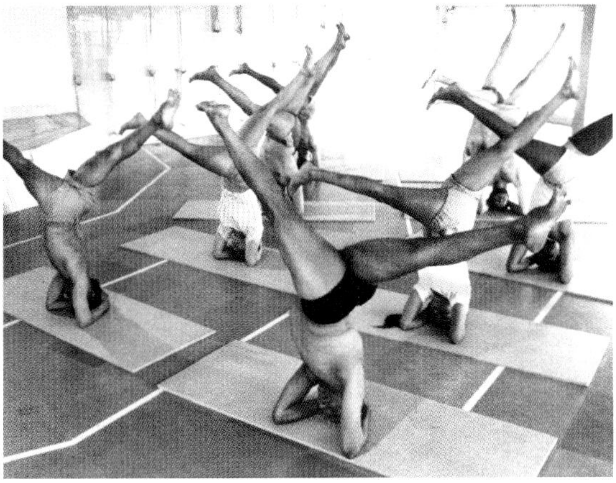

When teaching Parivrtta Eka Pada Sirsasana, Guruji demonstrates how the right and left sides of the body must speak to each other.

Observing Alignment

"I watch my right side, left side. I watch whether I am in the centre. I treat all the ten directions of my body – east, west, south, north, north east, north west, south east, south west, *ūrdhva* (upward), *adhara* (downward) evenly while doing any *āsana*. I bring the energy (*prāṇa*) to spread in all the ten directions of the body and make the awareness (*prajñā*) to flow evenly, concurring with energy (*prāṇa*). I make the self travel in each *āsana* to occupy even the remotest part of my body measuring from the centre – the real SELF. I embank (*digbandha*) all directions of my body for the self to rest in its abode in each *āsana* so that nothing enters in or goes out to disturb it. I make my body as a cave wherein I am alone and alive to everything."

Question from "The Strength of Yoga", interview by Roger Raziel in Paris, April 1984, first published in Le Monde Inconnu, *July 1984. Published in* Victoria Newsletter, *May 1991.*

Extract on this page from "What is Sthira Sukham Asnam?", talk on Hanumān Jayanti day 2007 in Pune.

Virabhadrasana I

Warrior Pose I

"Is your body stretching or your intelligence stretching inside your arms? What is stretching? You may stretch your arms physically, but are you aware of the other areas and other muscles of the arms co-ordinating evenly? Is there equanimity in the stretch? Did your mind go up with the arms? Did your mind reach there?"

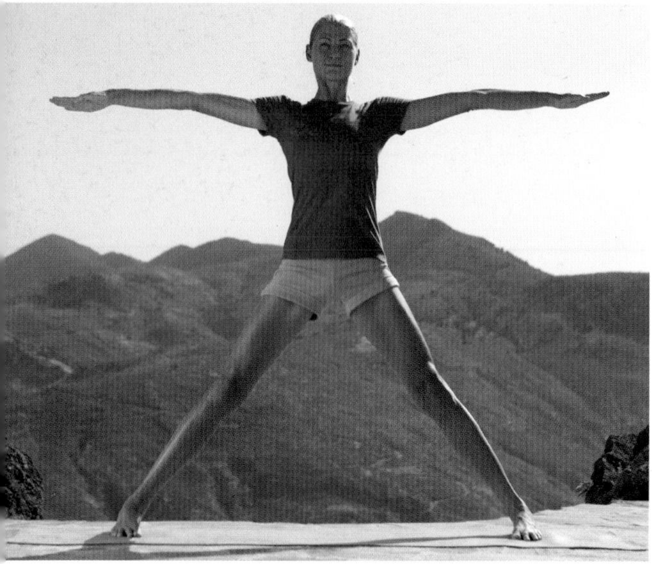

1 Begin in Utthita Hasta Padasana (see pages 108–109).

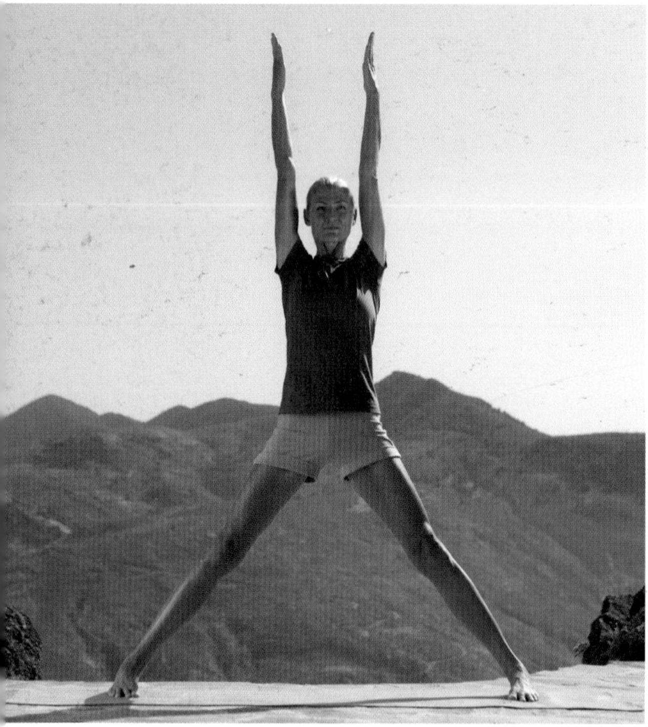

2 Turn your palms to face upwards. Inhale and raise both arms overhead, elbows straight, with your palms facing each other.

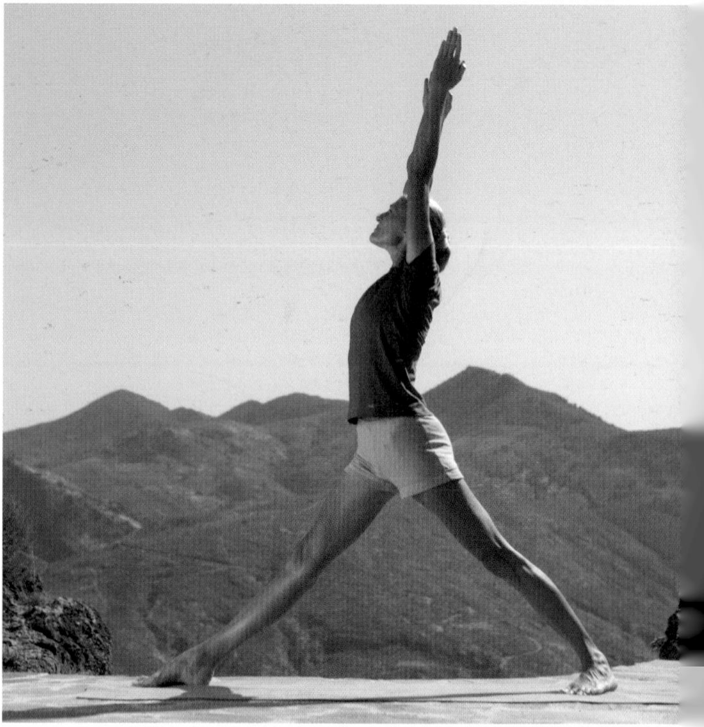

3 Turn your left leg and foot in by 60° and turn your right foot and leg 90° to the right. Inhale and rotate your entire torso to the right. Keep your arms extended and your chest lifted.

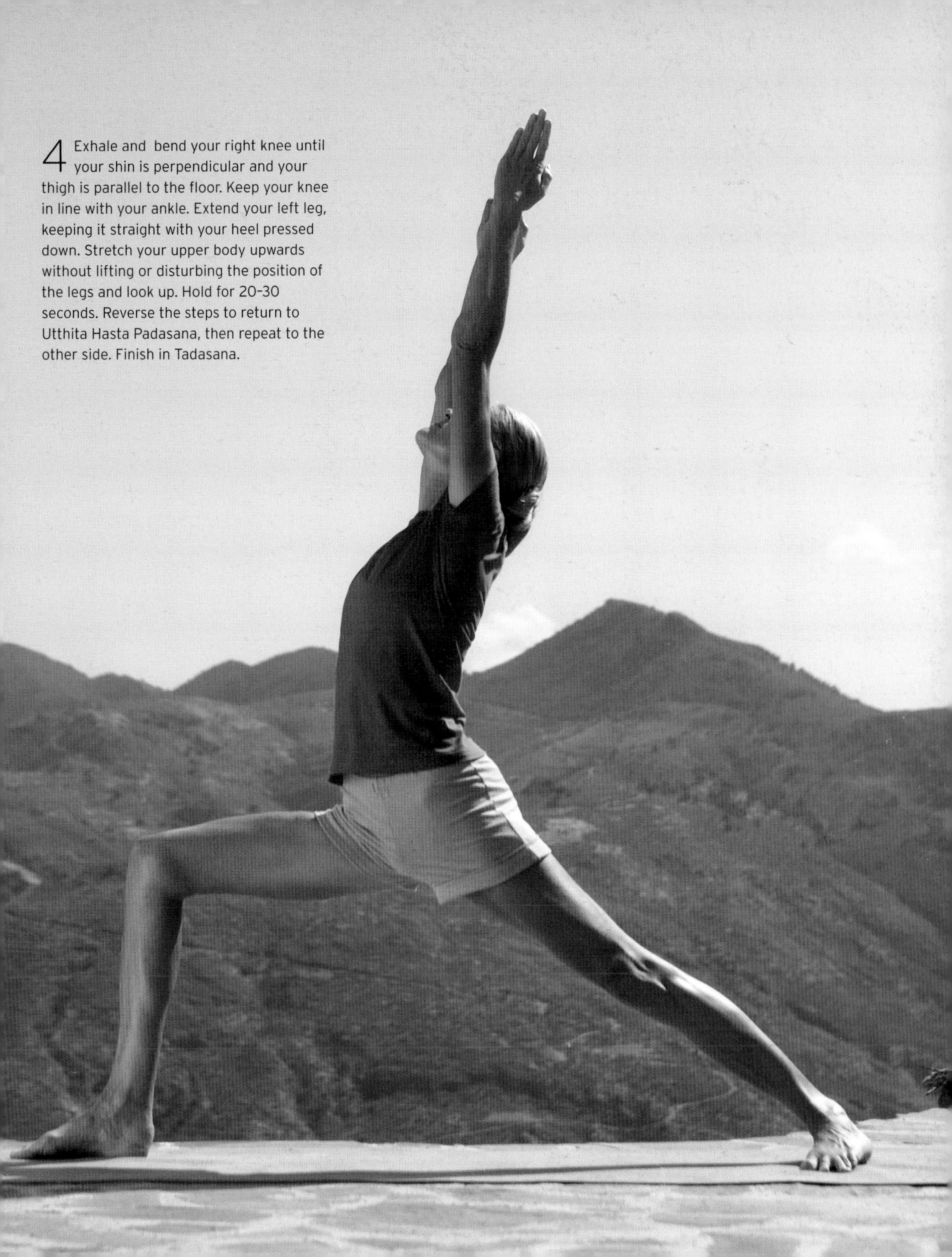

4 Exhale and bend your right knee until your shin is perpendicular and your thigh is parallel to the floor. Keep your knee in line with your ankle. Extend your left leg, keeping it straight with your heel pressed down. Stretch your upper body upwards without lifting or disturbing the position of the legs and look up. Hold for 20–30 seconds. Reverse the steps to return to Utthita Hasta Padasana, then repeat to the other side. Finish in Tadasana.

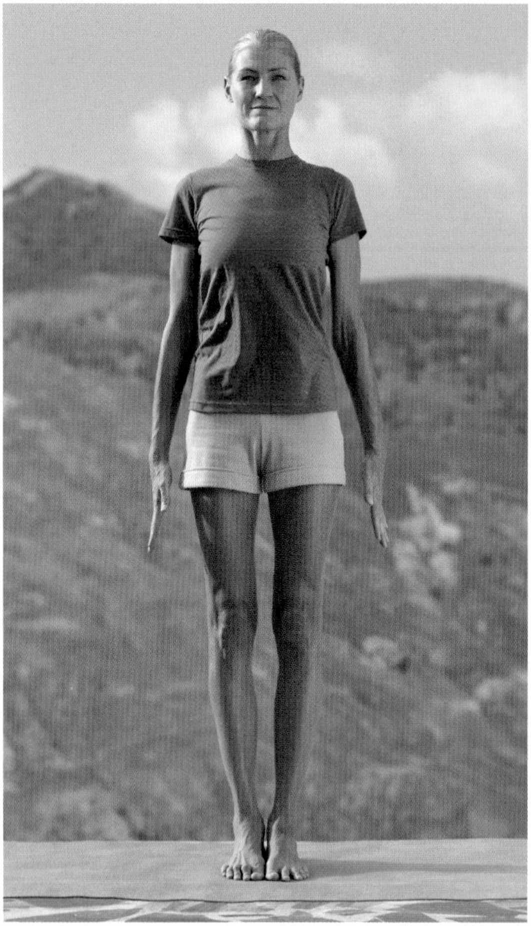

1 Stand in Tadasana (see pages 26-27).

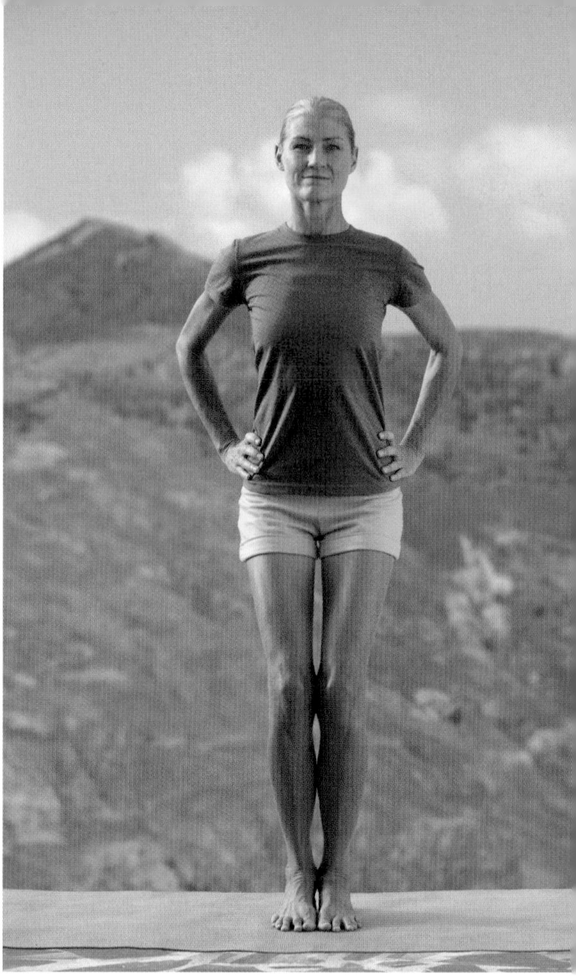

2 Place your hands on your hips and bend your knees. Keep your tailbone in.

Garudasana

Eagle Pose

"In order to adjust geometrically, we have to measure the dimensions of *āsana* so that we fit properly into it. Each *āsana* in its methodology has certain measurements of its height, length, width, and girth. Again there is a direction to the movement and action of the body which has to be followed properly. One has to analyze and realize the real shape and form of each *āsana* so that it is expressed and presented properly."

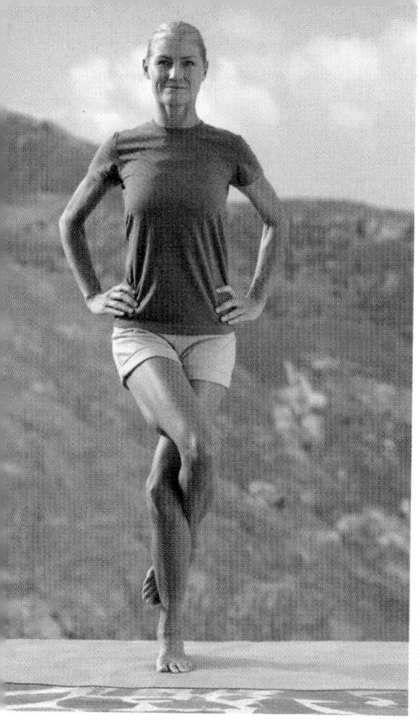

3 Cross your right thigh and knee over your left, taking the shin behind your left calf. Press your big toe into the leg.

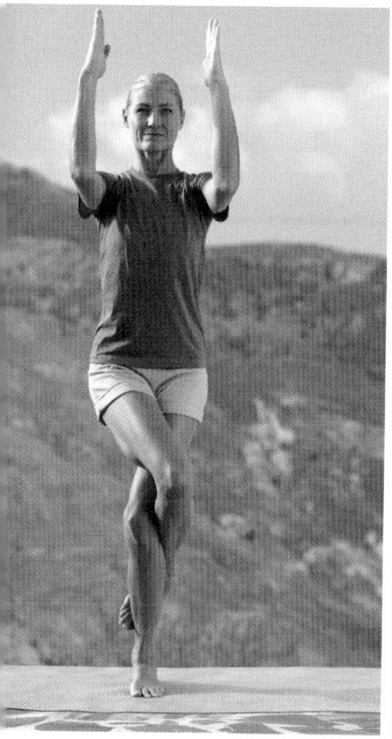

4 Balance on your left leg and raise your arms to chest level, elbows bent, and palms facing each other.

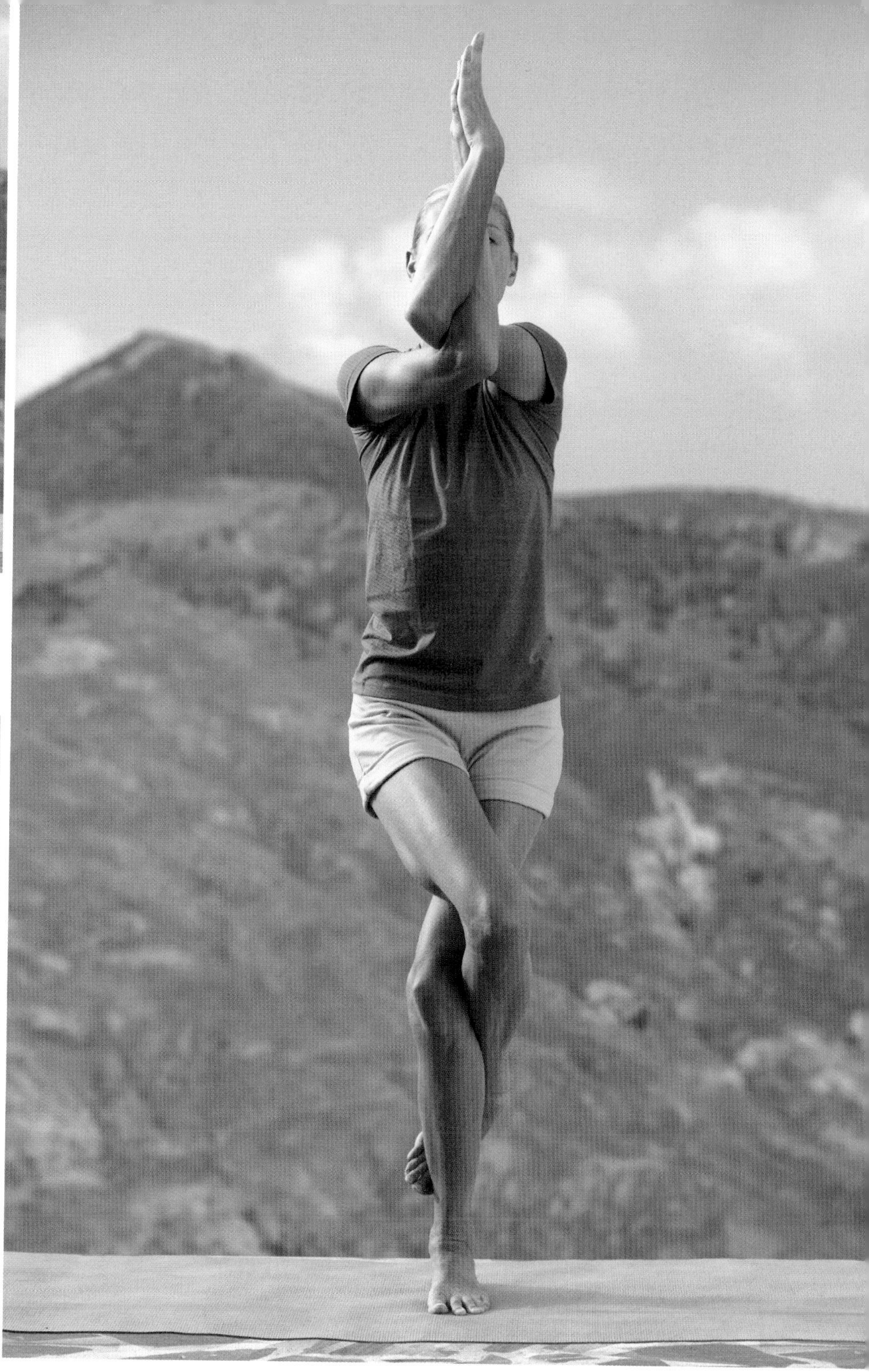

5 Cross your left elbow over your right elbow, tucking it into the elbow notch. Wrap your left forearm around the front of your right forearm and bring your palms together. Hold for 20 seconds, breathing evenly. Unwrap your arms and legs and return to Tadasana. Repeat to the other side. Finish in Tadasana.

"Whatever asana you do, see that your intelligence (prajna) is lighting each and every part of your body."

The Thread of Intelligence

" You know about the kites that children play with. There are different shapes of kites, each having a different form, design, thread, and person to play. As one observes children's kite games, the yogi learns by using his body as a kite. We have got hundreds of muscles and joints, thousands of fibres, millions and billions of cells and hence this body can be compared to a kite.

The Self, which is hidden inside, plays the kite; if the wind is not there, the kite cannot fly. As such, children move and pull the thread to make the kite fly by pulling and pushing the thread forwards or backwards until the kite catches the wind to soar up. Similarly, I use intelligence as a thread to act on the muscles to work properly and move evenly with rhythm. In the body, the calf or thigh muscles, or hinges, or ankles or heels are like different kites. To control these various muscles and structures that are like different kites, the thread of intelligence is made to be held by the holder – the Self (*sūtradhāra*) – to make the fibres, tissues, joints, and muscles move with control.

If the anatomical/physiological body is the kite, its thread is the intelligence and the Self is the holder of the thread. In order to adjust each muscle, joint, and fibre, the Self has to hold the thread and pull the intelligence in such a manner that all the various parts of the body are brought to a single state of stability like the kite that remains stable though soaring high in the sky. "

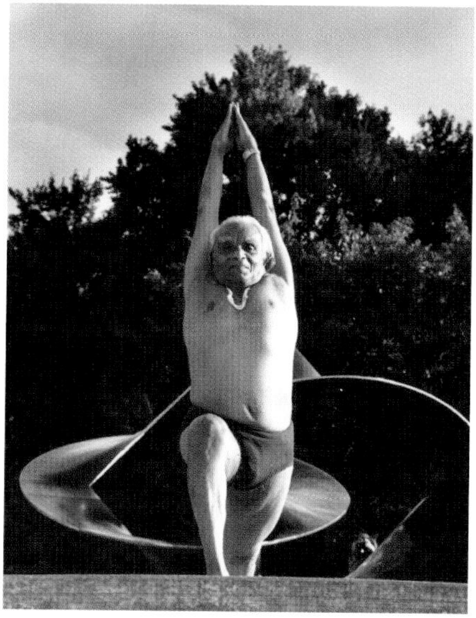

When performing asana, such as Virabhadrasana I, Guruji connects the periphery (the body) to the inner core (the Self) through the power of intelligence.

"The intelligence as thread grips the various parts of the body (the kite), so that the holder (the self) feels the oneness with the intelligence (thread), as if the kite, the thread and the self are one."

From a message at B.K.S. Iyengar's 79th birthday celebrations, December 1997, at RIMYI, Pune.

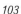

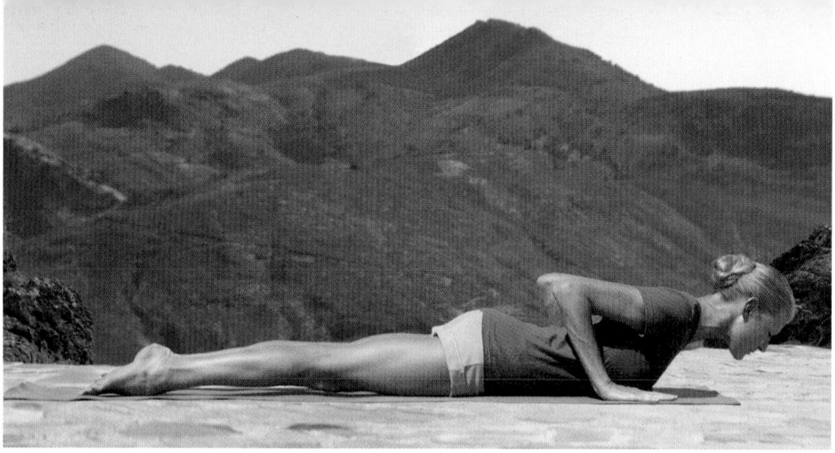

1 Lie face-down with your legs hip-width apart. Rest the tops of your feet on the floor with your toes pointing backwards. Place your palms beside your chest with your fingers pointing forwards.

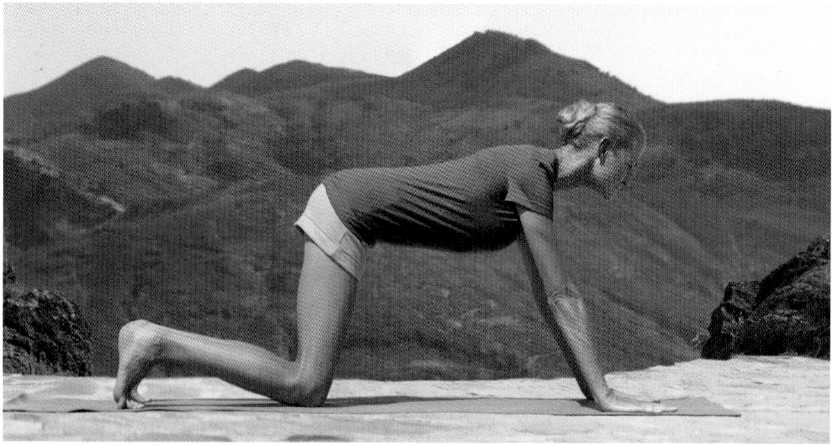

2 Turn your toes towards your knees. Press into your hands and straighten your arms to come to a kneeling position. Open your chest.

Adho Mukha Svanasana

Downward-facing Dog Stretch

"When you place your palms on the floor in *Adho Mukha Śvāṇāsana* you have to find where your energy is present and where it is absent, where the life force is active, or overactive, and where passive and inactive."

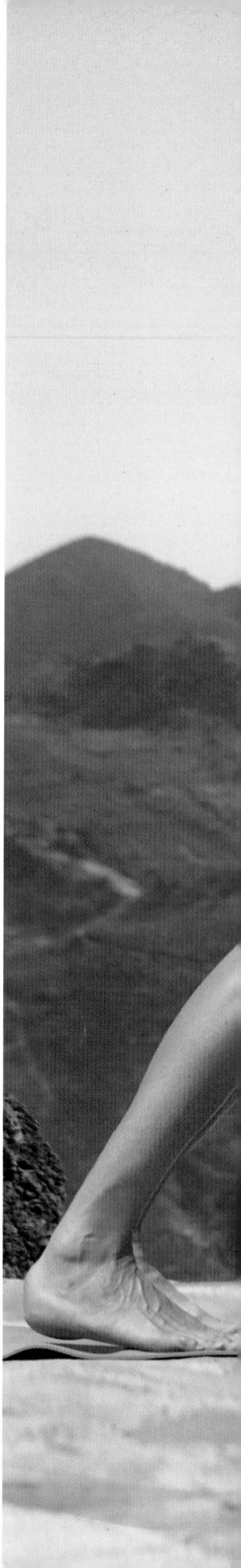

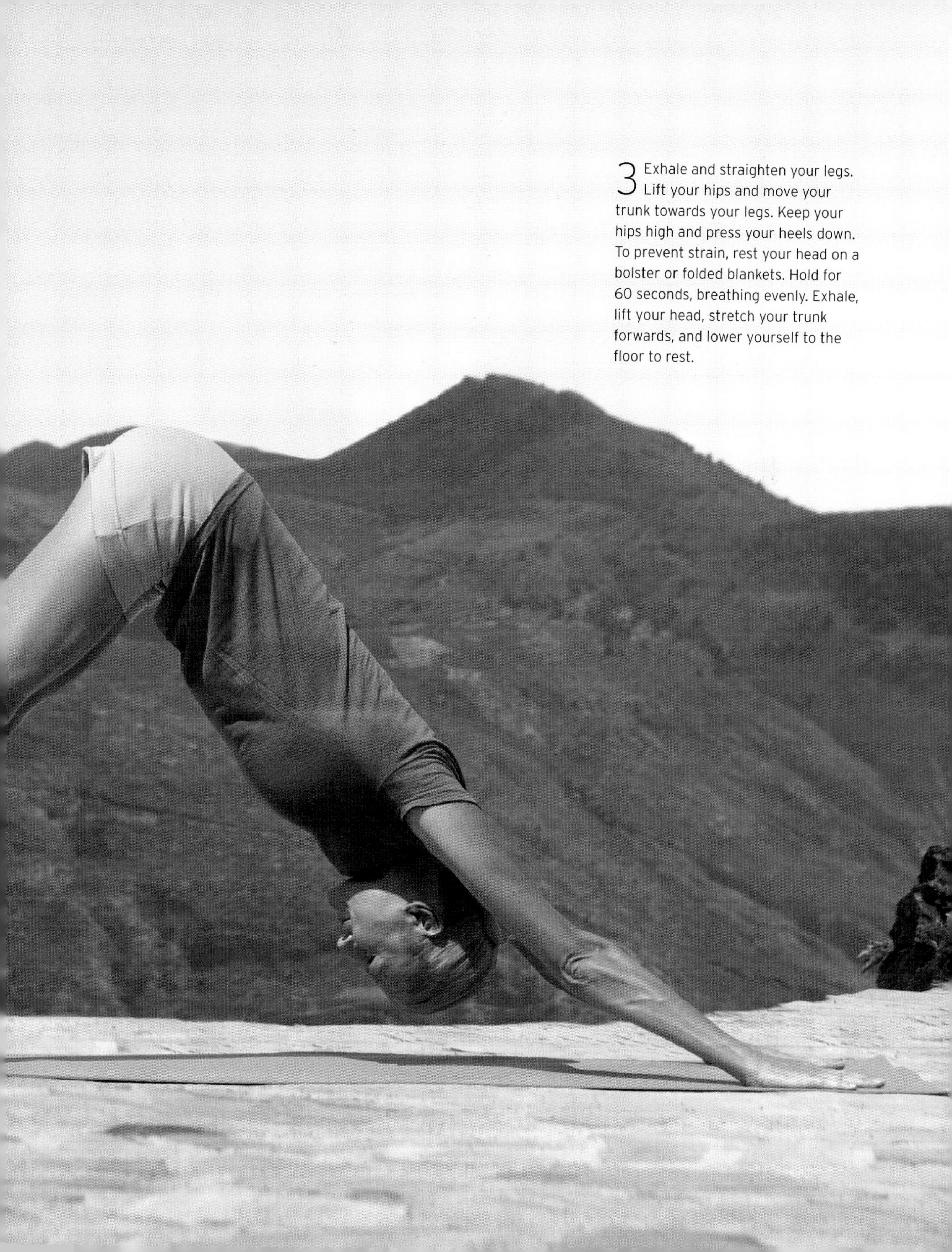

3 Exhale and straighten your legs. Lift your hips and move your trunk towards your legs. Keep your hips high and press your heels down. To prevent strain, rest your head on a bolster or folded blankets. Hold for 60 seconds, breathing evenly. Exhale, lift your head, stretch your trunk forwards, and lower yourself to the floor to rest.

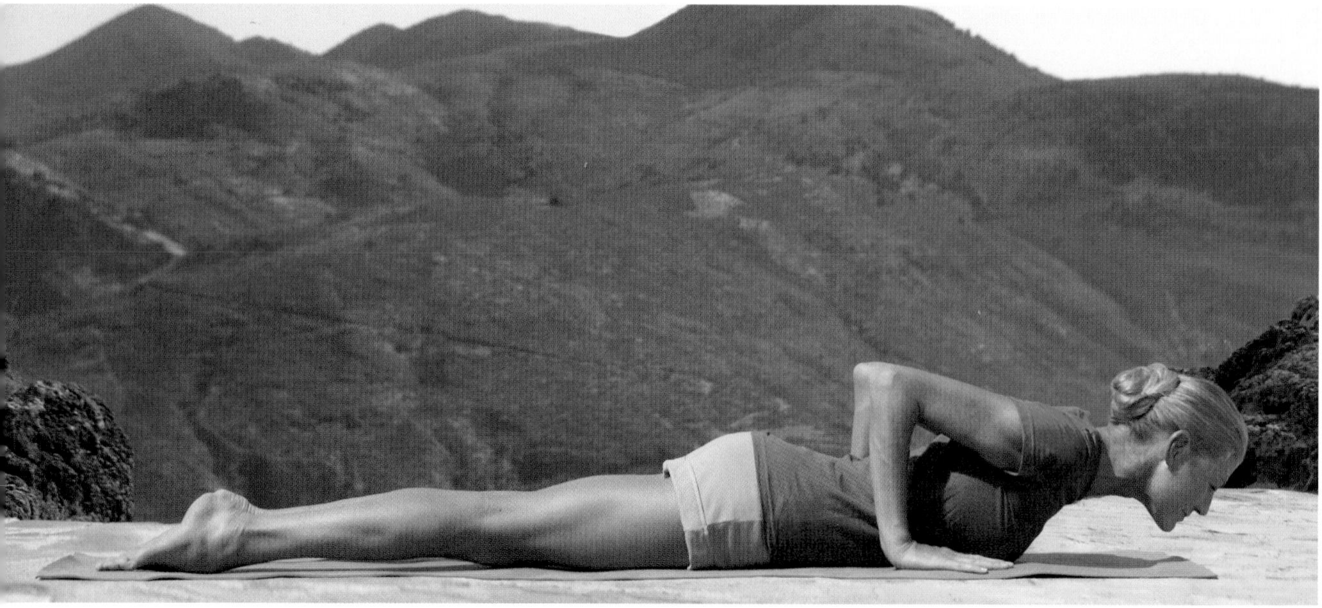

1 Lie face-down with your legs hip-width apart. Rest the tops of your feet on the floor with your toes pointing backwards. Place your palms beside your waist with your fingers pointing forwards.

Urdhva Mukha Svanasana

Upward-facing Dog Stretch

"In the practice of *āsana*, the mind is kept alert and the brain as a witnessing instrument, so the *sādhaka* realizes that yoga is not simply a physical discipline but a great mental discipline. Accurate performance of *āsana* heightens one's total awareness, reaching out to each and every pore of the skin, as it were. This way, the intellectual energy of the body is gradually raised to the level of the spiritual intelligence."

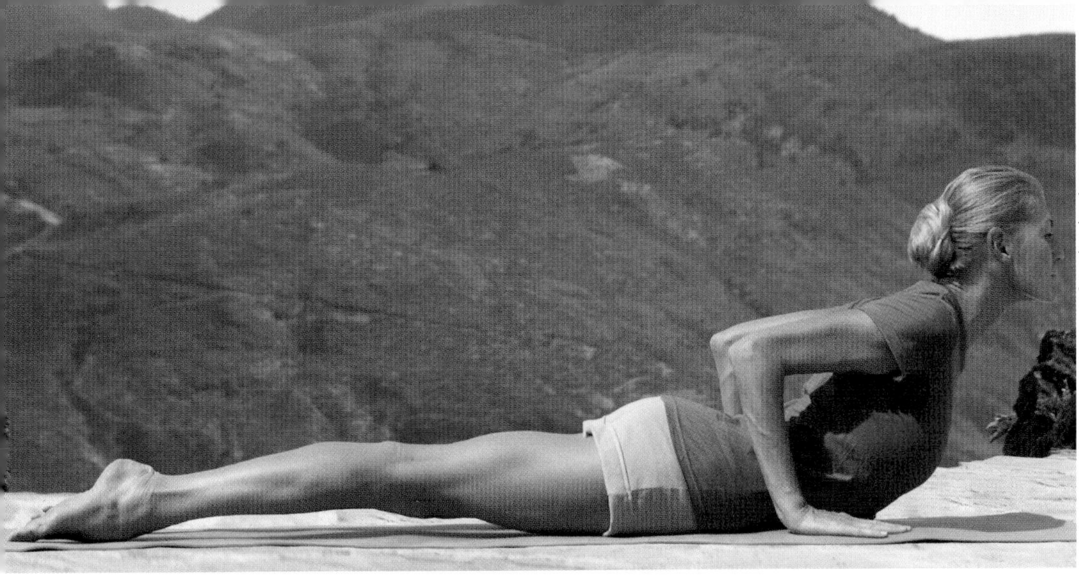

2 Inhale, press into the floor with your palms and the tops of your feet, then raise your head and trunk.

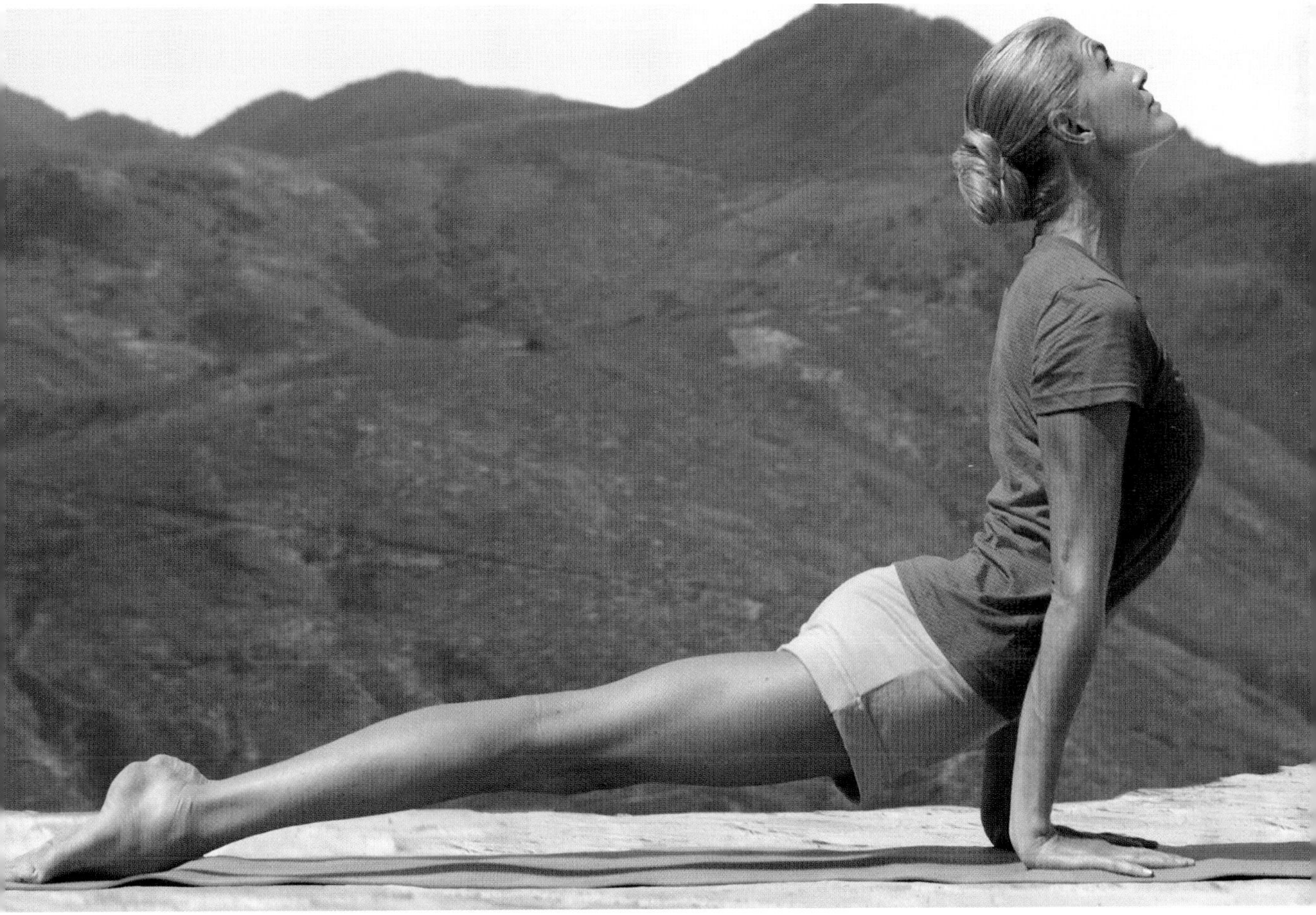

3 Straighten your arms and legs to lift your trunk and knees. Push your chest forwards and lift your sternum, feeling a stretch on the front of your body. Take your head back. Hold for up to 60 seconds. Exhale, bend your elbows, and lower yourself to the floor to rest.

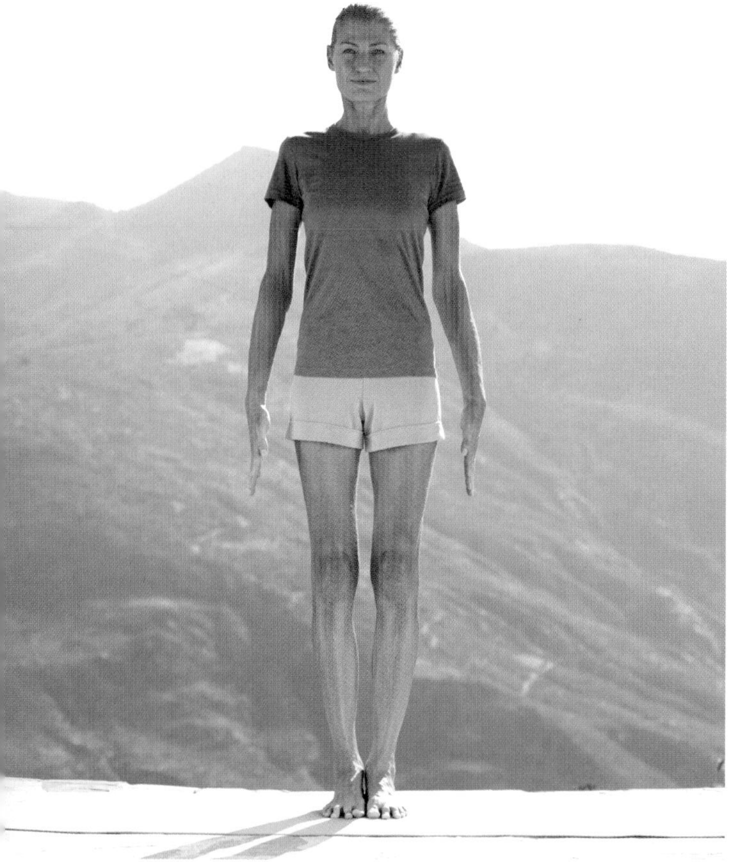

1 Stand in Tadasana (see pages 26-27).

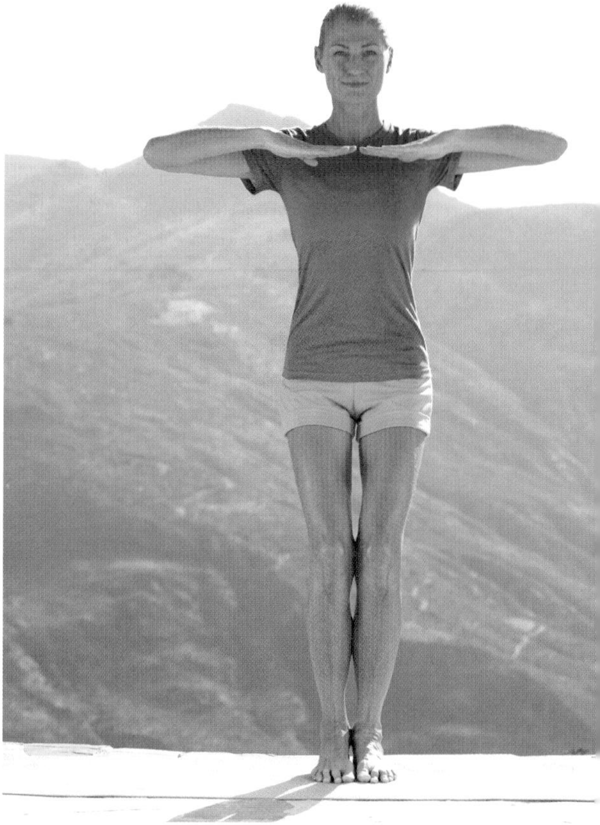

2 Bend your knees and bring your hands to your chest, keeping your elbows wide and in line with your shoulders.

Utthita Hasta Padasana

Extended Hand and Foot Pose

"Do you watch how the energy moves in the body?... See how the energy moves in your hands. Did you feel it when you were stretching or afterwards? Now slowly extend the hands without jerk or force and feel how and where the energy moves. This is how one has to notice the reflective action."

3 Exhale and jump your feet and arms apart. Land with your feet approximately 1.2m (4ft) apart and with your arms outstretched at shoulder-height, palms facing downwards. Ensure your feet are parallel to each other and pointing forwards. Lift your chest and look ahead. Hold for a few seconds, then jump back to Tadasana.

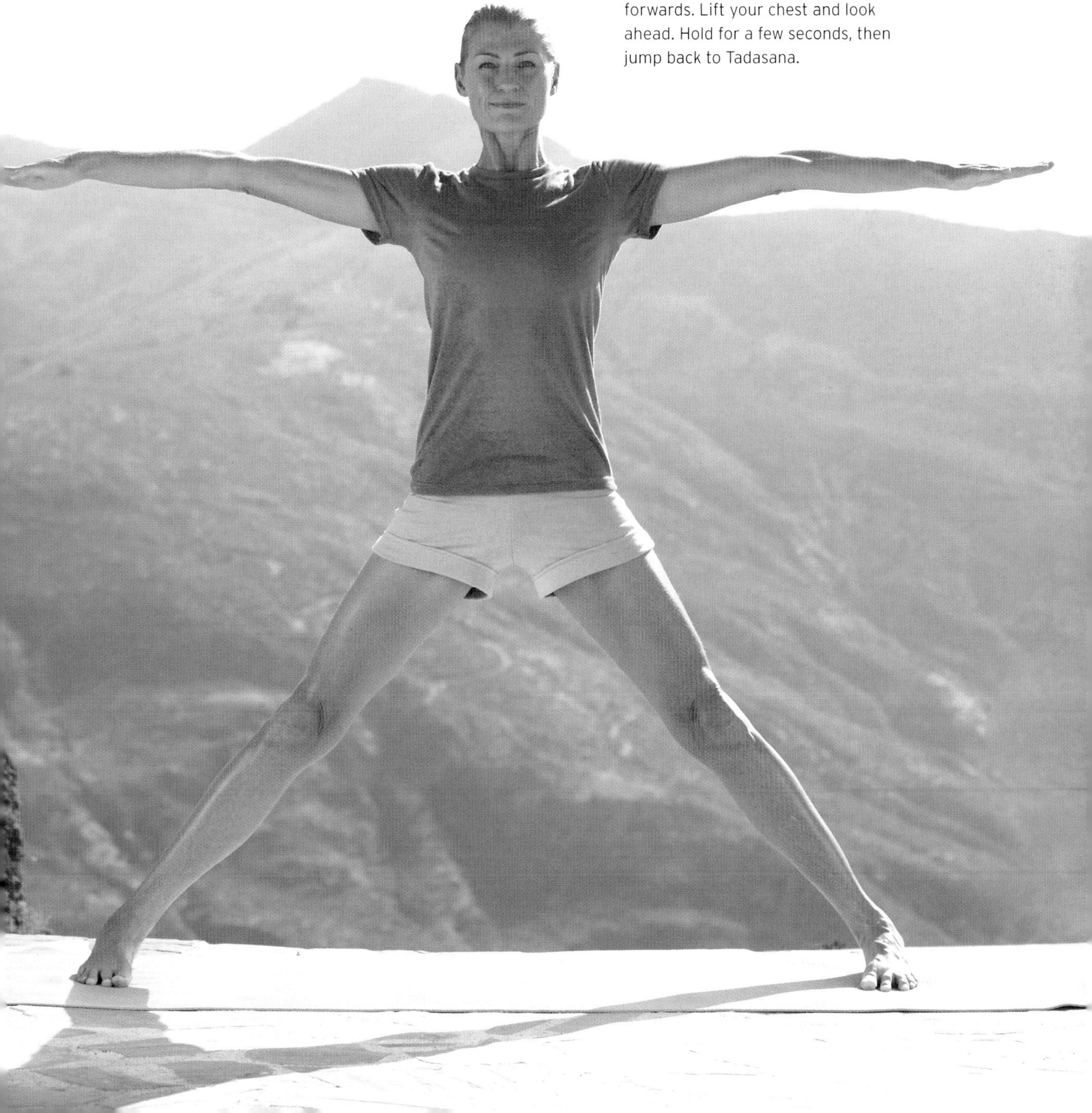

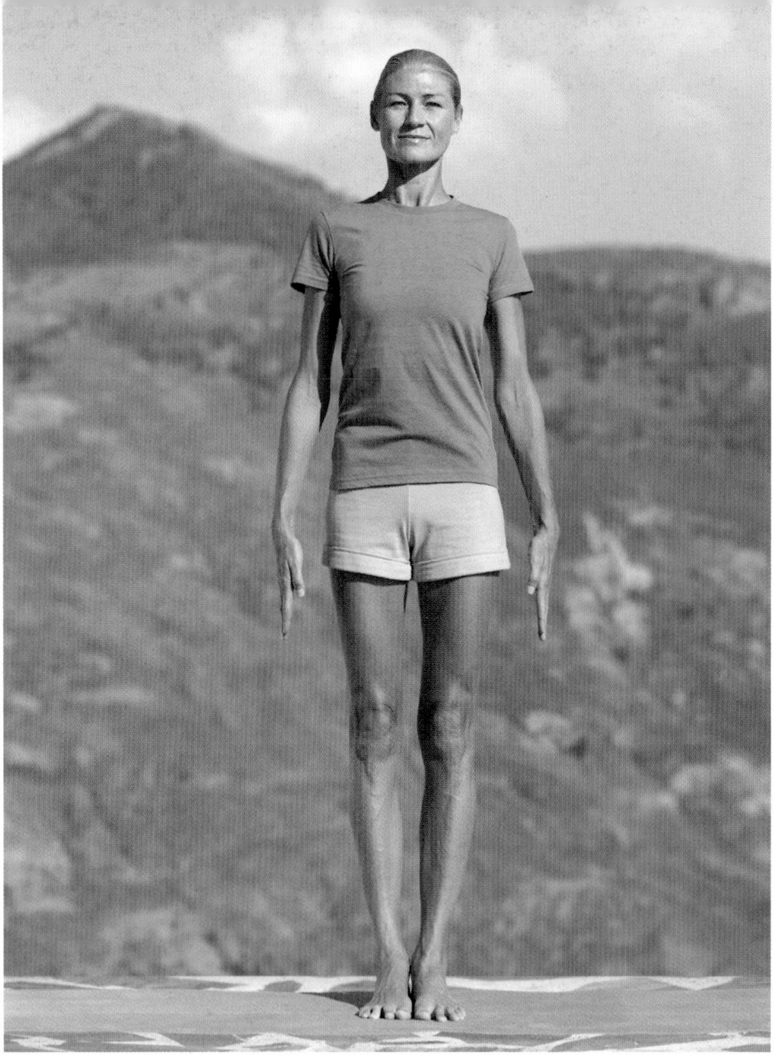

1 Stand in Tadasana (see pages 26–27).

Urdhva Hastasana

Upward Hand Pose

"Birds have two wings for flying higher and higher. For man, the shoulder blades are the wings to stretch higher and higher.... In order to stretch the arms above the head, one has to soften the skin on the outer side of the armpits and roll the shoulders backwards. Then, bringing the inner shoulder blades down, roll the shoulders in and stretch the arms up.... Often, I use a rod between the arms and the back of the head to get full extension of the arms."

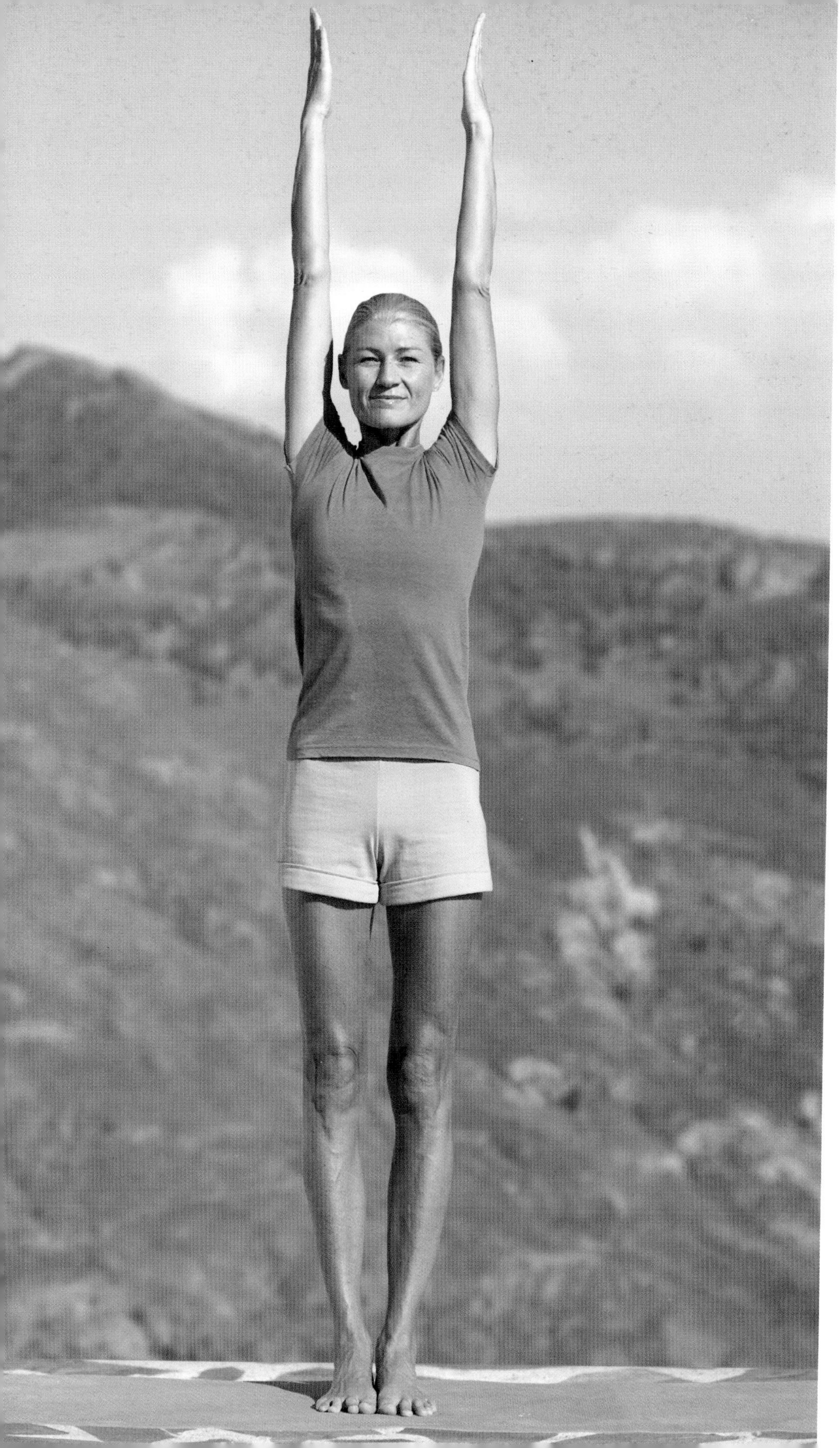

2 Inhale and stretch your arms forwards and overhead until they are perpendicular to the floor and parallel to each other. Keep your palms facing in and fingers together. Lift your sternum and side ribs and look ahead. Keep the back portion of the legs stable whilst stretching the arms up. Hold for 20 seconds, breathing evenly. Lower your arms to your sides to return to Tadasana.

"Though we use the word 100% perspiration...it refers equally to the body, mind and intelligence."

An Intense Practice

Q. Your teachings are based on an intensive practice of *āsana* and *prāṇāyāma*. This necessitates constancy and regularity. What is your advice for maintaining this practice?

"First of all, understand clearly the word 'intensity'. Intensity is not understood properly. Intensity is a mental attitude more than a physical attitude. Many people misunderstand what intensity means. They think it means straining and sweating. No! That is a wrong meaning of the word! Intensity is to get totally involved, fully immersed and absorbed in what one is doing. Intense practice means a fast and keen mode in adjusting, correcting, and progressively proceeding. When I say that I practise intensely, it means that my mental attitude and my mental disposition to the posture in *āsana* and the breath in *prāṇāyāma* are definitely deep inside. This I cannot express in words. Now, you say that you practise with an intensity of feeling. For me, *āsana* and *prāṇāyāma* blend my physical flow, emotional flow, intellectual flow, and the feel of the core evenly in my existence."

– Emotional? –

"Yes! Emotional. For me, emotional means a mental flow of equipoise, emotional equipoise. The mind is not focused on one thing, but exists everywhere, even in the corner of the fingernail. I have to feel that I am there, and that is known as intensity. When I say emotion, do not attribute emotions like love and sorrow to this state. What I mean to say is that when the mind is charged with an emotion like love, the whole mind is passionate and devoted to the subject. The mind undergoes certain qualitative changes when charged with such an emotional urge. Similarly, to me, the mind undergoes a qualitative change when I am doing *āsana* as well as *prāṇāyāma*.

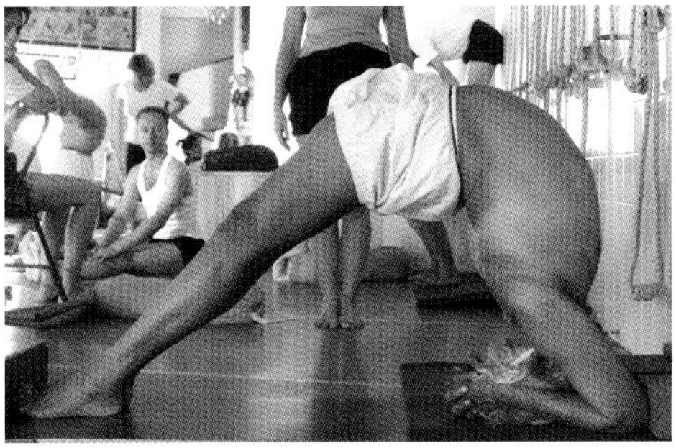

Guruji fully absorbed in intensive practice of Dwi Pada Viparita Dandasana. Students interrupt their own practice to look on.

I don't think anyone can understand the meaning of intensity so clearly unless and until there is devotion. The devotional practice is one thing and mental disposition is another, which changes from position to position in each *āsana*. The mind is not the same in each *āsana*, because the positioning being different, the approach too becomes different; the way of thinking differs; the way of action differs; the feel also differs. As each *āsana* varies in its presentation, so too the thinking and feeling process varies. As thinking varies, action varies. This totality of action and reflection changes the attitude of mind instantly from one *āsana* to other. It is a kind of mental and intellectual involvement. In your case, when you start, you are in the past and the moment you finish you are already in the future. You are never in the present. As emotion keeps the present moment lively, my mind remains alive with the moment, seeing its movements in that *āsana*. So, one has to see the way of thinking, the way of approach, and how it changes in a split second to come to the present moment. This observation teaches us to feel the freshness of mind, freshness of action, freshness of thought. And that is what I consider very important in the art of intense practice."

From "A Subject of the Heart", interview by Cathy Boyer, Johanna Heckmann and Anne-Catherine Leter, August 1995.

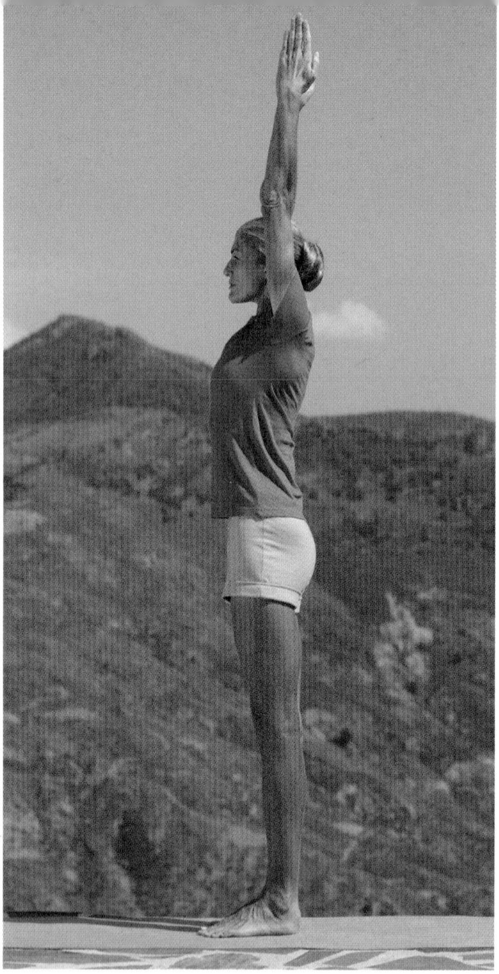

1 Stand in Tadasana (see pages 26-27). Raise both arms overhead until they are perpendicular to the floor and parallel to each other, palms facing inwards.

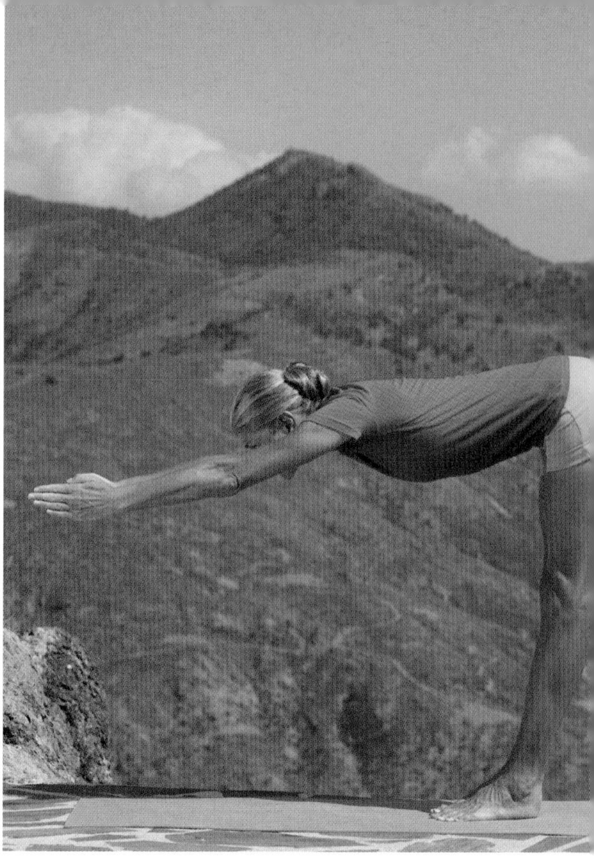

2 Exhale and extend forwards from your waist, stretching your trunk and arms forwards. Look slightly ahead.

Uttanasana

Intense Forward Stretch

"When you are asked to do *Uttānāsana*, have you ever studied the movement of energy? You only know that you are bending forwards and your hands are going down. But how do the energy and consciousness spread in the body? ...do you ever observe whether your consciousness expands from the back towards the sides, or do you only observe the vertical downward movement? When every *āsana* is multi-petalled, why do you make it single-petalled?"

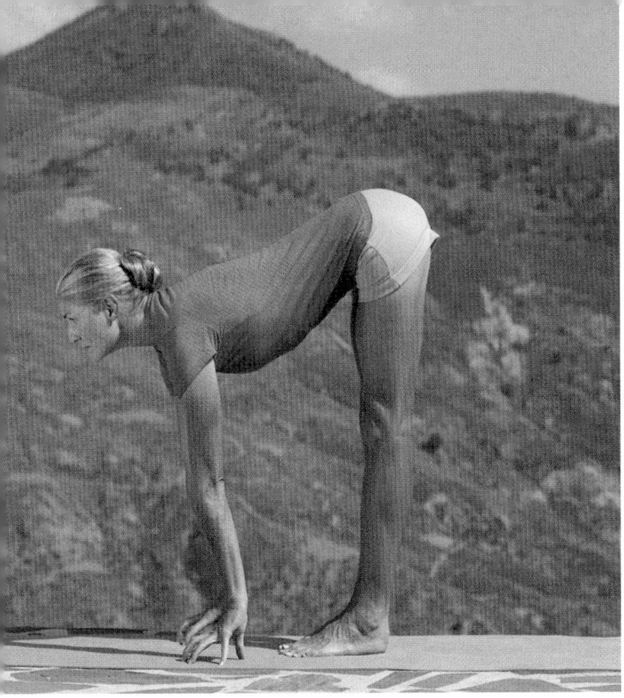

3 Keeping your spine and neck extended, bring the arms back, placing your fingertips beneath your shoulders. Lift your chest, look up and make your back concave.

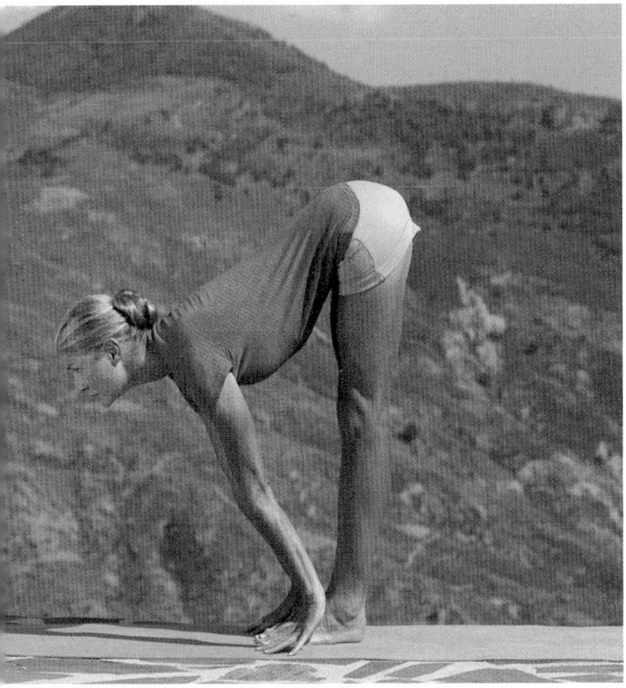

4 Stretch your arms back, placing your fingers in line with your toes on either side of your feet. Keep the backs of your knees and thighs fully stretched.

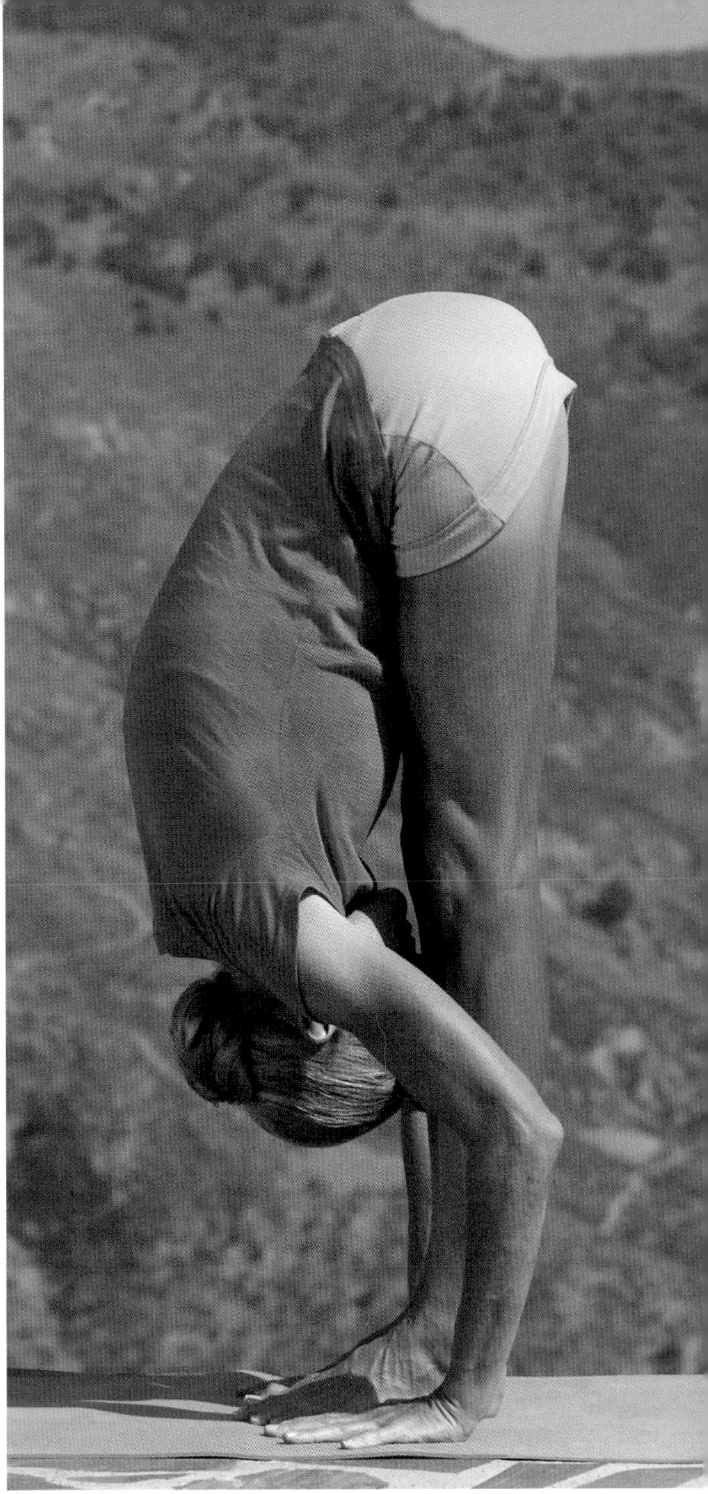

5 Exhale, bend your elbows, bring your head down, and move your trunk closer to your legs. Tuck your head in and try to rest your face on your knees. Hold for up to 60 seconds, breathing evenly. Inhale, lift your head and chest and, extending the spine, raise your trunk gradually, coming back to Tadasana.

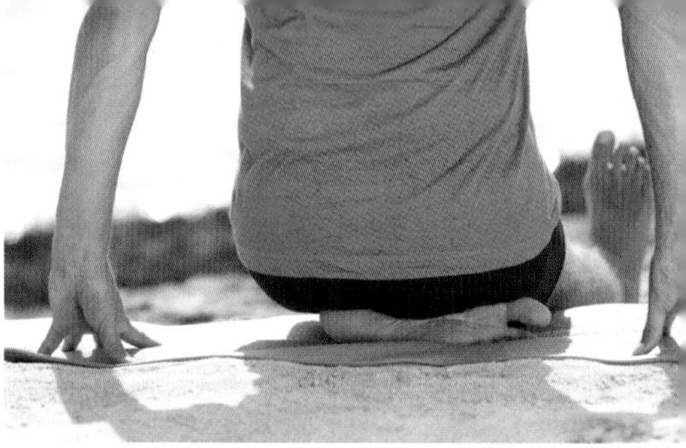

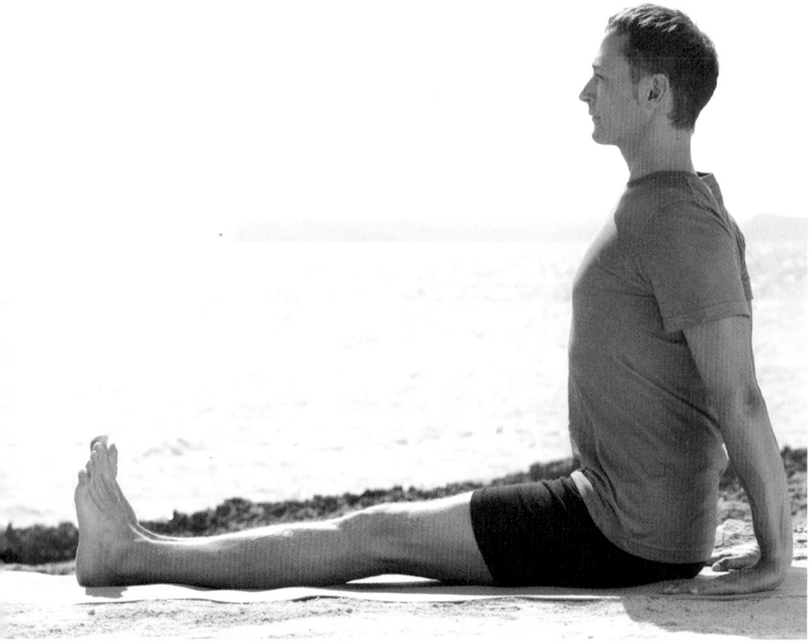

2 Bend your left knee, lift your buttocks, and position your left foot beneath them, heels and toes aligned. Lower your left buttock onto your heel and right buttock onto your toes.

1 Sit in Dandasana (see pages 14-15).

Ardha Matsyendrasana I

Lord of the Fishes Pose I

"When we do the *āsana*, we use what you call the four lobes of the brain: the right, the left, the front, and back.... Medical science speaks of the front brain as biological brain, and back brain as old brain. While practising the *āsana*, we need to trace how the back brain and the front brain react in keeping the discriminative faculty and serenity intact. When analytic and synthetic parts of the brain synchronize together, real sensitivity develops and leads us to experience a state of silence and stability."

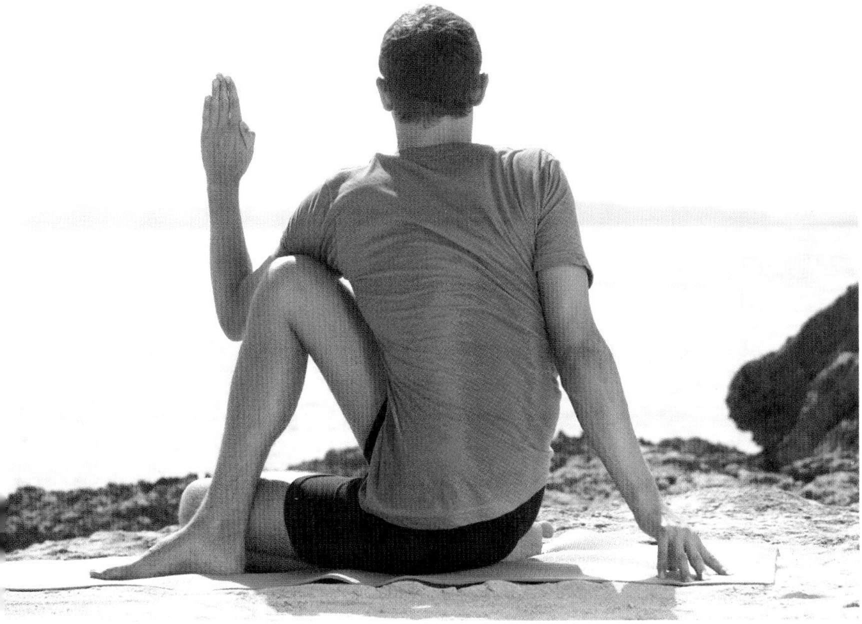

3 Bend your right knee and place your foot by the outer side of your left thigh, shin perpendicular to the floor. Turn your trunk 90° to the right, left armpit on the outer side of your right thigh, elbow bent, and palm facing forwards.

4 Exhale and wrap your left arm around your bent shin, reaching towards your waist. Take your right hand back and clasp the left wrist, palm facing outwards. Turn your head to look towards your right foot. Hold for 20-30 seconds. Release your hands, rotate back to centre, and straighten your legs into Dandasana. Repeat to the other side. Finish in Dandasana.

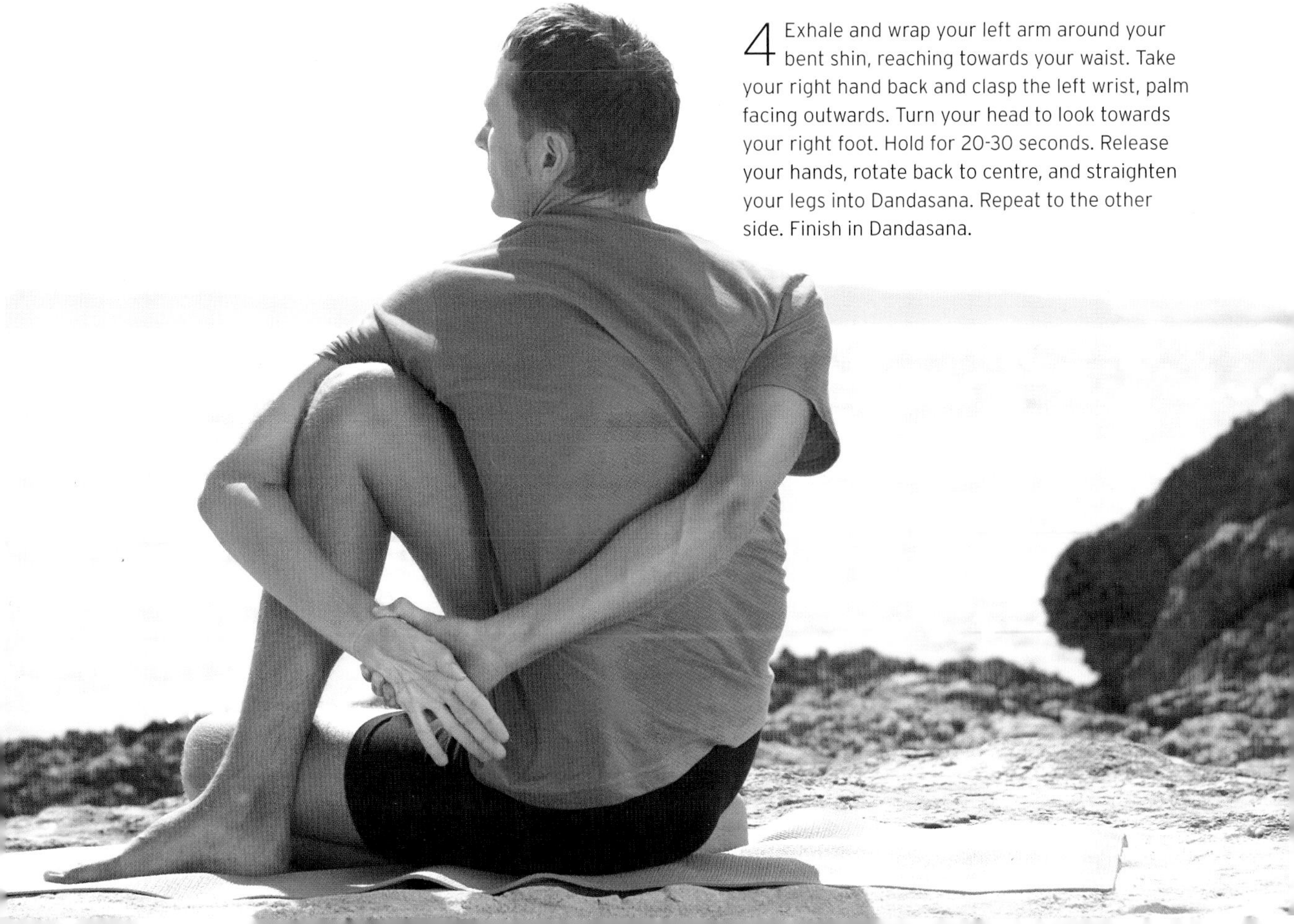

Finding the Centre of Gravity

“ As far as the *āsana* is concerned, the centre of gravity is not the same for each *āsana*, as each has a different position and hence the centre of gravity changes. If one stands on his legs and does *Tāḍāsana*, and if the weight on the legs is unequal, it means the centre of gravity has changed. In slanting the body, the gravity changes. One may not fall from the *āsana* , but one has to recycle the slant that is created by shifting to the other side so that one brings back the centre of gravity to the base.

As far as the presentation of *āsana* goes, if one adjusts the body with the right presentation, he experiences the feel of lightness. In this state know that the centre of gravity has changed in that *āsana*.

The *Haṭhayoga Pradīpikā* (1.17) says that the practice of *āsana* has to be such that it should bring levity in the body and mind (*aṅgalāghvam*). The body has to feel the lifefulness and lightness in a perfect presentation. In order to bring this lightness, one needs to work in a particular way to ensure that the body does not become heavy, or sway or sink. In each *āsana*, one has to feel the sense of ascendance and upliftment in the body and intelligence. This firm presentation brings lightness and one feels the elevation in mind.

If the body in each *āsana* is properly adjusted, the centre of gravity shifts and this causes emotions and intelligence to change for the better in the *āsana*. While doing the *āsana*, if the chest sinks one feels emotional disturbance. This is particularly felt when one is depressed or in a state of loneliness. Sometimes even fear complexes sink the body's position, changing the centre of gravity. The moment the chest opens in back-bends, the emotional centre opens, the body changes its shape, and one feels

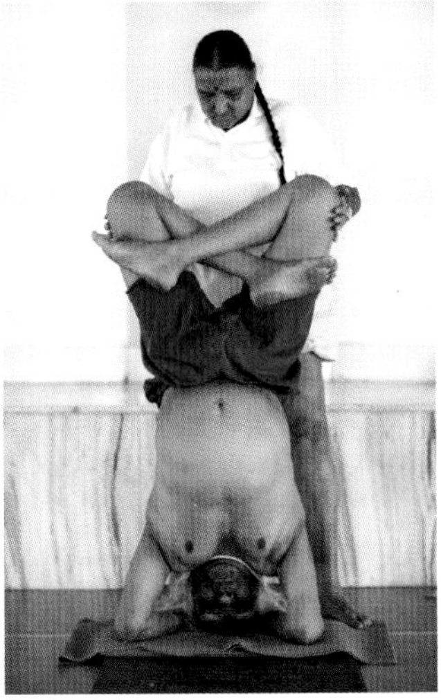

"All the āsana *have to be practised to be in line to the core to experience the infinite that is within" states Gurujī. Here, his daughter Geeta helps him to establish such centring to the core during a morning practice of Padmasana in Sirsasana.*

elated. But if the chest gets collapsed, then the mind sinks and the emotional weather becomes heavy, which means that the gravitational force has changed.

If the position of the body is corrected in *āsana* emotional stability occurs, which makes one to understand the trueness of the *āsana*.... The centre of gravity of the body and the mind as well as the emotional and the intellectual centres should remain aligned. Then one finds the correct centre of gravity in an *āsana*. This way, one has to find the centre in each *āsana*.

When Patañjali mentions *ananta samāpatti* in *āsana*, it means that in each *āsana*, the body and mind have to gravitate towards the centre of the soul. To touch that infinite within, the finite body has to work through *āsana* to develop sharpness of intelligence. This is the way one has to rectify and perfect each *āsana* in order to gravitate towards that right centre. It depends not only upon one's intellectual calibre, but also on the devotional approach in his endeavour.

The true centre of the body is the Soul or the Core of the being. Whichever may be the *āsana*, the contents of the body, right and left sides, are to be measured and balanced evenly in line with the Soul or the Core. ”

From " On On Aṣṭāṅga Yoga – Centre of Gravity in Āsana", Aṣṭadaḷa Yogamālā *Volume 7, pp121–24.*

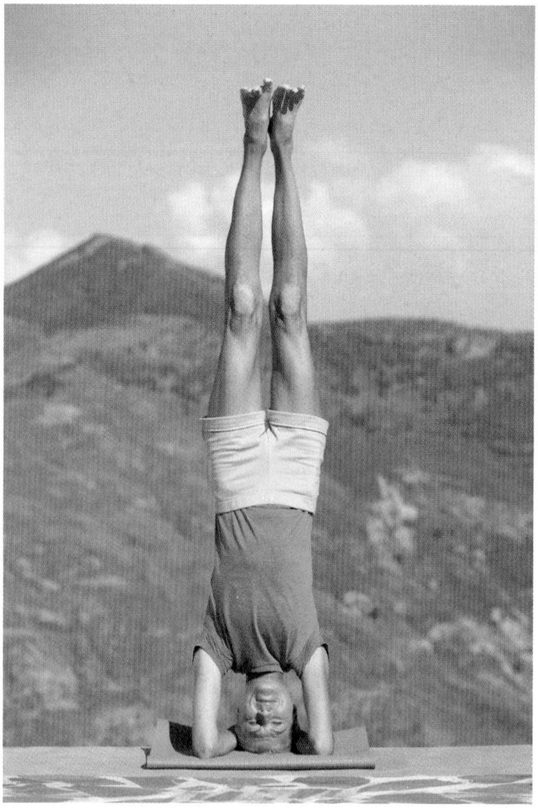

1 Begin in Salamba Sirsasana (see pages 72–75). Keep your head, arms and shoulders in this position throughout.

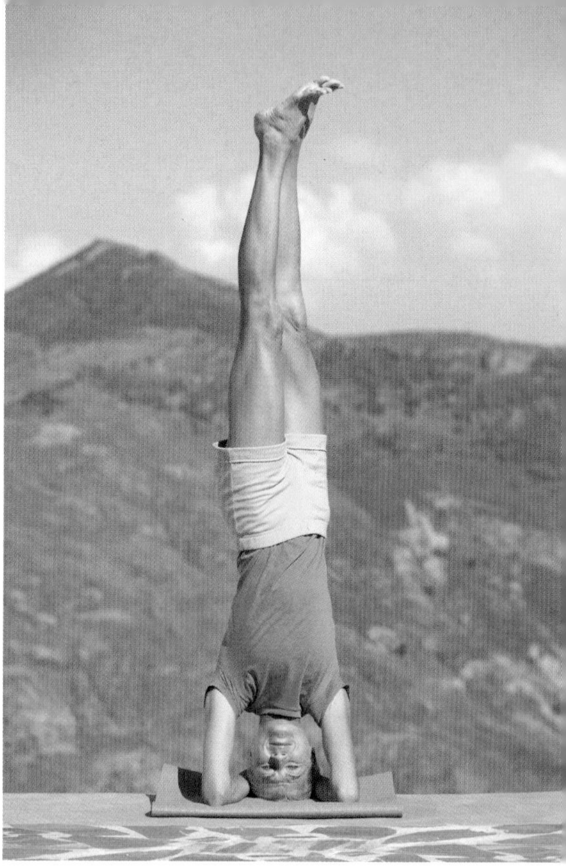

2 Exhale and turn your legs and trunk to the right. Keep your shoulders lifted and stretch upwards. This is Parsva Sirsasana. Hold for 20 seconds. Exhale, rotate back to centre, then repeat to the left. Return to centre, lower your legs, and rest, or begin step 3.

Sirsasana Variations

Asana Sequence

"Do you not concentrate continuously in order to maintain the balance by raising your shoulders and keeping them parallel? Think about this and you will realize that you are doing something which is more than physical. You are working for the mind and body to unite as a single unit, by igniting the light of the Self."

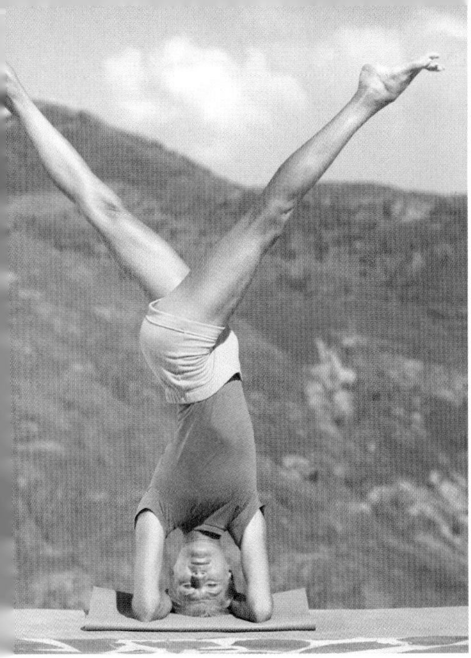

3 In Salamba Sirsasana, stretch your left leg forwards and right leg back. Exhale, revolve your trunk right and turn the legs 90° (Parivrttaikapada Sirsasana). Hold for 20 seconds. Exhale and turn back to centre, legs together. Repeat with your right leg forwards and left leg back. Return to Salamba Sirsasana. Come down or begin step 4.

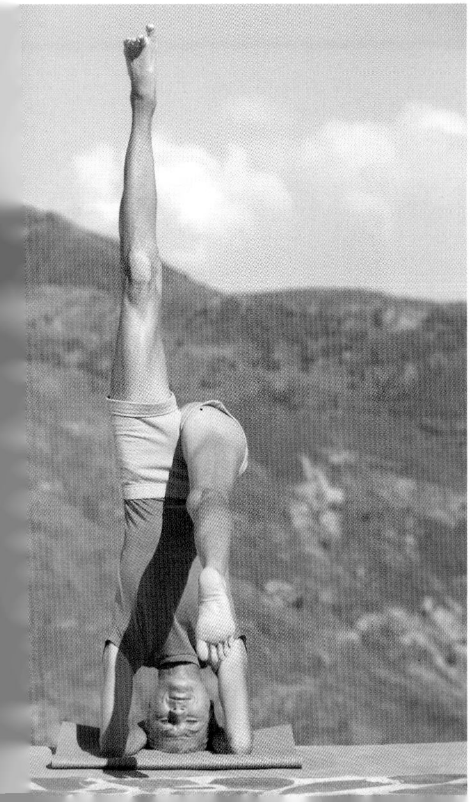

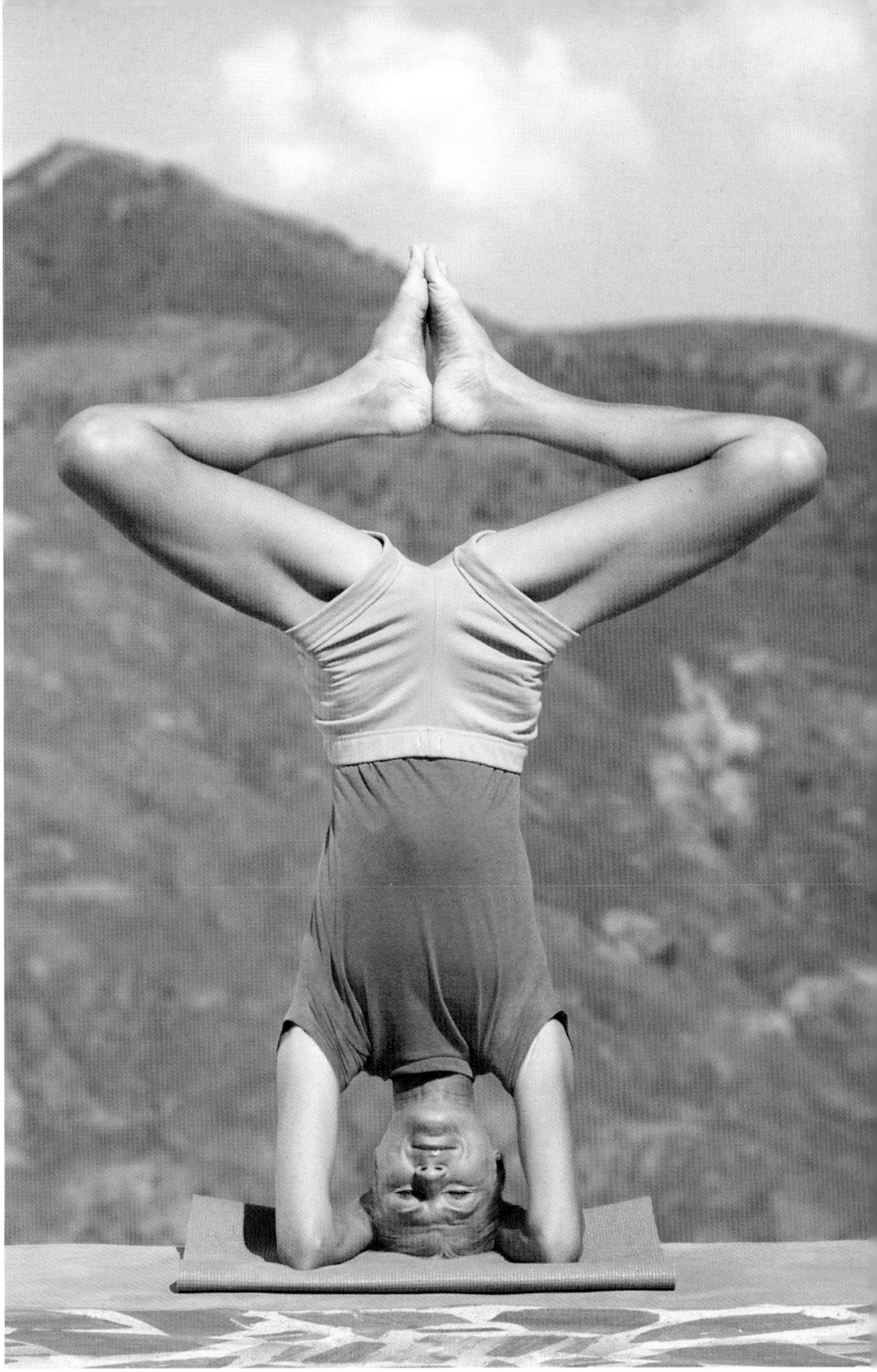

4 In Salamba Sirsasana, exhale and lower your right leg towards the floor. At the same time, extend your left leg vertical. Keep both legs in line and straight (Ekapada Sirsasana). Hold for 20 seconds. Exhale, lift your right leg back to your left, then lower your left leg. Return to Salamba Sirsasana and come down or begin step 5.

5 In Salamba Sirsasana, exhale and bend your knees to the sides, pressing your soles together. Keep your knees in line with your hips and lift your spine (Baddha Konasana in Sirsasana). Hold for 20 seconds. Straighten your legs, exhale and come down. Rest for a few seconds with your forehead down before sitting up.

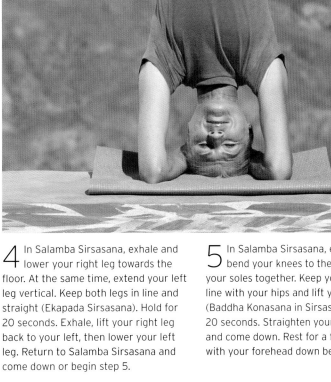

"The skin has this special sense of touch which is nothing but the touch of the inner intelligence."

The Sensitivity of Skin

" *Yogasādhanā* needs a tremendous inward penetrative and introverted state of mind. You have to be very, very sensitive to the inside body. Look at a leaf. See its end and its middle. When there is a gentle breeze, the middle of the leaf may shake or not, but the end of the leaf vibrates because that part is not only thin but very sharp and sensitive. Your intelligence should be sharp like the thin edge of the leaf.

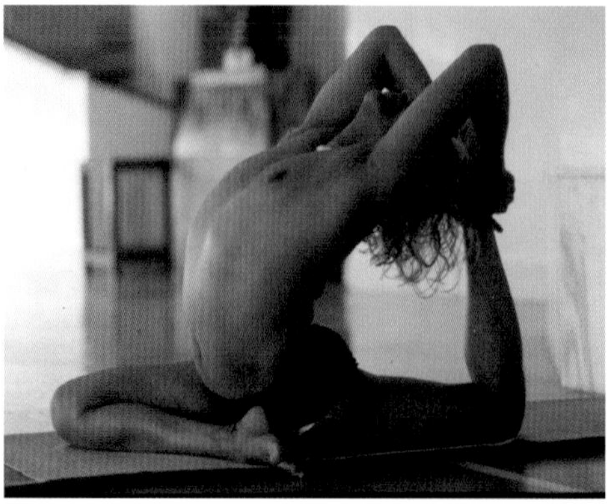

In Eka Pada Rajakapotasana Guruji reveals the skin's incredible powers of expansion.

If your intelligence is as sensitive as the thin end of the leaf, I am sure you will understand the presentation of the *āsana* far better than now. The skin at the corners of our torso, legs or arms is like the thin edges of the leaf. Skin has the power to contract (*sunkucita*) or expand (*vikāsata*). If the skin has no power to contract or expand, neither can the muscle. Medical science only speaks of the muscle contraction and expansion. Nobody thinks that the skin has the power to accommodate the muscles. If skin was incapable of expansion and contraction, it would have torn easily, ruptured easily, and blood would have oozed out. Skin creates the space for the inner body. Skin is infra-structurally ether. This ethereal body, the skin, has a tremendous touch-sensitivity (*sparśa*).

The *āsana* teaches us the subtle (*sūkṣma*) element of the ether through skin. Each and every part of our body has a certain amount of ether, which expands and contracts. For example, when you do *Utthita Trikonāsana* on the right side, the ether expands on this leg while it contracts on the left. That is why you move the right leg easily for adjustment. In the left leg, the earth element is strong and hence you cannot adjust and move your left leg with ease. So learn to change the earth element in the left leg into the ether element to adjust. In the right leg, you change the ether element into the earth element to gain stability. ”

From "The Gem of Life is In Your Hands", Gurujī's message 14.12.1999 at RIMYI.

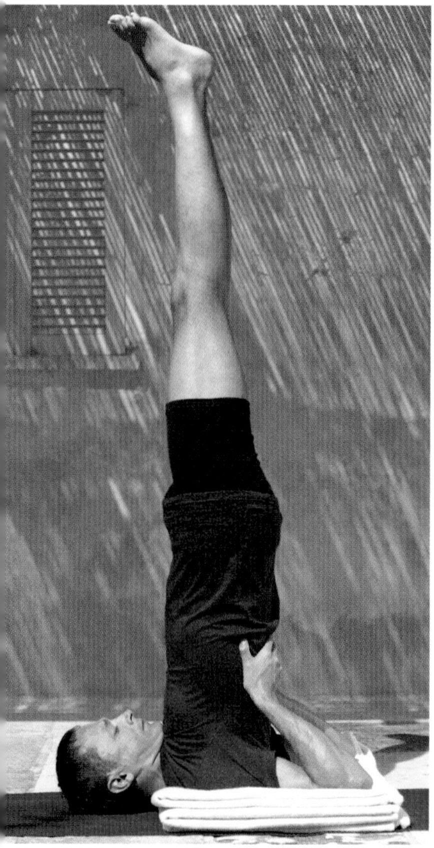

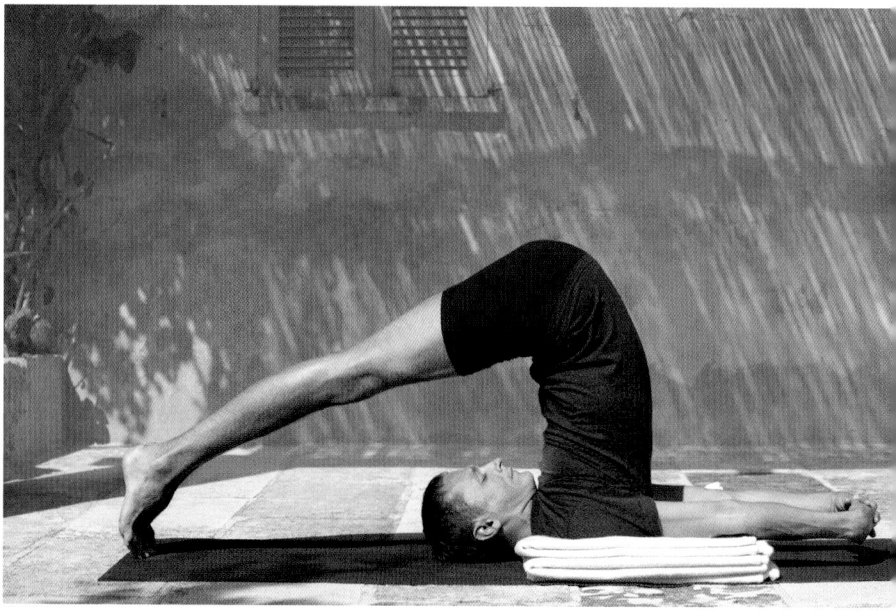

1 Begin in Salamba Sarvangasana (see pages 128–29). Keep your palms pressing against the middle of your back as you move into step 2.

2 Exhale and lower your legs, taking your chest and hips slightly back, until your toes touch the floor. Stretch your arms and interlock your fingers. Hold for 1–5 minutes (halfway through, change the interlock of your fingers). Release your hands and reverse the actions to return to Salamba Sarvangasana. Gradually slide your spine to the floor, then lie back and relax.

Halasana

Plough Pose

"Don't you experience serenity when you are resting very well in *Sarvāṅgāsana, Halāsana,* or *Setubandha Sarvāṅgāsana*? That means you are doing meditation even though you are in the *āsana*. You are connected to the body and at the same time you are detached. Meditation, as it is ordinarily taught, leads you to emptiness. There is a disconnection between the body and the soul, and in-between there is emptiness. But when you do *Halāsana*, the mind is not distracted from the body or from the soul and that is known as fullness."

Karnapidasana

Ear-pressure Pose

"In backbends your mind is in a full state of awareness and sharp. If your intelligence is not sharp, you collapse. In *Sālamba Sarvāṅgāsana* or in forward bends, you can relax a bit here and a bit there. In *Halāsana* and *Karnapidasana* you can completely relax. So you can learn from different *āsana* the three states of consciousness, *jagrata, svapna*, and *susupti* (wakeful, dream, and sleep)."

1 Begin in Halasana (see opposite). Support your back with your palms as you move into step 2.

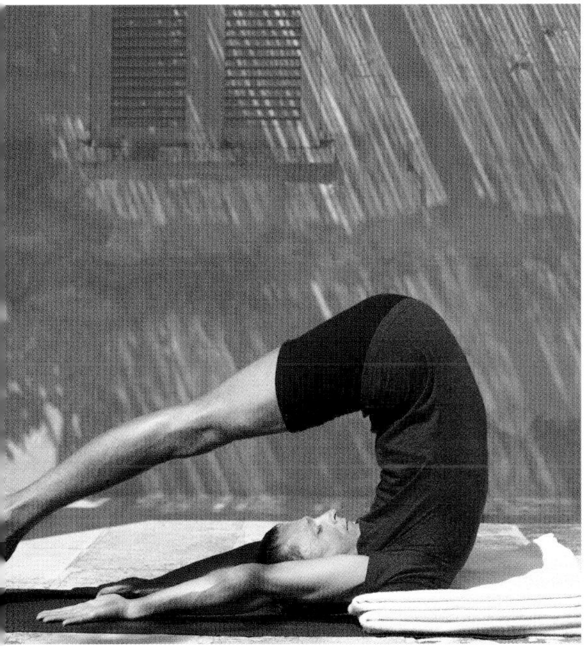

2 Bend your knees and lower them to the floor on either side of your face. Lift your back. Hold for 30-60 seconds. Raise your knees back to Halasana. Bend your knees and roll down to rest on your back.

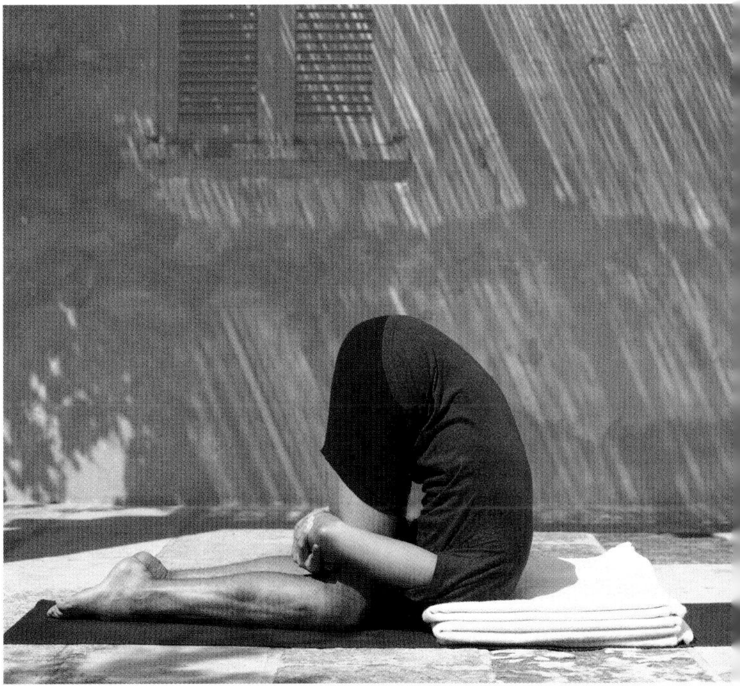

"The feeling in the spiritual heart must be, 'I am not separate from asana, asana is not separate from me, I am asana and asana is me.'"

I Am Asana

Q. *Sthira sukham āsanam* is usually translated as: "sitting comfortably in a posture" but you offer us the spiritual aspect of the *āsana* practice when you interpret this *sūtra* as: "I am the *āsana*, *āsana* am I", from your knowledge and experience. Could you please explain it further?

"This 'I am the *āsana* and *āsana* I am' is experienced in every *āsana*, but how can I make you to experience it? It has to be in your qualitative experiential practice. You have to bring that state of activity in your intelligence and consciousness, but it is impossible for anyone to imprint this feeling on you.... You have to observe and get absorbed. In this way, I am sure these questions would be answered by your own self rather than listening to me. (*Gurujī* smiles and then suddenly says: 'Here I got the clue'. *Gurujī* takes a book and puts it vertically on the table.)

See: this is the front page, this is the back page. Imagine that the back page is the back of the calf muscle, and the front page is the front of the calf muscle, is not the front page parallel to the back page? Similarly, you have to observe the length and touch of the back muscle and feel the even contact with the skin. Then adjust the length of the front muscle with the bone to be evenly in its contact. This is how the study should be done. Now take the width of the calf. Does your intelligence flow on the inner side of the calf or on the outer side? If intelligence touches both the parts, then it is a perfect positioning of the intelligence of the calf with the intelligence of the seer. Then you are in *āsana* and *āsana* you are. This is *sthira sukham āsanam*. It means like this you have to adjust each and every part of the body parallel to each other and the seer has comfortably settled in each cell and in each part of the body. (*Gurujī* smiles.)"

Āsana as worship

"In a perfect *āsana*, the consciousness tends to go inwards. It is under a centripetal state. The efforts end at this stage and awareness begins to spread all over like water spreading evenly on the floor. This is the centrifugal state of consciousness. In *āsana* one has to get glimpses of this feeling by connecting the entire frontier of the body towards the core and vice-versa. If the centripetal state is *dhāraṇā*, the centrifugal state is *dhyāna*. So diffuse the centripetal state harmoniously everywhere turning *dhāraṇā* into *dhyāna*.

The practice of *āsana* for me is like worship. Saints worship God. In my practice, I worship *āsana* as my deity. If one can understand what I am saying, then he may go beyond the realm of the physical frame with clear intelligence and clean consciousness to experience the essence of life."

Question from "The Inward Path for a Better World", interview by Vicky Alamos, Xavi Alongina and Jose Maria Vigar in the Library at RIMYI, December 1998, first published in Yoga Jwala, *the magazine of the Spanish Iyengar Yoga Association, no.1, 2000.*

Extract this page from "On Aṣṭāṅga Yoga – Āsana", Aṣṭadaḷa Yogamālā *Volume 7, p121.*

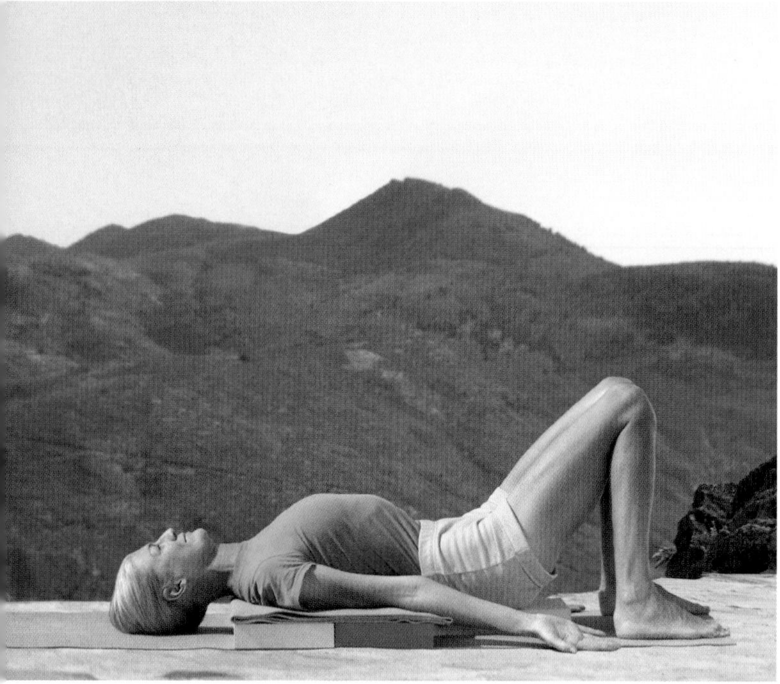

1 Arrange four blocks side by side and a fifth in front of them. Place a folded mat over the four blocks. Lie over the mat with the tops of your shoulders 5cm (2in) from the edge. Bend your knees and place your feet near your buttocks, hip-width apart. Rest your arms by your sides, palms up. Roll your shoulder bones back and down and lift your chest.

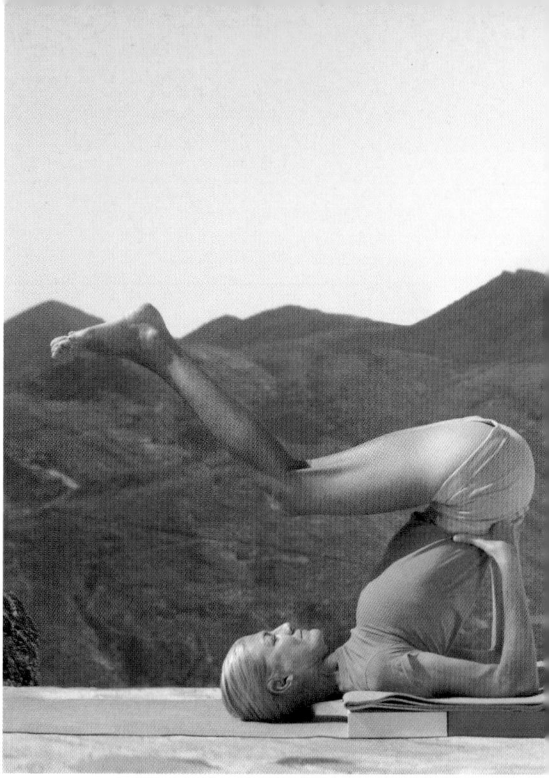

2 Turn your palms down, press them into the floor and, exhaling, swing your legs overhead, raising your hips and trunk and supporting your back with your hands.

Salamba Sarvangasana

shoulderstand

"Patañjali wants you to discover this silent space. You have to watch this space and learn to prolong this silent moment of pause. Only then do you draw near to *samādhi*. In this pause you have a glimpse of tranquillity. Instead of concentrating on restraint, concentrate on this silent moment. Develop this in your practice of *āsana* and *prāṇāyāma*."

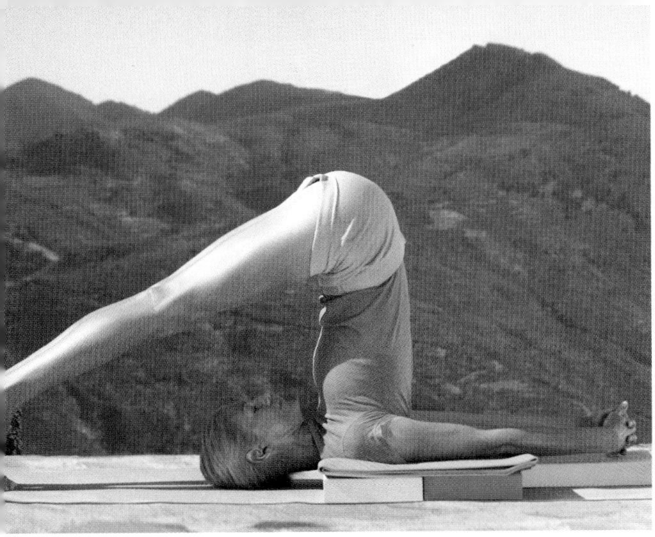

3 Drop your feet and stretch your legs, pressing your toes down. Clasp your fingers, extend your arms, and lift your chest and hips, making your trunk vertical.

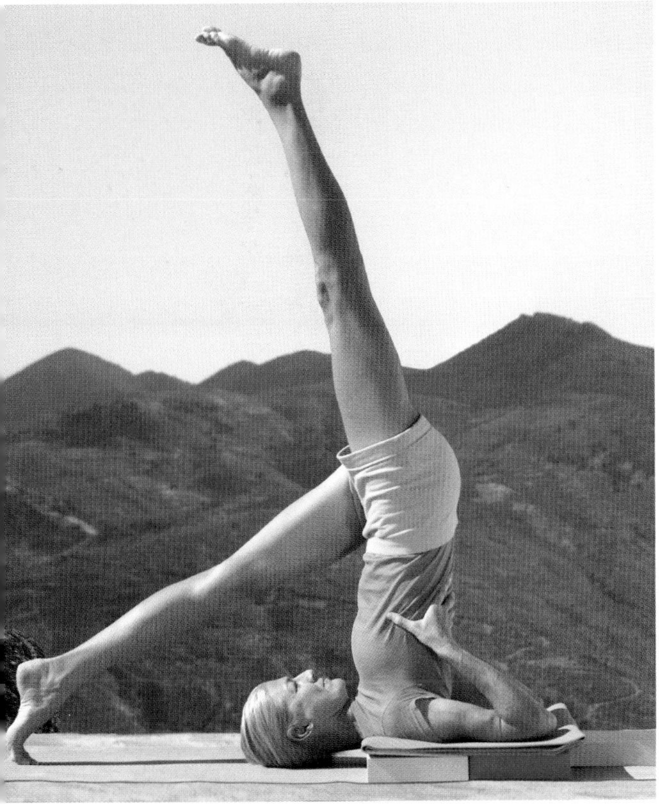

4 Place your palms on your back and lift your spine even more. Then exhale, raise one foot, and lift the leg in line with your trunk (see above). Once it is perpendicular to the floor, follow with the other leg, keeping both legs straight, until your legs are together.

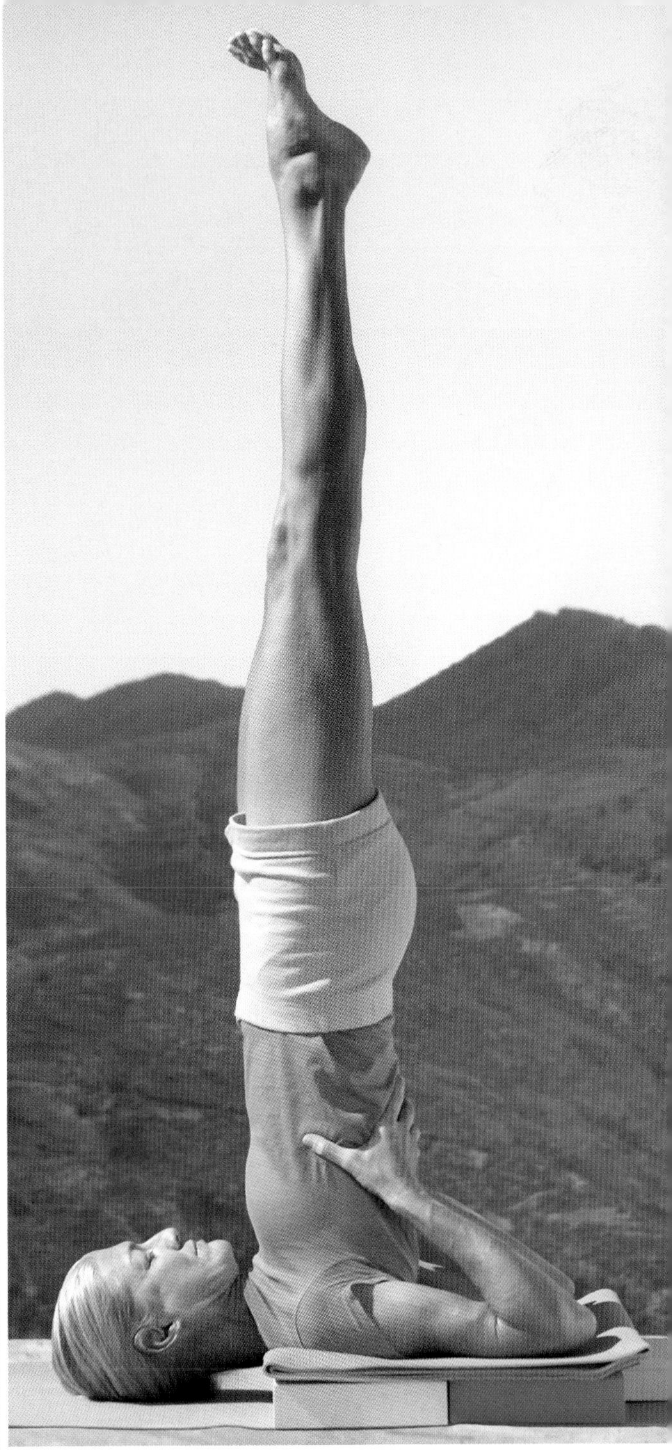

5 Extend your heels and stretch your toes up, keeping your knees firm, and elbows in line with your shoulders. Hold for up to 5 minutes, breathing evenly. Exhale, bend your knees, bring your thighs to your chest, then lower your buttocks and back, releasing your hands. Lie over the support to rest, feet on the floor and knees bent.

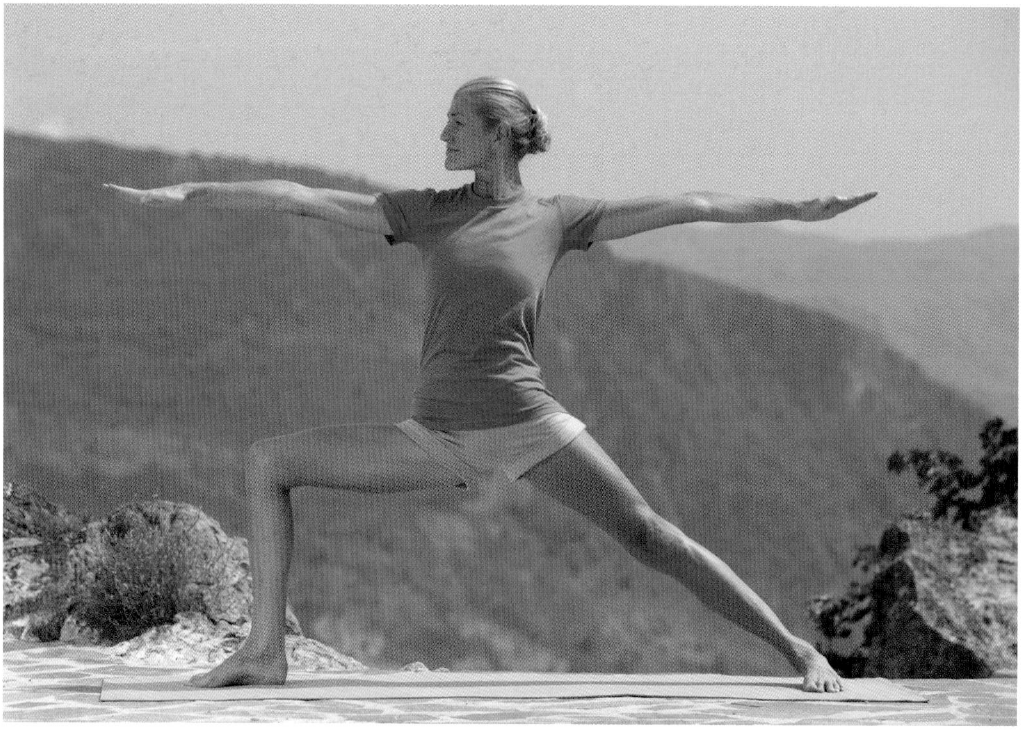

1 From Tadasana jump into Utthita Hasta Padasana (see pages 108–109). Then come into Virabhadrasana II (see pages 32–33).

Utthita Parsvakonasana

Extended Lateral Angle Pose

"When you do *Vīrabhadrāsana* II you want to extend your armpits while stretching both hands. When the teacher says go to *Utthita Pārśvakoṇāsana* from *Vīrabhadrāsana* II, you forget the attention on the armpits. Watch your inattentive mind at that moment to understand how *āsana* teach you to sharpen your intelligence. You lose your attention to extension on the side you are doing. You do not know how the mind which existed in the armpits of *Vīrabhadrāsana* II disappeared when you went to *Utthita Pārśvakoṇāsana*. Mind is also *brahma*. One should not shrink it."

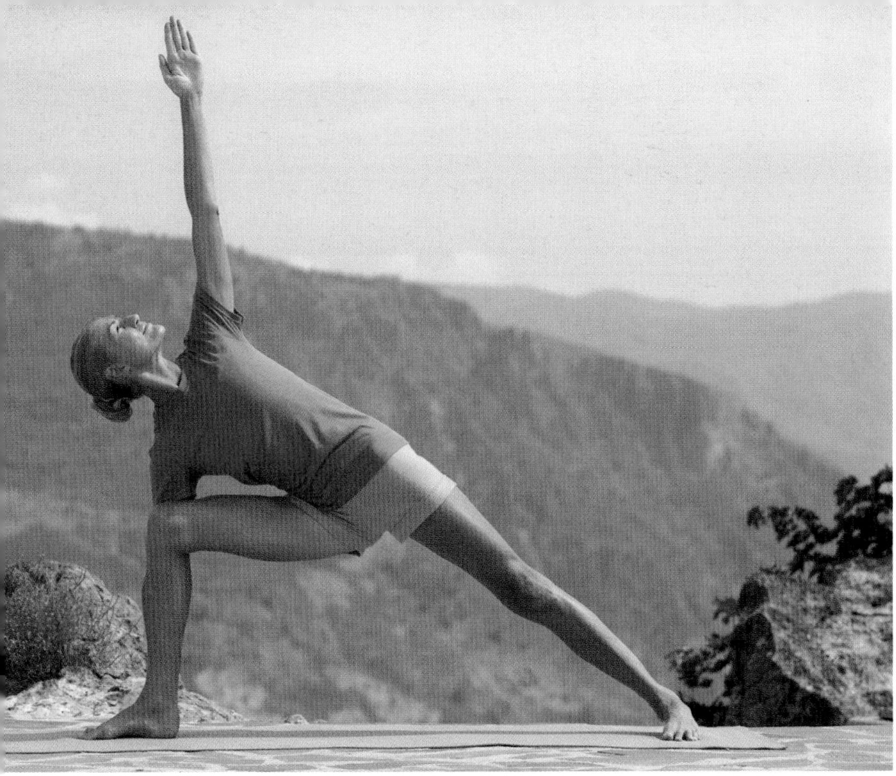

2 Exhale and place your right hand on the floor beside the outer side of your right foot. Stretch your left arm up, in line with your shoulders. Keep your chest facing forwards and your chest, hips and left leg aligned. Ensure that your left knee is firm and left leg straight.

3 Extend your left arm over your left ear and try to rest the right side of your trunk along your thigh. Turn your head to look up and open your chest. Stretch the spine. Hold for 20–30 seconds, breathing evenly. Inhale and reverse the steps to return to Virabhadrasana II. Straighten your right leg and turn your head and feet forwards into Utthita Hasta Padasana, then repeat to the other side. Finish in Tadasana.

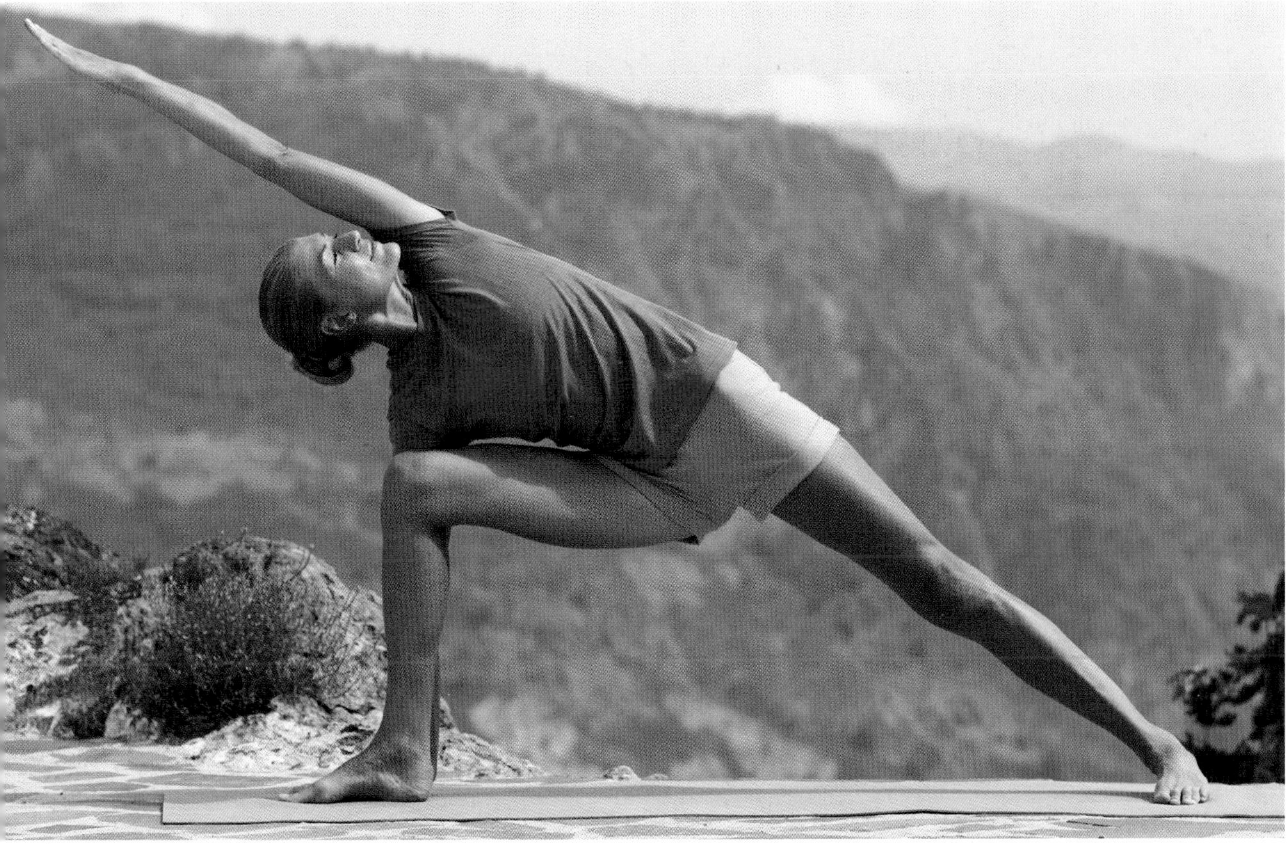

The Art of Sitting

“Before sitting for *prāṇāyāma*, you should know how to sit, so that turbulence in the body does not take place. Know exactly the end-middle portion of the tailbone and sit in such a way that it runs perpendicular to the floor. Treat this point as the South Pole, and the centre portion of the head of the spine as the North Pole.

Jālandhara Bandha [*see pages 148–49*] helps to spot this area to adjust clearly for the rest of the spine to float in line, as if you had placed one vertebra of the spine over the other, like a mason planting one brick over the other.... In order to learn *Tādāsana* [*see pages 26–27*] we place and spread the bottom mounds of the feet evenly. Similarly, we have to learn to use the buttock bones as if they are the mounds of the seat in the sitting position. Do not strain but relax the groins. Position the centre of the buttock bones and the crown or the middle portion of the ankles that touch the ground, so that the water element of the body finds its level on the seat, groins, and feet. In the same way, keep the back and front of the floating ribs running parallel to each other.”

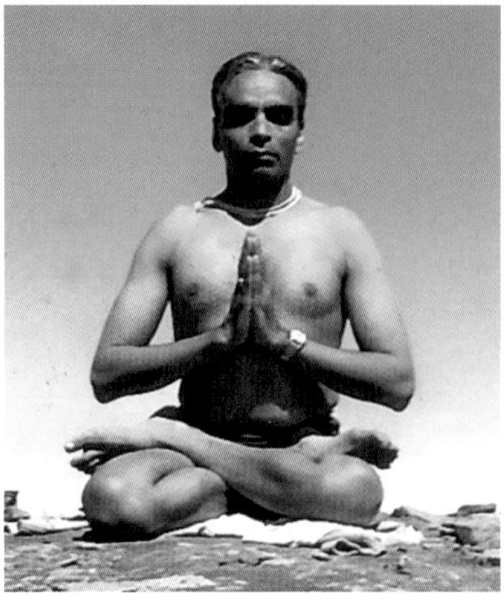

Guruji meditates in Padmasana on a mountain top.

Q. What is the role then of seated meditation, especially sitting in *Padmāsana*. Is there a purpose for that?

"For meditation one has to be essentially in a sitting *āsana*. Meditation is not possible in sleeping or standing *āsana*. In supine or *supta* position one is likely to go to sleep. In standing *āsana*, one cannot stand too long on the legs which causes strain. Meditation is done only in a sitting posture since one has to sit for a long time for the transformation of consciousness to occur.

The best of all *āsana* is *Padmāsana* for meditation. In *Vīrāsana*, the lower lumbar moves deep into the frontal body so the spine can never be straight. In *Siddhāsana* the lower portions are completely inert, only the thoracic-dorsal spine will be active. Whereas in *Padmāsana* the entire spine from the tailbone to the brain is made to be kept alert and active. Only *Padmāsana* does this, no other *āsana*. That is why *Padmāsana* is considered the best of all *āsana*. Most people cannot do it, because they have lost the habit of sitting on the ground.... Because of squatting, people were getting the rotations in their groins, legs, and knees easily, so they could do *Padmāsana* easily. Now people have only restricted movements. They don't use their joints to the optimal level, therefore the joints are rusted. Hence I say that one can take any sitting *āsana* such as *Svastikāsana*, *Siddhāsana*, *Vīrāsana*, *Baddha Koṇāsana*, provided the sitting is correct."

Extract opposite from "Practice of Praṇāyāma", also published as "Introduction to Praṇāyāma", Yoga Rahasya, *July 1994.*

Question from "The Journey from Conative Action to All-Pervasive Awareness", the Iyengar Yoga Institute Review, *San Francisco, Winter 1992.*

Svastikasana

Auspicious Pose

"Regarding *prāṇāyāma,* first learn to sit correctly. The spine should be straight and firm. The respiratory organs should be free from stress. The spine must be ready, the nervous system must have the power to endure and the lungs the capacity to bear the load of sustained deep inhalation and exhalation."

1 Sit in Dandasana (see pages 14–15). Place blankets beneath your buttocks if your knees are stiff. Extend the spine and open the chest.

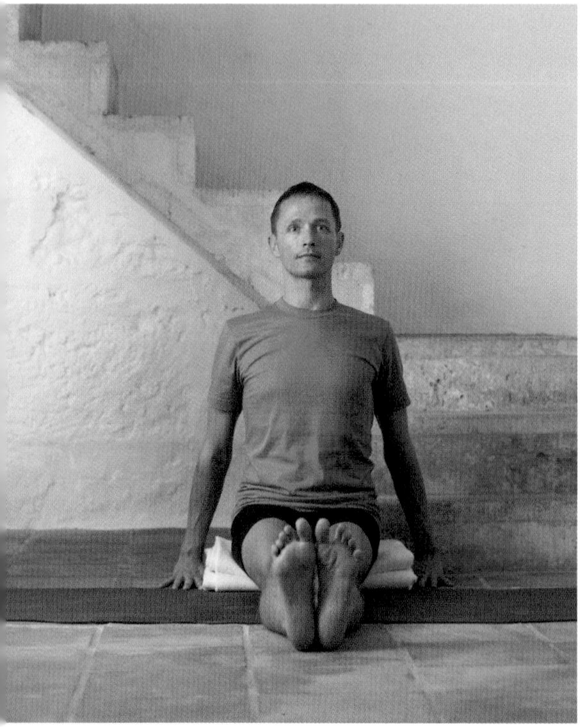

2 Bend your left knee and place the foot beneath your right thigh. Bend your right knee and place the foot beneath your left thigh. Rest your hands on your knees, palms up, or join your palms at your chest. Hold for 30–60 seconds. Return to Dandasana and repeat to the other side. Finish in Dandasana.

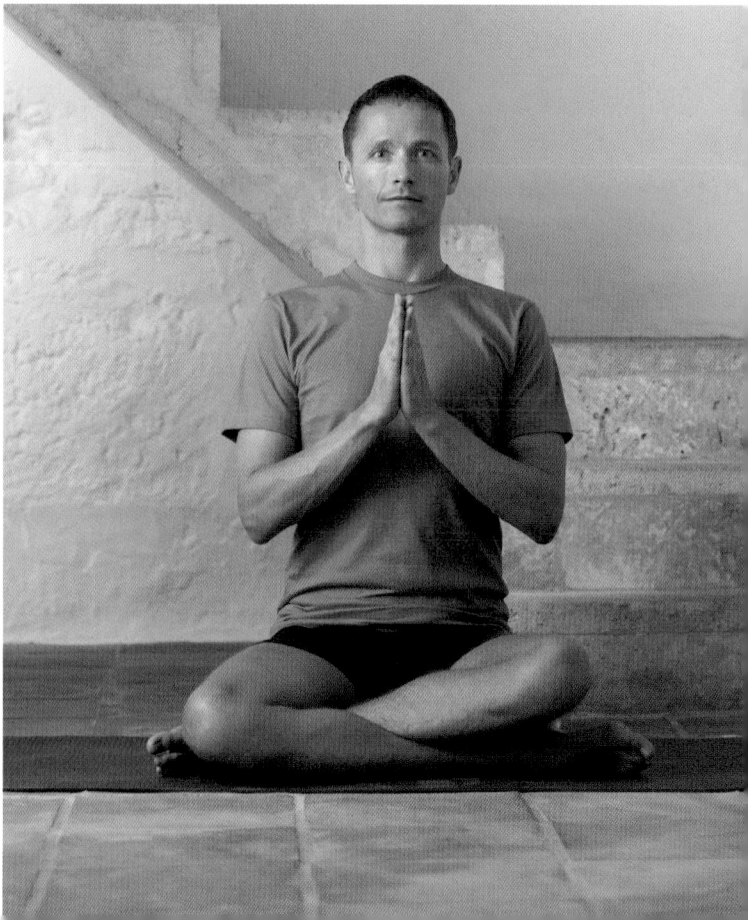

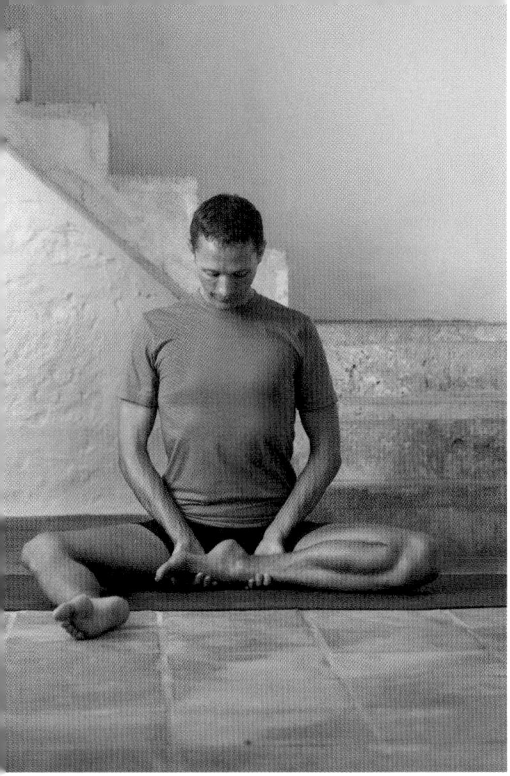

1 Sit in Dandasana (see pages 14-15). Place blankets beneath your buttocks if your knees are higher than your hips in step 2. Extend your spine and open your chest. Bend your legs and draw your left heel to your perineum. Rest the sole against your right thigh.

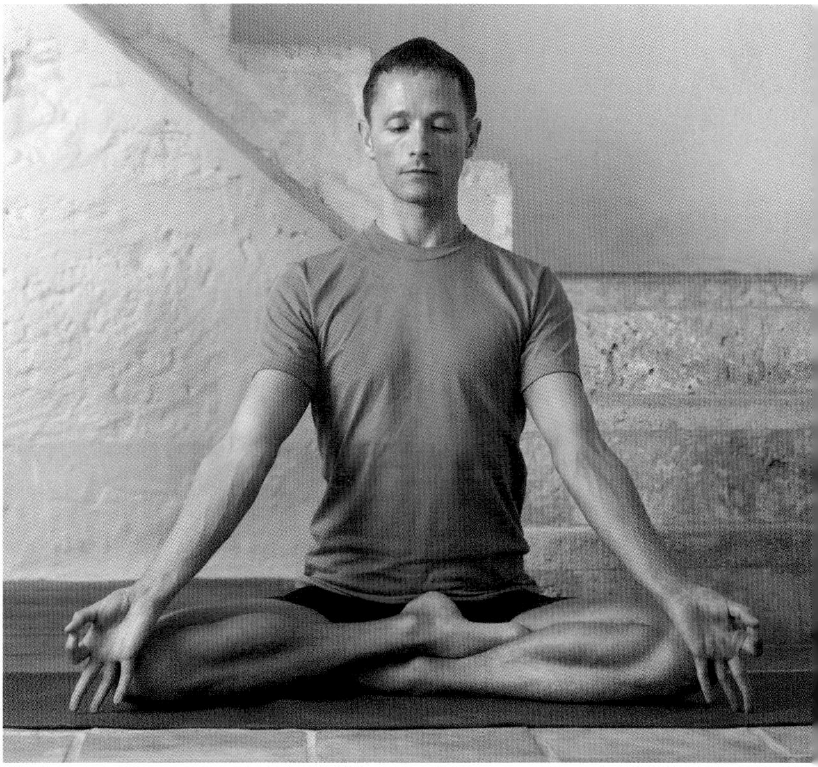

2 Place your right foot over your left ankle, heel touching your pubic bone and sole between your left thigh and calf. Rest the backs of your hands on your knees and join the tips of your thumbs and first fingers, extending the other fingers (Jnana Mudra). Keep your head level and look at the tip of your nose. Hold for 30-60 seconds. Return to Dandasana and repeat to the other side. Finish in Dandasana.

Siddhasana

Perfect Pose

"The most important thing is to acquire correct position of the *āsana.* It is essential to attend to the *āsana* with a measured freedom of extension, expansion, and contraction in the muscles and joints. By this measured attentive practice a balanced state in *āsana* is earned for the energy to flow without interruptions and break in the body. Accurate *āsana* is when each and every cell of the body responds harmoniously with life-full-ness flowing evenly and smoothly."

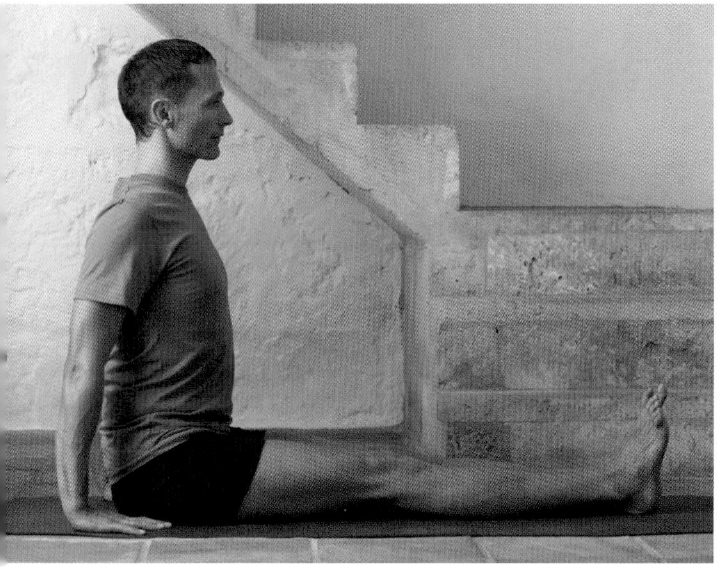

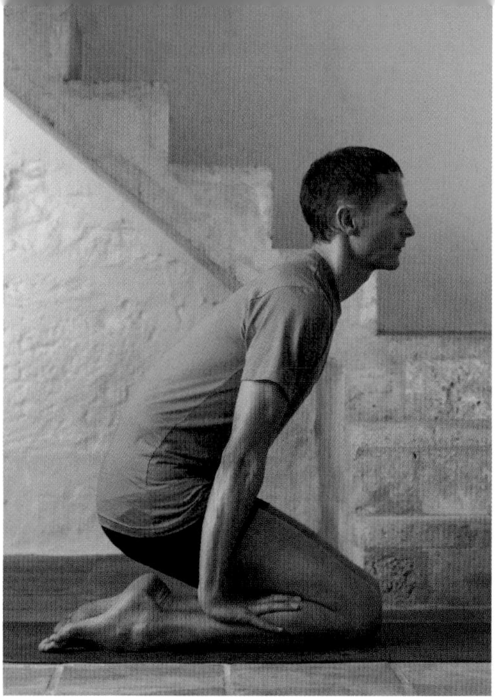

1 Sit in Dandasana (see pages 14–15). Have blocks or a blanket ready if your buttocks do not touch the floor comfortably in step 3.

2 Kneel with knees together and feet 45cm (18in) apart. Use your thumbs to turn your calf muscles towards the outer side of your legs.

3 Rest your buttocks on the floor (or a support) between your heels, toes pointing backwards. Your inner calves should touch your outer thighs with the thighs parallel. Rest your palms on your knees. Hold for 1–5 minutes. Kneel up and stretch each leg in turn, then finish in Dandasana.

Virasana

Hero Pose

"Sometimes, legs may ache, and the mind might say, 'Miss yoga'! But an intelligent mind has to find out why they are paining and work out how to remove that pain. One finds means to escape, but to persist and pursue needs a strong mind. Practice is like using a pin to remove a splinter in the hand. In the same way, one has to learn to use the intelligence to practise to remove so-called pains and reform the practices so that these pricks do not occur at all."

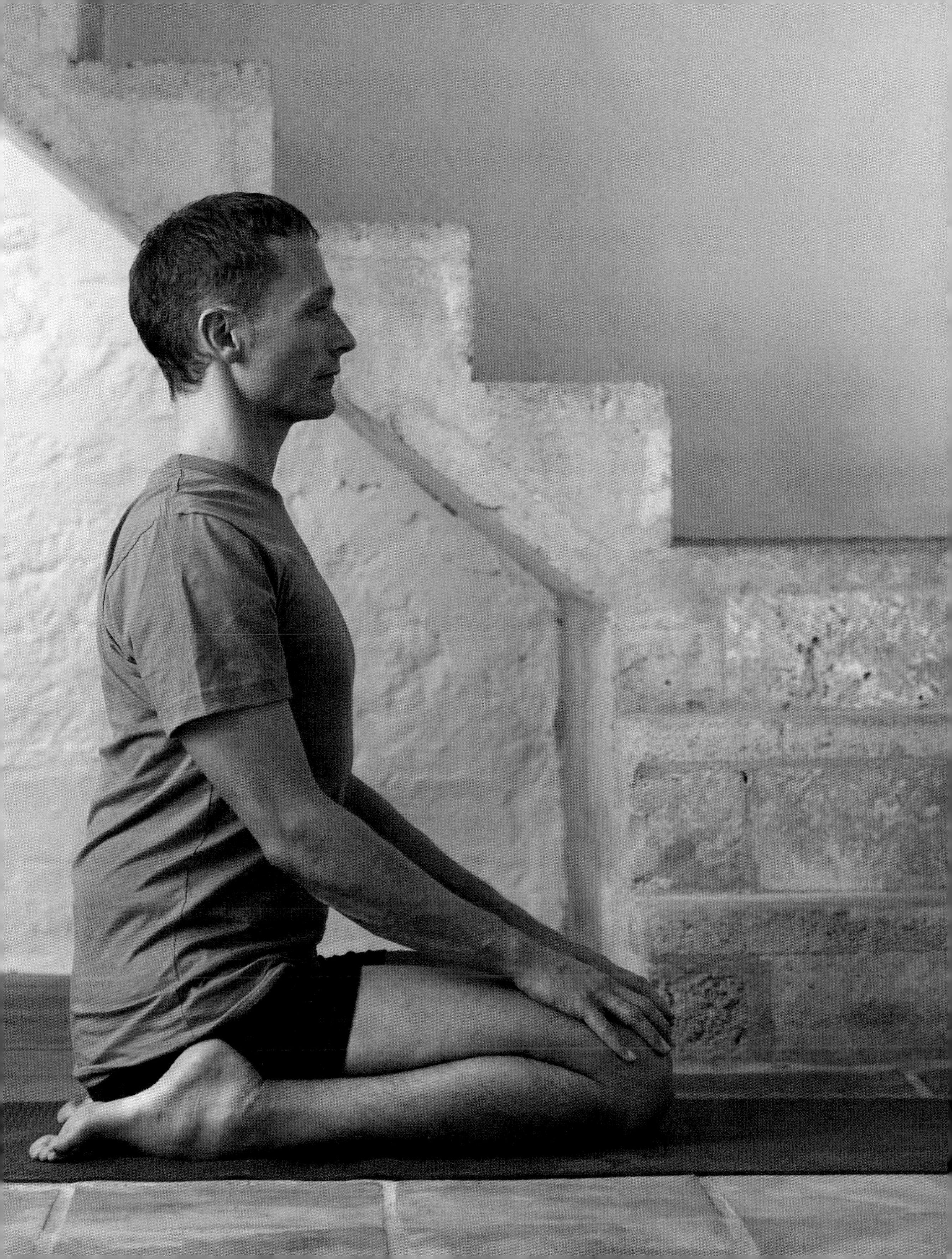

Bhadrasana

One-leg Padmasana

"Each individual should know his own capacity and how much the body can take. You are not going to get into the lotus pose, *Padmāsana*, by the brain.... One needs to study and judge judiciously how much movement there is in the knees, how much are the muscles extending to get the *āsana.* If one cannot sit in *Svastikāsana*, how can one perform *Padmāsana*? At least one can try to do one leg *Padmāsana*, known as *Bhadrāsana*."

1 Sit in Dandasana (see pages 14-15).

2 Bend your knees. Hold your left foot and draw it in until the heel is near your perineum and the sole against your right thigh.

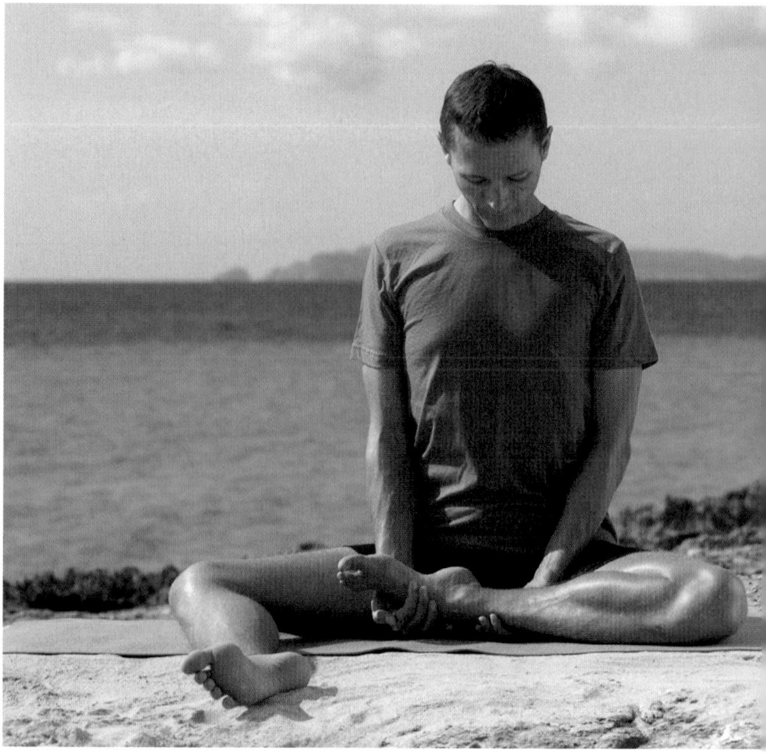

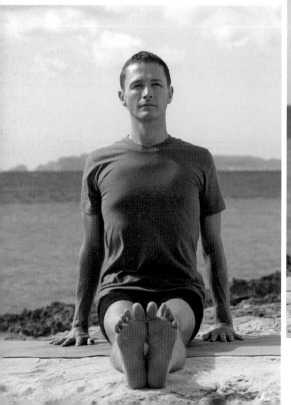

3 Using both hands, lift your right foot and place it on your left thigh, heel near your navel and sole facing upwards. Rest your hands in Jnana Mudra (see page 135). Hold for 30 seconds. Release your hands and legs, return to Dandasana, and repeat to the other side. Finish in Dandasana.

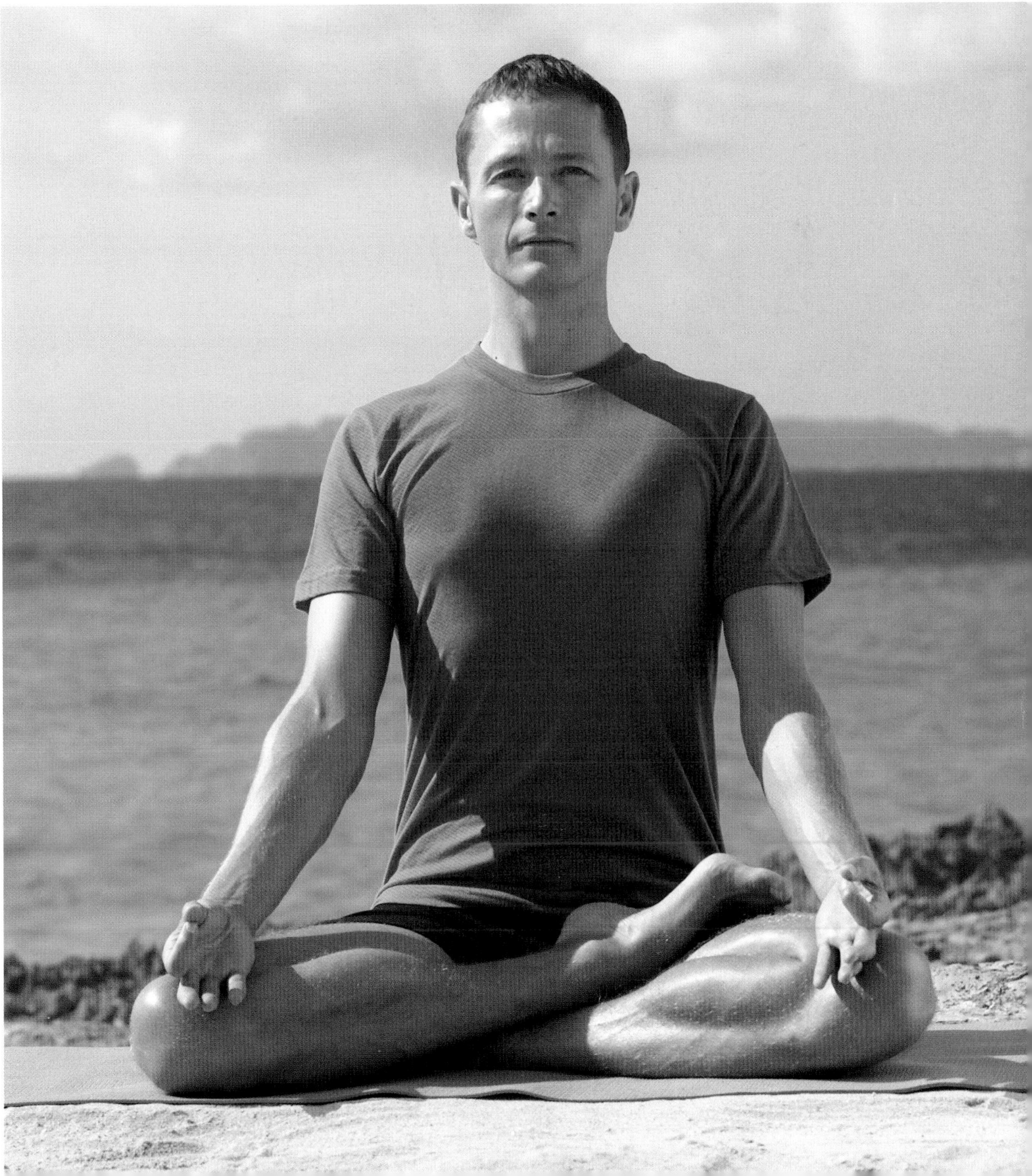

How I Began Pranayama

"In 1941, I went to Mysore. I requested *Gurujī* that he should teach me *prāṇāyāma*. Knowing the capacity of my lungs and my under-developed chest, *Gurujī* said that I was not fit for *prāṇāyāma*. Whenever I approached him to teach me *prāṇāyāma* his answer was the same.

Again in 1943, I visited Mysore for a few days. As I was staying with my *gurujī* and knowing that he would not teach me *prāṇāyāma*, I thought of watching him while he practised *prāṇāyāma* in the mornings. *Gurujī* was a regular practitioner of *prāṇāyāma*, always practising at a fixed time in the mornings, but he was never regular in his *āsana* practice. He was in the habit of getting up very early, but my sister was a late riser, so nobody knew that I was up to observe his practices. I wanted to see how he sat and what he did with his facial muscles. I stealthily peeped through the window and observed his movements very carefully. I wanted to learn to sit, to stretch the spinal column, and relax the facial muscles. Each morning I watched his adjustments and movements, the dropping of the eyeballs, the closing of the eyes, movements of the eyelids, lift of the chest, movement of the abdominal organs, maintenance of the waist, the sound and flow of his breath. Having observed his practice minutely, I was tempted, approached him with humility and pleaded him to teach me *prāṇāyāma*. He said that it might not be possible for me to do *prāṇāyāma* in this life. His refusal to ṭeach me was the seed for me to start the *prāṇāyāma* practices myself. Though I was determined to do it, it was not as easy as I had thought it to be. I struggled the same way to do *prāṇāyāma* as I struggled to learn the *āsana*. With failure after failure, dejection and discontent, I restlessly persisted with the practice of *prāṇāyāma* from 1944. The pains and struggles of 1934 reappeared even in the *prāṇāyāma* practices. The end of struggle, dejection, and the state of restlessness came only in 1962–63 and not before, though everybody was proclaiming that yoga brought poise. I was laughing at their statements and thought it all to be nonsense.

"I began practising all the asana meticulously to straighten my spine. When I felt strong in the spine, I again began my pranayama."

Restlessness and unhappiness prevailed over me for decades. In the beginning, I could not do even one breath with any rhythm. If I took one deep inhalation, I had to open my mouth for the exhalation, as I could not release the breath through the nose. If I inhaled normally to master deep exhalation, I could not draw in the next breath due to the laboured releasing of the breath. I was under constant pressure. I was not finding the cause of this problem and my *Guru*'s words that I was an unfit student for *prāṇāyāma* were ringing in my ears, bringing a negative state of mind in me.

Like a religious person, each morning I would get up early for *prāṇāyāma*, and after one or two attempts I used to lie down, thinking within myself, 'I cannot do it today, let me try tomorrow.' This process of getting up in the early morning and not practising after one or two attempts continued for years. Then one day I made up my mind to do at least one cycle before losing heart in between. Then, after an interval, I followed with a second cycle with great difficulty. I used to give up for the third cycle, as it was next to impossible. In this way, I pursued the practice daily, but it was ending in failure; yet I succeeded after eight to ten years to sit for one hour at a stretch for *prāṇāyāma*. Many may not believe that it took me such a long time. The reason why it took me so long is on account of my spine, which could not take the load of sitting straight. ”

From "My Yogic Journey", talk given on B.K.S. Iyengar's 70th birthday at Tilak Smarak Mandir.

Patanjali on Pranayama

"Practice of *prāṇāyāma* not only removes the veil of haziness covering the light of intelligence, but makes the mind a fit instrument for meditation.

Normal breathing flows irregularly according to one's physical and emotional state. So one has to deliberately regulate this zigzag flow of breath with attention. When this attention is brought in the flow of the inbreath and outbreath know that *prāṇāyāma* has begun.

Prāṇāyāma consists of inhalation (*pūraka*), exhalation (*recaka*), and retention (*kuṁbhaka*). Elongation and prolongation of *pūraka* and *recaka* is time (*kāla*). The inhalation-retention and exhalation-retention is done by the torso (*deśa*), while precision of movement (*saṁkhya*) is maintained through the rhythmic, smooth flow of breath. Please know that in *pūraka* the causal body (*kāraṇa śarīra*) moves from the inner depth towards the vastness of the body, covering the entire place of the gross part of the torso (*deśa*) with space (*ākāśa*). Retention (*antara kuṁbhaka*) is to hold on to that created space as long as possible without shrinking the place. In *antara kuṁbhaka* the causal, the subtle and the gross bodies are merged into a single unit. In *recaka* the gross body (*deśa*) moves closer to merge with the inner most body via the inner body without shrinking in place but receding the space. In *bāhya kuṁbhaka* there is the feel of that state of oneness where the gross and subtle bodies unite with the causal body. This is *prāṇāyāma*.

"In puraka it is not the air inhaled, but the very Lord Himself who enters in the form of breath."

From the deliberate *prāṇāyāma*, (*Yoga Sūtra* II. 49 & 50) Patañjali adds one more *prāṇāyāma* that transcends the deliberately modulated method; namely, inhalation (*pūraka*), exhalation (*recaka*) and retention (*kuṁbhaka*). Here, the breathing is done by the breath itself, in an unpremeditated way. ”

Pranayama as Prayer

"The Infinite Lord is outside our finite body as well as in the depth of the core of the body. The *sādhaka* inhales the infinite and holding it (*antara kuṁbhaka*) becomes completely merged with the *jīvātman* (individual soul). He does not allow any thought to intrude or create disturbance while the Infinite is communing with his individual self. In exhalation (*recaka*) the *sādhaka* adjusts his thoughts by allowing the self to surrender, through his outgoing breath, to the Lord. He places his very essence of life through the conditional process of exhalation as a devotee places the garland of flowers at the feet of his chosen deity (*Iṣṭa Devatā vigraha*). In the exhalation-retention (*bāhya kuṁbhaka*) he waits for the Lord to accept his deep surrender and remains throughout that retention with humble serenity and oneness with Brahman.

Pratyāhāra is hidden in the very process of *prāṇāyāma*. The mind drawn by senses goes out and hankers for worldly pleasures. By the practice of *prāṇāyāma*, the senses are drawn in the reverse gear and their energies are made to flow back towards the inner fullness of the mind so that they are detached from the objects of pleasure. In *pratyāhāra* the senses are trained to be yoked to the inner light that is ever pure, real, and one without a second."

Extract opposite from "Yogānjali", 70 Glorious Years of Yogacharya B.K.S. Iyengar, *published by Light on Yoga Research Trust.*

Extract on this page from "Yoga and Dharma" also published as "Yoga and Religion", Aṣṭadaḷa Yogamālā *Volume 1, pp165–66.*

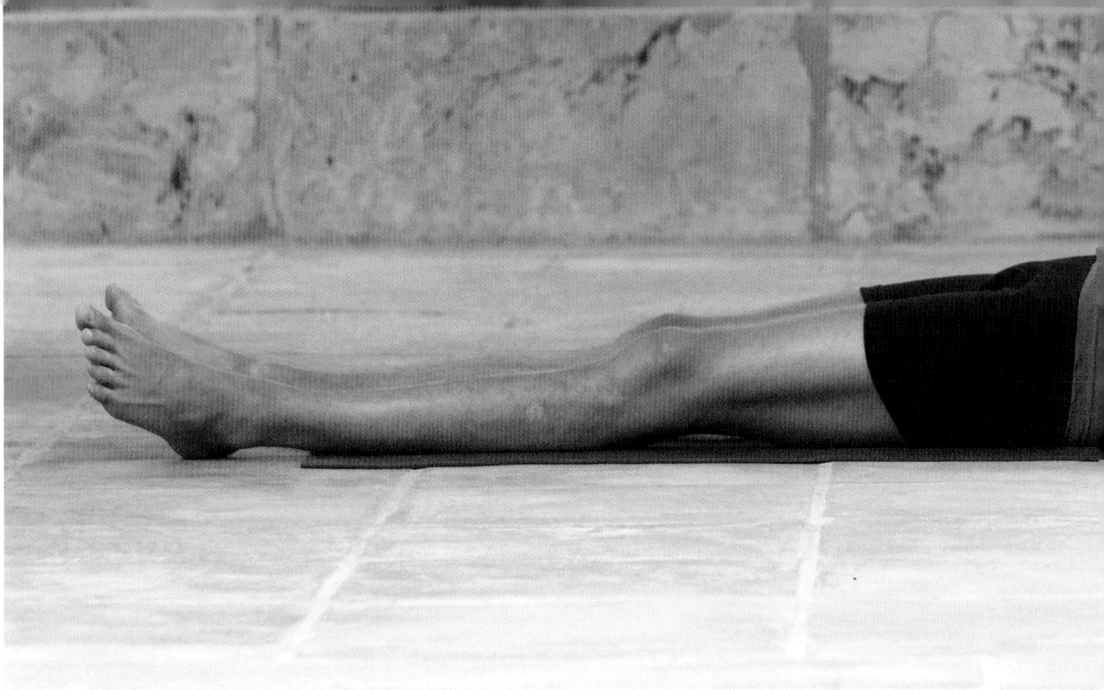

Savasana

Corpse Pose (with support)

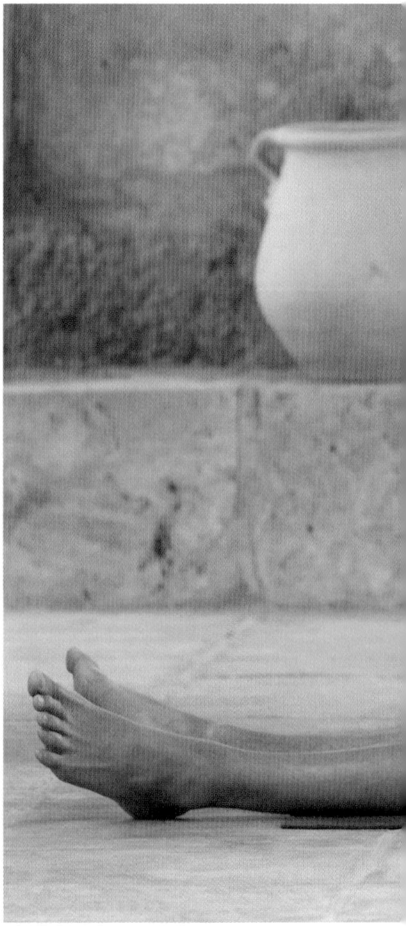

"The beginners have to open the chest physically, particularly the sternum and ribs. There are various ways of working with pillows placed underneath the trunk to open different parts of the torso. For example, lying over a horizontal pillow makes the abdomen soft and lying over a longitudinal pillow helps the sternum and chest to spread and open well. This way one can learn to adjust pillows to get the right feel, which enhances not only the physiological body, but the mental body too."

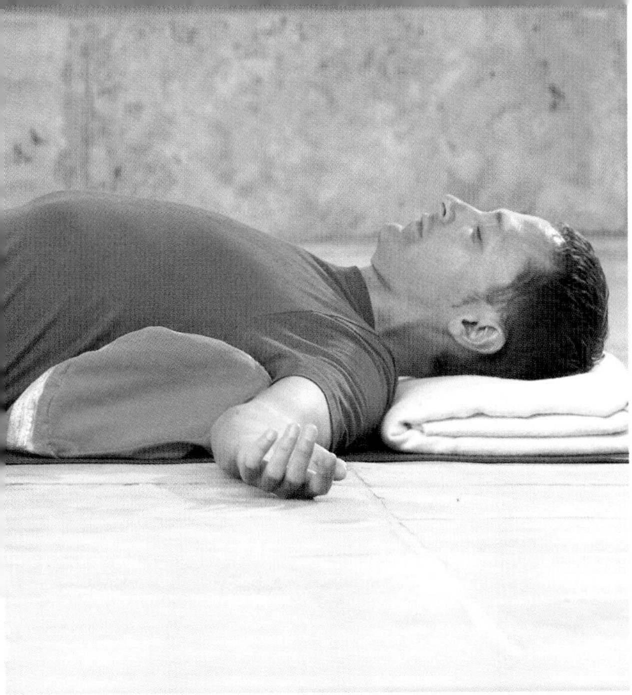

1 To prepare for pranayama, place a folded blanket at one end of your mat and a pillow horizontally across it. Recline over the pillow so that the blanket supports your neck and head and the pillow your dorsal spine. Spread your arms at shoulder-height, palms up, and separate your legs, toes dropping outwards. Observe the lift in your chest and broad collarbones. This aids inhalation. Hold for at least 5 minutes. Roll to one side to rest and then the other before sitting up.

2 Repeat with a vertical pillow positioned to support from the bottom of your trunk, buttocks on the floor, without touching your waist. Rest your arms away from your sides, palms up, and separate your legs, toes dropping outwards. Observe how the vertical lift rests your spinal muscles and helps exhalation, enhancing relaxation. Hold for at least 5 minutes. Roll to one side, then the other before sitting up.

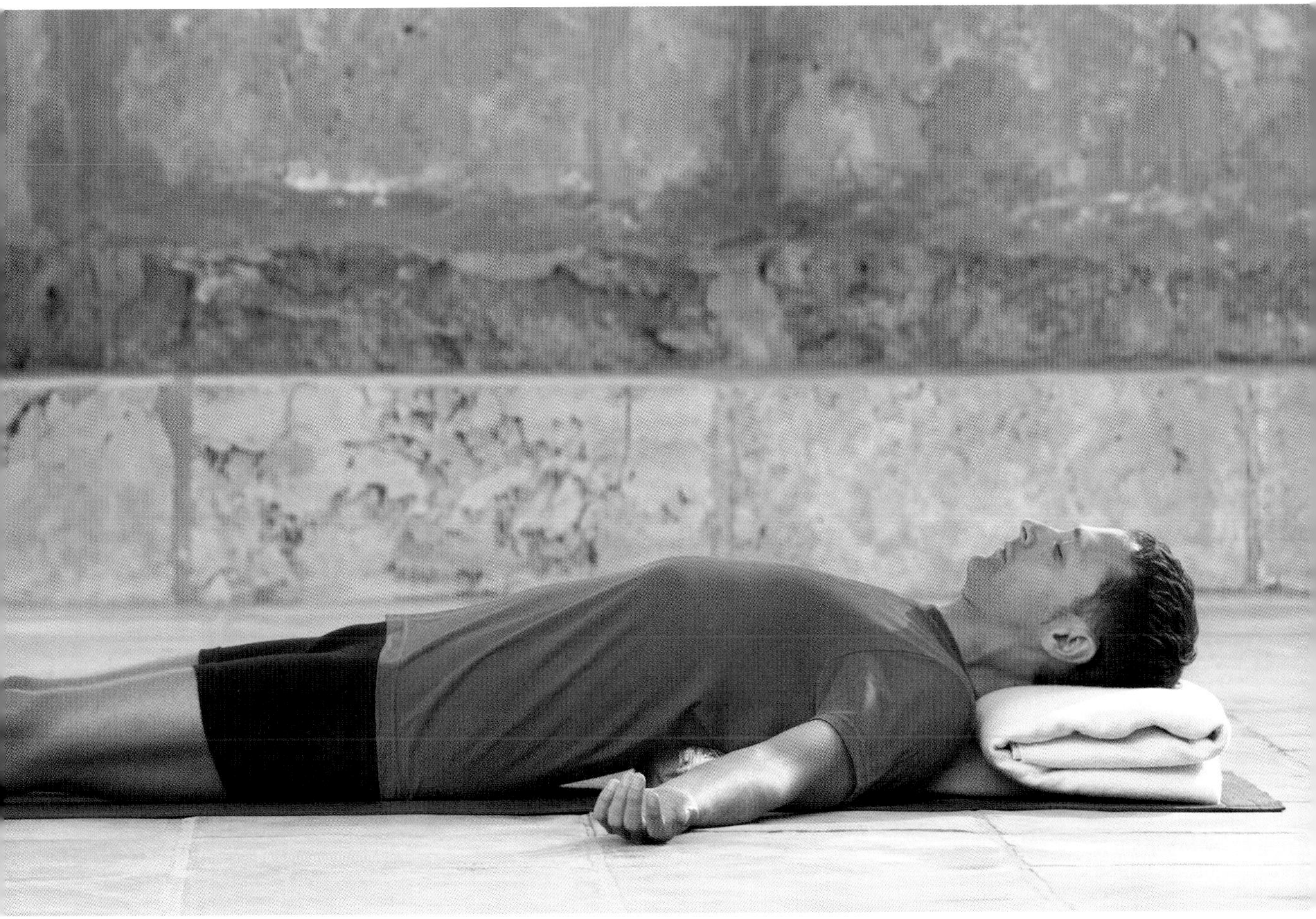

The Importance of Chinlock

“In order to build natural dykes for *prāṇāyāma* practices, *Jālandhara Bandha* or the chinlock was introduced by the yogis. This judiciously helps the *prajñā* of the inner *prāṇa* to receive the incoming *prāṇa* as well as check the incoming *prāṇa* to flow in rhythmically and later on be distributed.

In controlled nostril or digital *prāṇāyāma* such as or like *Anuloma*, *Pratiloma*, *Sūrya Bhedana*, *Chandra Bedhana*, and *Nāḍī Śodhana*, the practitioner has to construct the dykes at the inner edge of the roof of the nostrils for inhalation and the outer edge of the roof for exhalation. He has to know these above mentioned places in order to form the dykes before beginning digital *prāṇāyāma*.

If the breath deviates from its conditioned paths, it enters forcibly and goes out forcibly. This type of deep breath cannot be termed *prāṇāyāma*. In *prāṇāyāma*, the job of the *sādhaka* is to see that in inhalation the energy gets filled in deeply and soaked into the body and in exhalation, the energy is released through the sluice gates of the nostril formed by the fingers and the thumb so that time is given for it to be absorbed and stored in the system.”

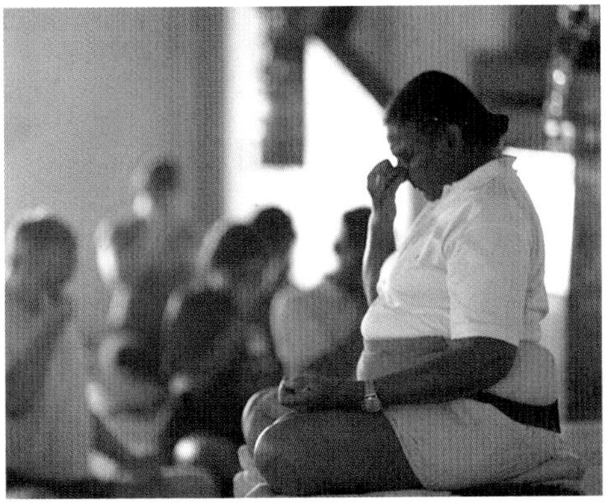

A class of students practises chinlock and the precise placement of fingers for digital pranayama with Geeta Iyengar.

"Jalandhara Bandha... automatically makes the brain become reflective and pensive."

Extract opposite from "Introduction to Praṇāyāma", Yoga Rahasya, *July 1994.*

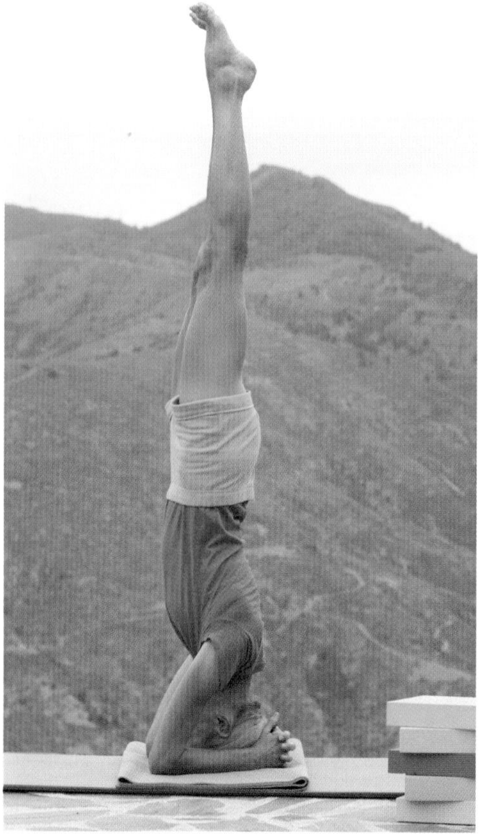

1 Fold a mat into four and come into Salamba Sirsasana (see pages 72-73). Hold for up to 5 minutes. Come down and rest.

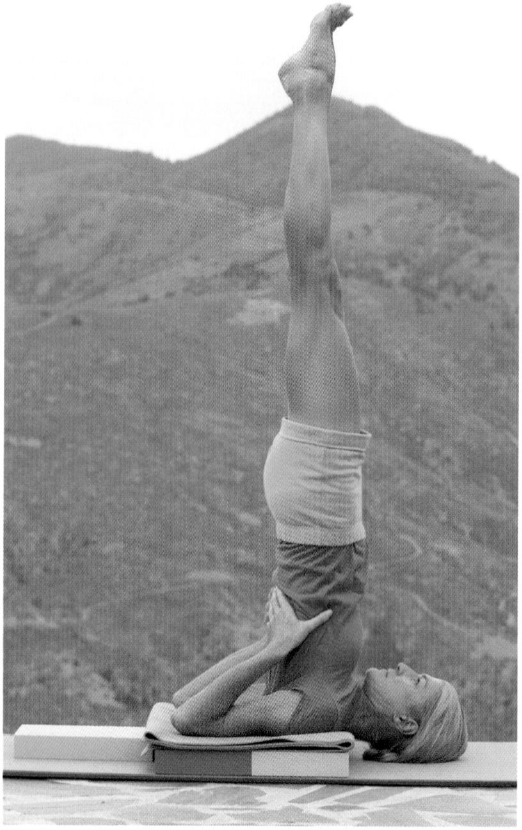

2 Arrange five blocks with a folded mat on top, then come into Salamba Sarvangasana (see pages 128-29). Hold for 5 minutes.

Preparation for Bandhas

Asana Sequence

"Before thinking of *prāṇāyāma*, it is essential to learn *Sarvāṅgāsana* and *Halāsana*. As *Jālandhara Bandha* is essential in *prāṇāyāma*, *Sarvāṅgāsana* creates a natural chin lock (*Jālandhara Bandha*). In *Śīrṣāsana* automatic *Uḍḍīyāna Bandha* takes place. These *bandha* are essential factors in *prāṇāyāma*. They keep the brain free from stress and protect the heart and blood vessels...."

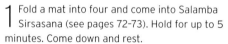

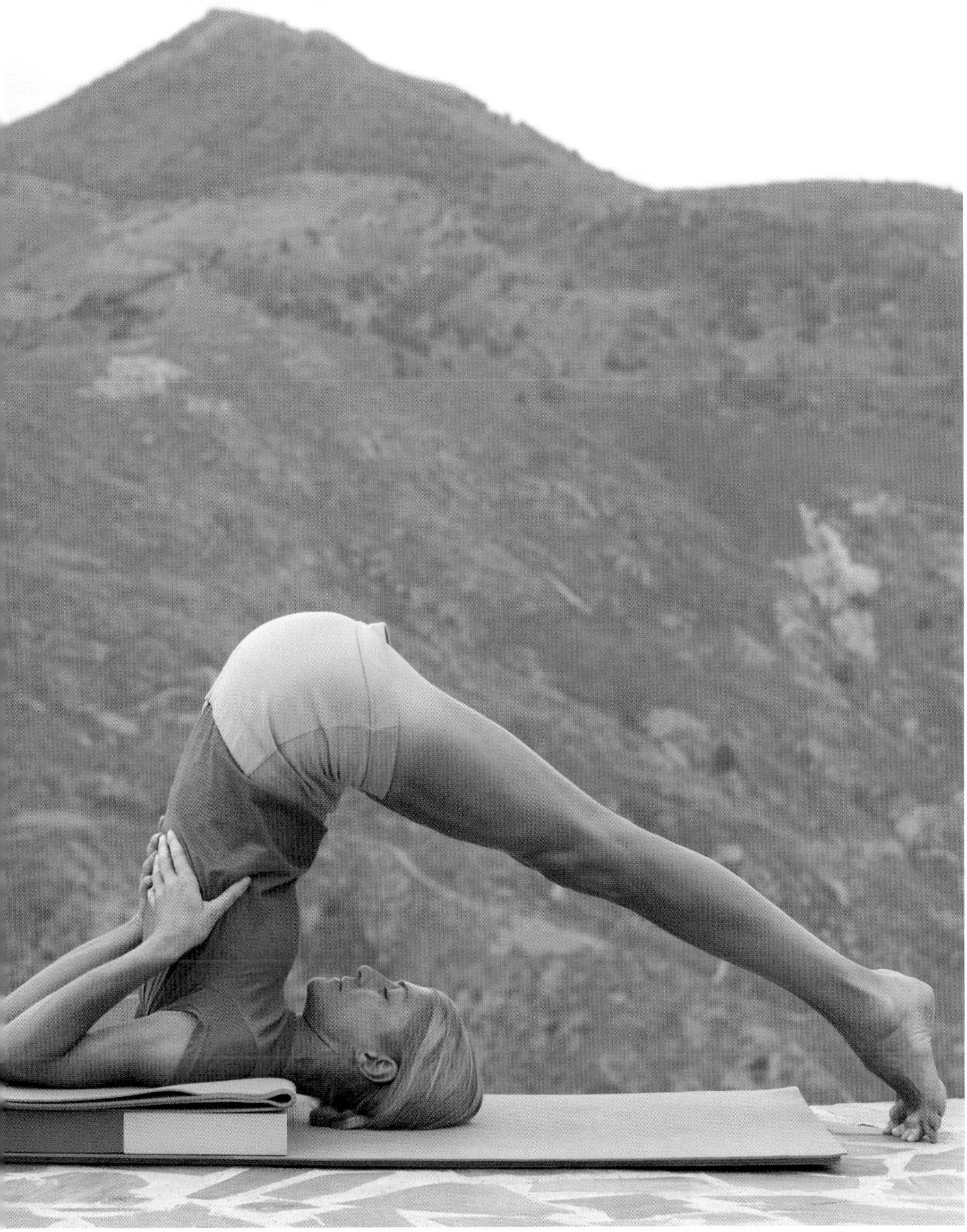

3 Keeping your legs straight, exhale and lower them over your head until the tips of your toes rest on the floor in Halasana (see page 124). Hold for 3 minutes, breathing evenly. Release your hands, lift your feet, bend your knees, and bring your thighs towards your chest. Push your buttocks back and lower them to the floor. Lie over the support to rest, feet on the floor and knees bent.

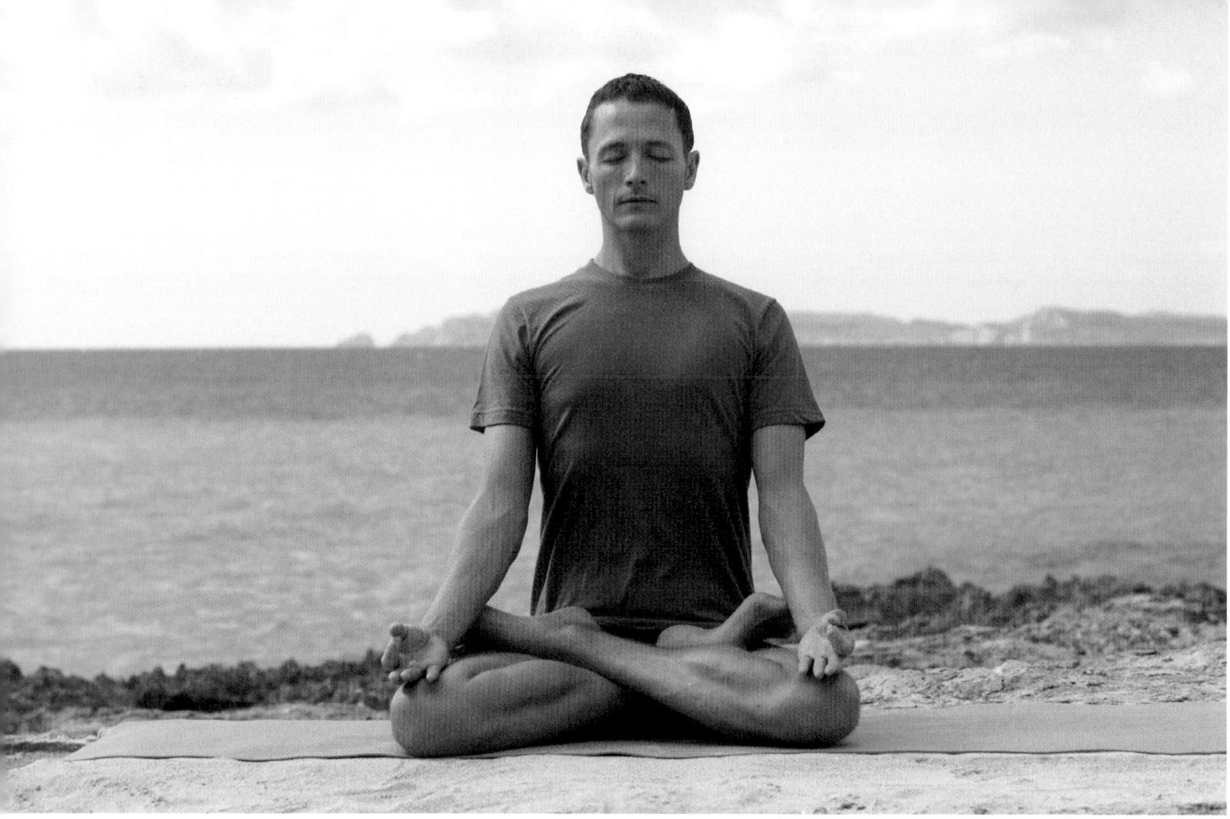

1 Sit in Padmasana (see pages 162-63). If your thighs, knees, or ankles are less flexible, sit in Svastikasana (see page 134), Siddhasana (see page 135), Bhadrasana (see pages 138-39), or Virasana (see pages 138-39). Rest your hands in Jnana Mudra (see page 136-37).

In all the poses, check that your spine is well stretched and concave and that your legs are as immovable as a root so that the trunk above remains firm. Push your lower shoulderblades into your chest and broaden your thoracic area. Lift your front ribs and your sternum from base to top.

Jalandhara Bandha

Chinlock

"When you do *Jālandhara Bandha* you are not putting any extra strain on the brain while retaining the breath. If you hold the breath without *Jālandhara Bandha* your eyes turn red, your ears get blocked, a load of tension is felt in the electrical nerves of the brain. With *Jālandhara Bandha* these loads of strain are not felt on the brain. The load is shifted from the brain to the chest."

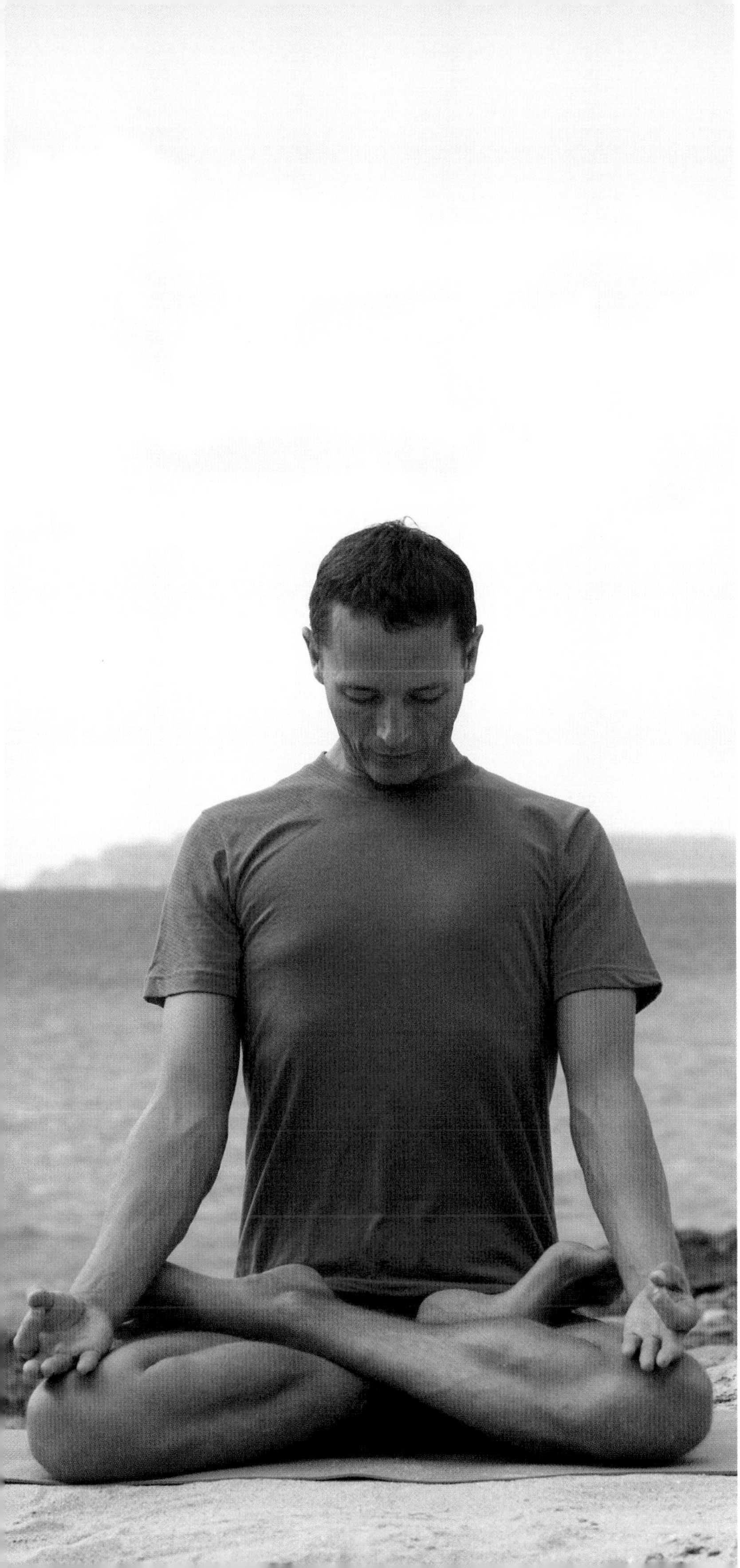

2 Lower your head from the nape of your neck to meet your ascending sternum. Do not force the neck muscles to rest the chin in the collarbone notch; simply lower the neck as far as it will comfortably go. Begin your pranayama (see pages 154–55). After finishing, lift your head, release your hands, and stretch out your legs.

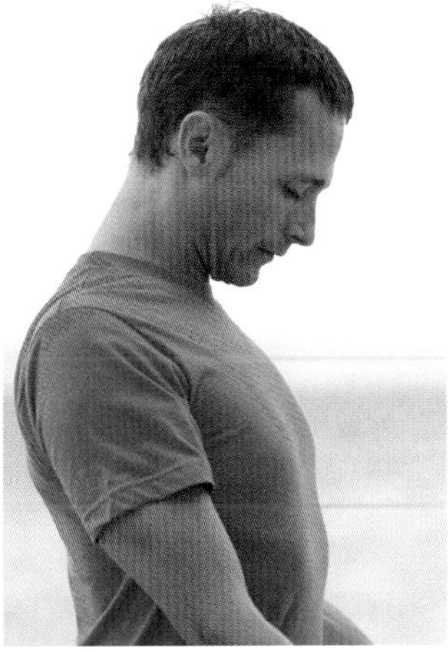

Position of chin and chest viewed from the side.

Pranayama and Deep Breathing

“If you keep a vessel under a tap, the water that flows, touches the bottom of the vessel and moves to the sides to accommodate the water as it comes. Unless and until the first water which dropped into the vessel finds a surface, the vessel does not fill at all; there will be air gaps. So if you open the tap very heavily, it will seem that the water has come to the top, but if you slow down the flow, the water descends to find its level.

If the water gushes from the tap, the vessel cannot be filled at all to the brim. It is the same in deep breathing. Though it appears that one has filled the lungs, the vessel of the breath remains empty. Secondly, if the tap is opened fully, the force of the water from the tap makes the vessel vibrate and distort its position. The same happens for the torso in deep breathing and one will not know whether the drawn-in breath is absorbed or not by the lungs.

If the tap's opening is narrowed, the water that drips into the vessel does not disturb, and when the vessel receives the water, the level rises smoothly, rhythmically, covering the surface of the vessel evenly. So also in *prāṇāyāmic* breathing, you make the upper palate open in such a way that the air that is drawn in is not made to gush, but flow into the narrow passage through the half closed palate.

One can measure how much one wants to open or close the upper palate to allow the breath to go in smoothly through the windpipe to fill the lungs. The windpipe bifurcates into two branches, which further branch off. The tissues open out tremendously in *prāṇāyāmic* breathing. This way the drawn-in breath goes toward the extremities and feeds the alveolar cells. The alveolar cells absorb the drawn-in air without any disturbances, vibrations, or leaving any gap between the air cells and the bronchioles. The drawn-in air is not released without feeding those areas. In deep breathing, they do not feed because the walls harden. The intercostal muscles of the chest become hard, therefore that breathing does not supply the needed energy to the extremities.

If you see the surface of water in a lake or sea, you can observe how gently, how subtly the water wets the sand without disturbing it. So our inhalation has to move in such a way that the energy, which is drawn, wets the air cells so that they can absorb the energy. ”

Breathing in Asana

"If you carefully observe the contact of the breath in different *āsana*, you observe that the breath touches different parts in different *āsana*. It means that breath moves and touches the body. Even if you take a deep in-breath or a deep out-breath, the touch of each breath in the torso differs each time and will not be the same. Each breath touches sometimes the inner parts and at other times the outer parts or the middle parts. When a deep inhalation or a deep exhalation is taken, you like to be in touch only with that part where the breath touches and neglect the other parts allowing these areas to remain dry and senseless. If the land is dry, it cracks. The same thing happens here: wherever the breath touches, that part gets nourished and the non-attended parts remain undernourished. It means there is progression on one side and regression on the other. While doing the *āsana* learn to observe that the breath taken in or out touches the torso evenly."

First extract from "Iyengar on Praṇāyāma", Iyengar Yoga Institute Review, *San Francisco, October 1984.*
Second extract from "Youth's Inquisitive Interest in Yoga", questions asked at RIMYI's Annual Day 2008.

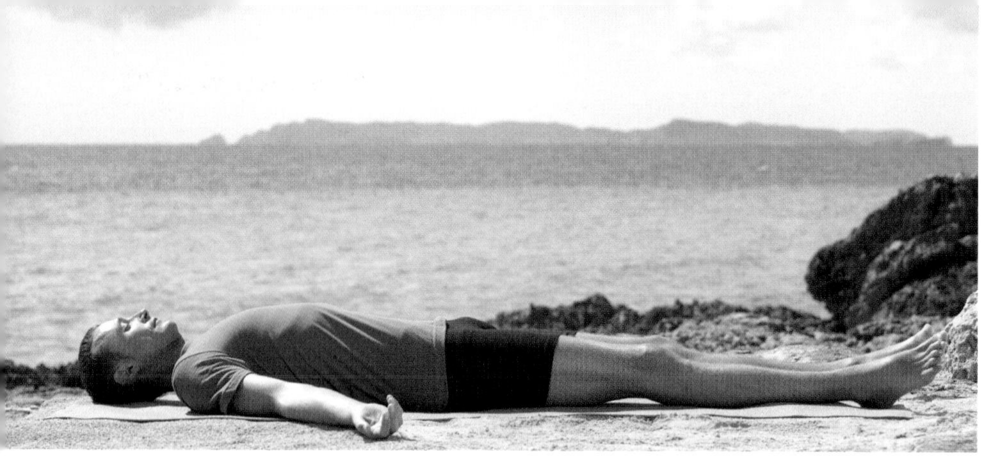

1 Lie in Savasana (see pages 62–63), eyes closed. Exhale, relax your diaphragm, and deflate your abdomen towards your spine. Take a slow, steady inhalation through both nostrils. Feel the air on the roof of your palate and hear its sibilant "sa" as you fill your lungs. Hold for a second or so.

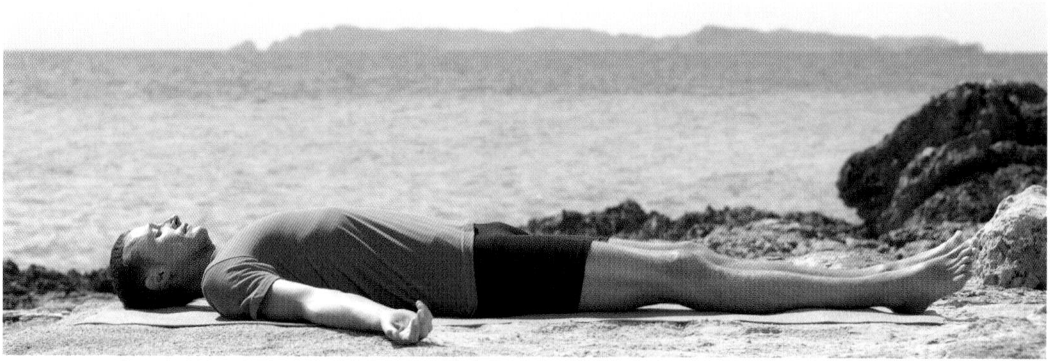

2 Exhale steadily until your lungs are empty. Feel the outgoing air on the roof of your palate and notice the aspirate sound "ha". Wait for a second before inhaling again. This completes one cycle. Repeat 8–10 cycles. Roll to one side to rest and then the other before sitting up.

Ujjayi Pranayama

Conquest of Energy

"When you begin practice, it is important to observe first the flow of exhalation. The exhalation leads towards quiet relaxation. Here, you experience the neutral state of body and mind. Know that proper exhalation leads towards proper inhalation.... For some, exhalation is more difficult than inhalation and for others the reverse. In exhalation, you have to meet the one who resides inside. You are made conscious of your existence. In inhalation, you get to know yourself."

Viloma Pranayama

Against the Natural Order

"If one does the *prāṇāyāma* hurriedly or hastily, one will find that the flow of the breath gets disturbed. The direction of avenues inside changes. This way one disturbs the channel of the breath. As one gets better, one can reduce normal breathing between *prāṇāyāma,* as the channels get opened."

1 First master Viloma lying in Savasana (see pages 62–63). Then sit in a comfortable sitting pose, such as Svastikasana (see page 134). Rest your hands in Jnana Mudra (see page 135). Lift your sternum, then lower your chin to your collarbone notch in Jalandhara Bandha (see pages 150–51).

2 Exhale until your lungs are empty. Inhale for 2 seconds through both nostrils, feeling the air on the outer nasal membranes. Hold the breath for 2 seconds. Inhale for 2 seconds, hold for 2 seconds, and continue this process until your lungs are full. Then retain the breath for 3–5 seconds. Exhale slowly until your lungs are empty. This completes one cycle. Repeat 6–8 cycles, then lie in Savasana to rest.

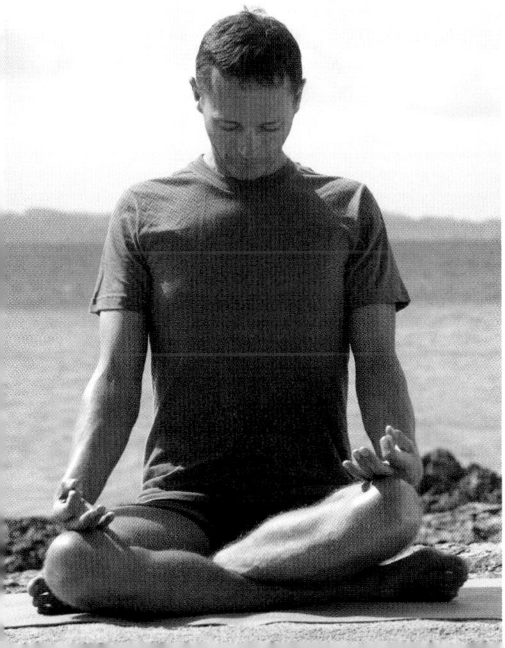

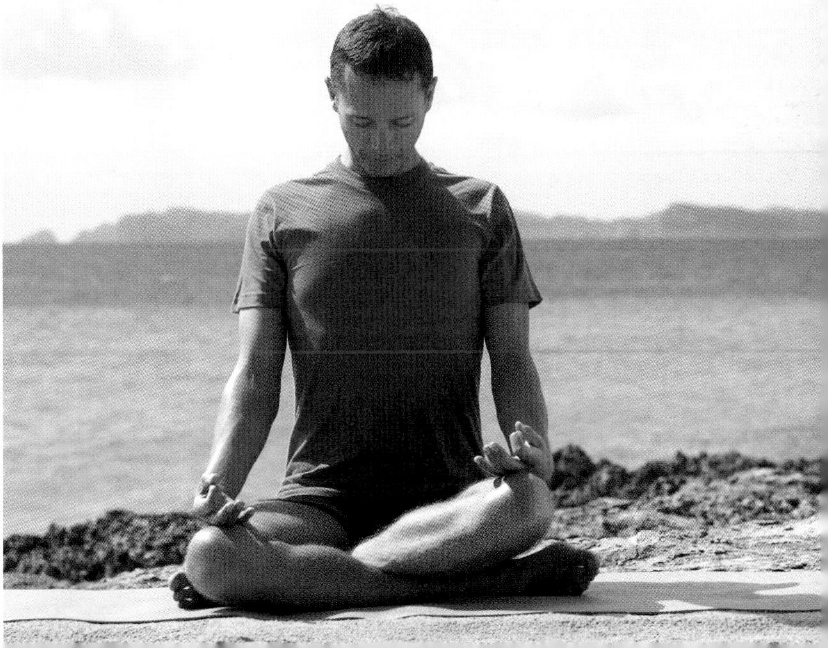

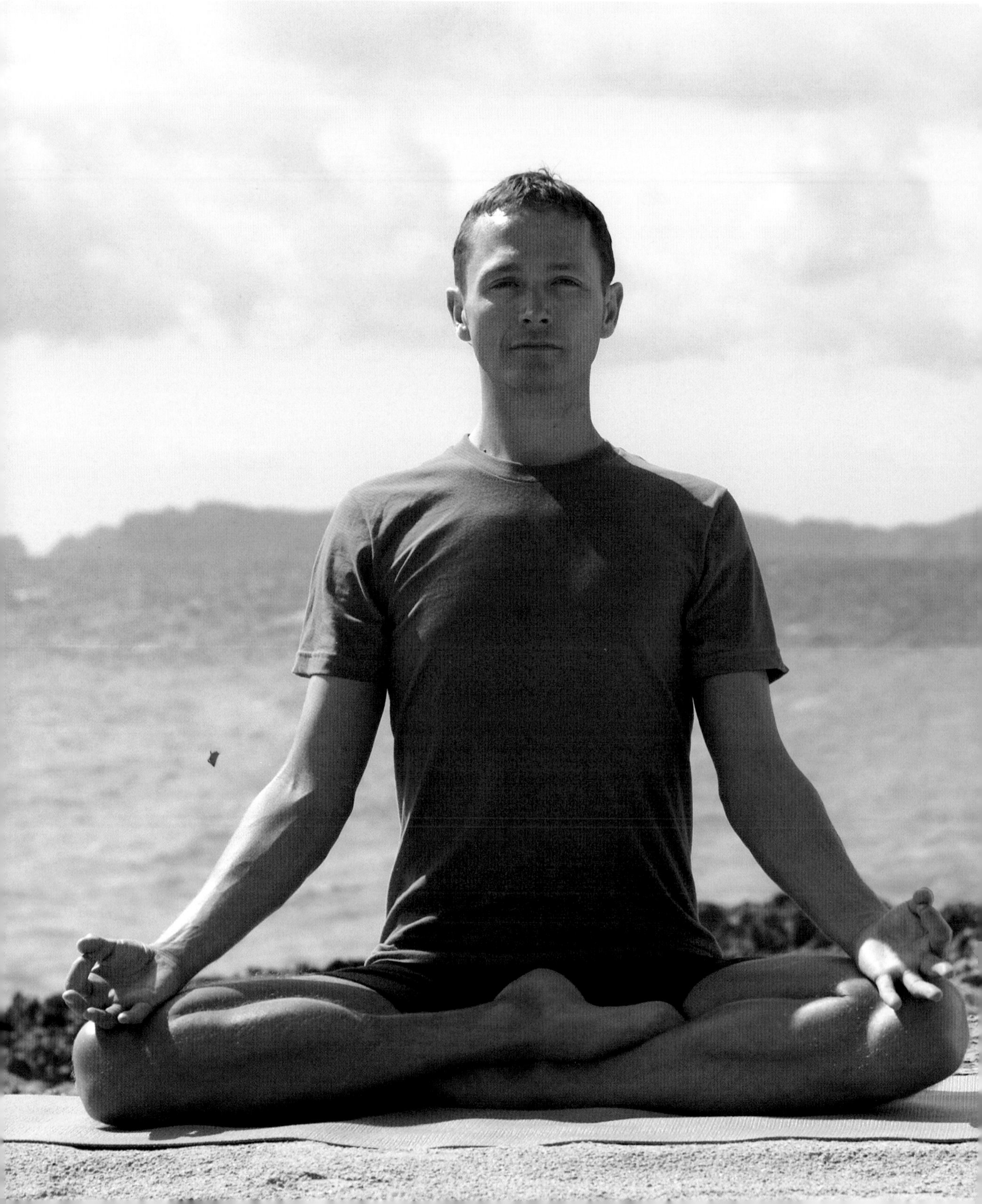

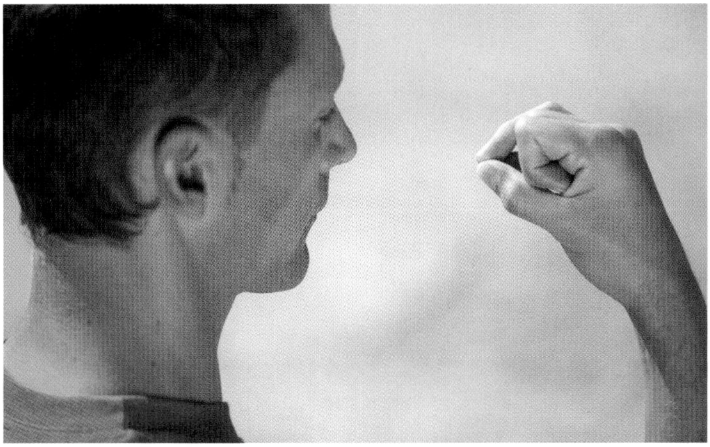

1 Sit in any comfortable sitting pose. Rest your hands in Jnana Mudra (see page 135).

2 Take the first and second fingers of your right hand into the base of your thumb and extend your fourth and fifth fingers. Bend the first and second fingers towards the palm, then form a circle by joining the tip of your thumb with the tips of the little and ring fingers. Raise the fingers towards your nose.

Nadi Sodhana

Purifying Breath

"My own student Yehudi Menuhin, to some extent, was an indirect *Guru* from whom I learnt the placing of the fingers very accurately on the nostril passages.... I observed his fingering work, the mobility of the knuckles on the violin strings, and the placement of the tip of the thumb on the bow and fingers on the strings. This gave me the clue of placing the thumb and fingers on the nose to control the inner carpet of the membranes and to trace the exact air passage for my *prāṇāyāma*."

→ continued

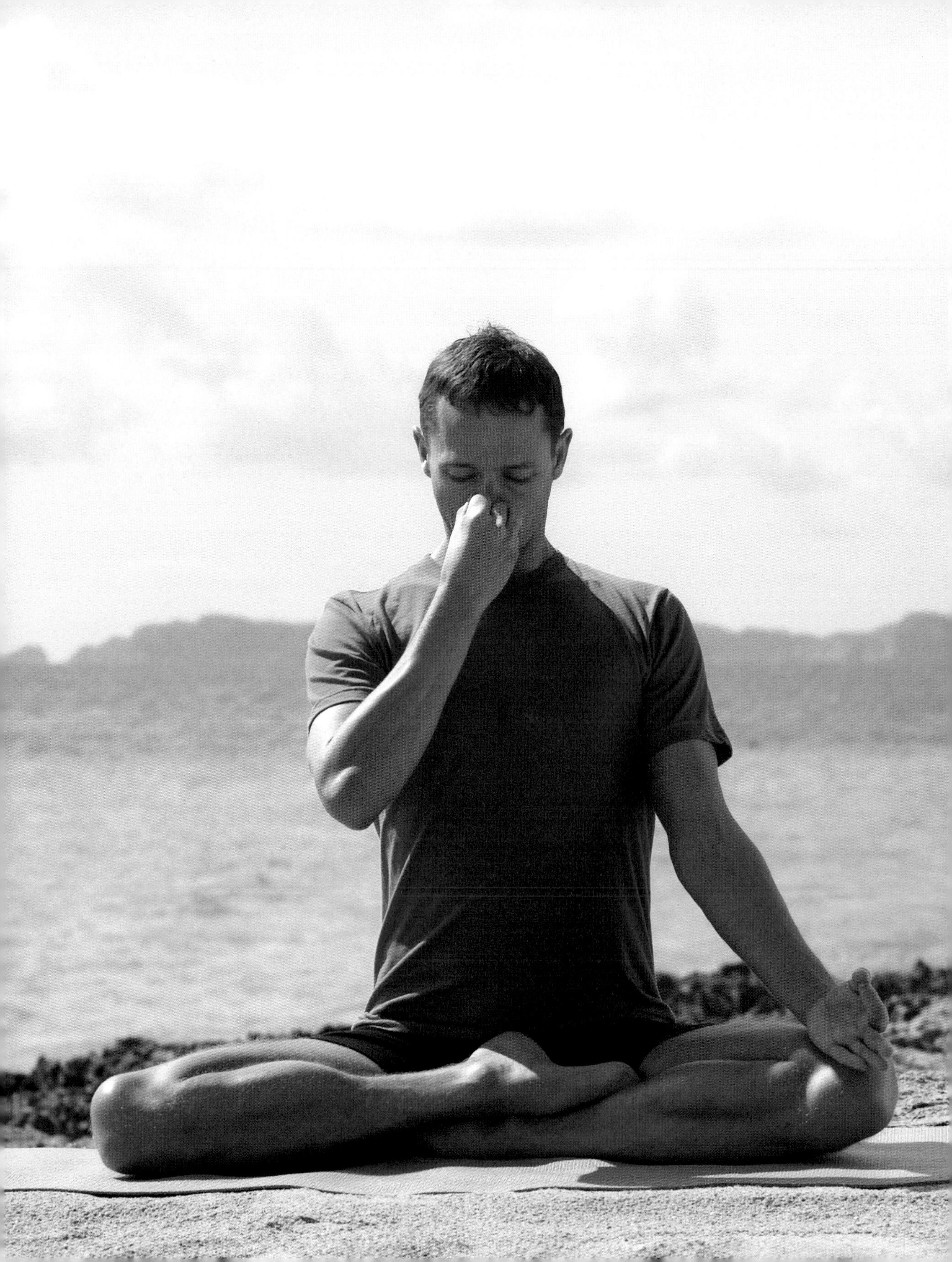

3 Lift your sternum and lower your chin in Jalandhara Bandha (see pages 150–51). Press the tip of your thumb into your right nostril, on the soft cartilage below the bone; press the ring and little fingers into the left nostril at the same level. Exhale through your half-open right nostril.

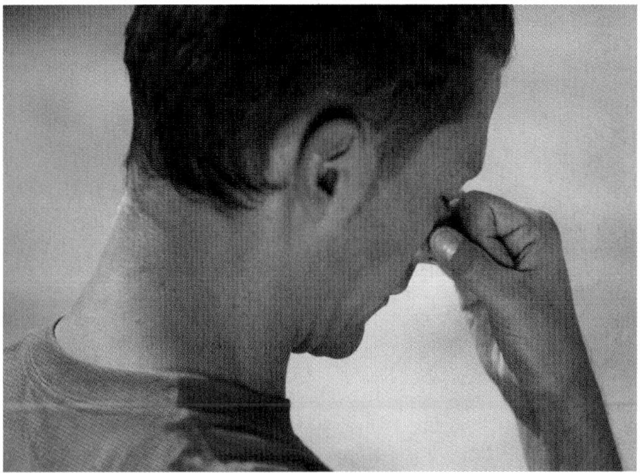

4 Keeping the left nostril blocked, inhale through the right. Close the right nostril with your thumb tip. Release your fingers to partially open the left nostril. Exhale through it. Pause, then inhale through this nostril. Close your left nostril, open your right nostril partially and exhale. This completes one cycle. Inhale through the right nostril to start the next cycle. Complete 8–10 cycles.

Patanjali on Meditation

“The moment the word ‘meditation’ is introduced, the present generation thinks that this is an easy method. When you ask them what they are doing, they all say, ‘I am meditating.’ Patañjali gives a variety of methods because he knows that meditation is not possible for all....

Patañjali offers various methods for those who cannot meditate on God and begins with:

- *Maitrī karuṇā muditā upekṣānāṁ sukha duḥkha puṇya apuṇya viṣayāṇām bhāvanātaḥ cittaprasādanam* (*Yoga Sūtra*, 1.33): If these above guidelines of friendliness, compassion, and joy are built up in a *sādhaka* towards his fellow beings, and if he cultivates indifference in himself towards his pleasure and pain, good and bad, then his consciousness gets favourably disposed to live in serenity. As a yoga practitioner, I have learnt how one has to behave with people and how one has to handle oneself when one is confounded by the hindrances of body, mind, and consciousness that come in the way of spiritual evolution. He wants each one of us to study the hindrances judiciously, so that one knows when to observe friendliness and compassion, feel gladness in progress and to show indifference to the things which disturb one's *sādhanā*.

- *Pracchardana vidhāraṇābhyām vā prāṇasya* (*Yoga Sūtra*, 1.34). Another alternative way is by maintaining the pensive state felt at the time of soft and steady exhalation and during passive retention of the breath after exhalation.

- From the exalted state of meditation (*dhyāna*), Patañjali comes down to *prāṇāyāma*. Can you see the significance? One who suffers from a disease has only two choices, to accept his illness and surrender to God, or to challenge the disease and to fight it out with positive thoughts. Both acceptance and surrender are a form of meditation. However, as meditation is not possible to all, he wants us to watch the outgoing breath and to hold it passively. In this process, the consciousness moves into a passive state and deepens into a quiet state before inhalation. This state of quietude is *praśānta citta* or tranquil state as the thought waves are made to fade at least during and after exhalation.

- Then, he says, 'go wholeheartedly into whatever subject that attracts one.' (*Yoga Sūtra*, 1.35). (I follow this guidance and get fully and totally absorbed in the *āsana* and *prāṇāyāma*. By this statement of Patañjali, one cannot call the *āsanas* physical exercises). Any ideal thought that attracts one totally to get absorbed in it, moves naturally towards the higher plane of consciousness. For twenty-four hours a day, great scientists' minds and bodies are fixed with dedication on one subject. By this total involvement, focus and absorption on their subject, they may be considered as yogis.

- Now, he shows another alternative: *Viśokā vā jyotiṣmatī* (*Yoga Sūtra*, 1.36). Contemplation on the serene and luminous light of the spiritual heart. This sorrowless light is the *ātman*. But can we directly reach the *ātman*? Can you imagine how difficult it is?

- So, he guides in the next *sūtra*, 'Take those who have experienced and transcended sorrows as objects of your concentration.' (*Yoga Sūtra*, 1.37). He says, 'Take ideal persons such as Ramana Maharshi, Ramakṛishna Paramahamsa, Christ, Buddha or any other. Take them as examples. Develop character by studying their ways of behaviour and see that they help to quieten the consciousness.'

- He suggests we study, recollect, and compare the states of consciousness during the wakeful state, the dream-filled and dreamless sleepy states, in order to live and experience steadiness throughout (*Yoga Sūtra*, 1.38).

- At the end, he says to contemplate on a pleasing object, conducive to the steadiness of the consciousness, for serenity (*Yoga Sūtra*, 1.39). ”

From "Pearls of Yogic Wisdom", Aṣṭadaḷa Yogamālā *Volume 1, pp243–46.*

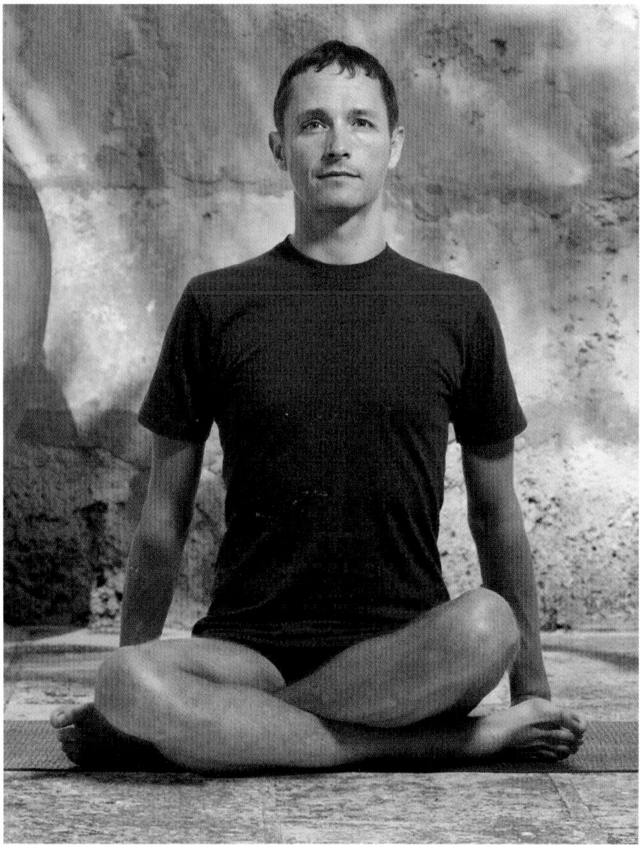

1 Sit in Svastikasana (see page 134), then place your hands beside your hips.

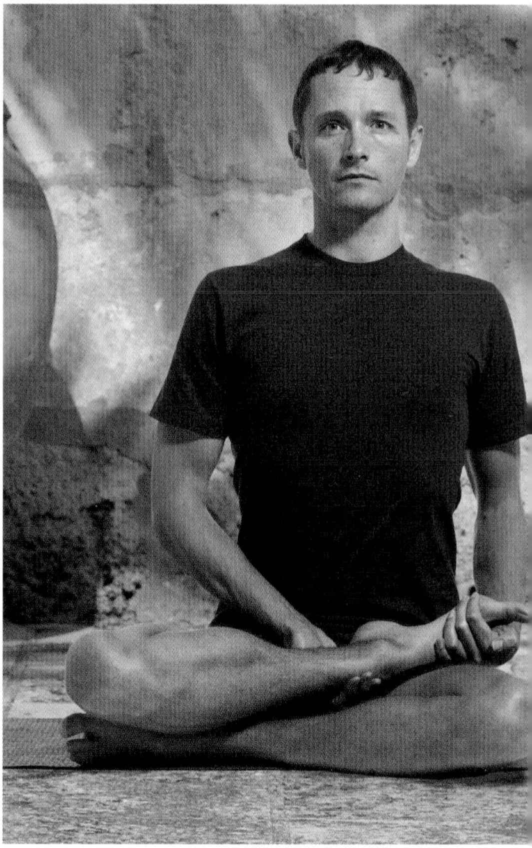

2 Using both hands, lift your right foot up and onto the root of your left thigh, with the toes touching your groin.

Padmasana

Full Lotus Pose

"Can one do an *āsana* without meditation? An *āsana* without meditation becomes an exercise. An *āsana* with meditation brings poise, pensivity, and serenity. Patañjali says, *Deśa bandhaḥ cittasya dhāraṇā* (*Yoga Sūtra* III.3) – i.e., one can concentrate inside the body as well as outside the body.... I teach *āsana* in such a way that each mental part and each cell of the body becomes the object of concentration."

3 Lift your left foot onto your right thigh. Extend your spine and the sides of your trunk and broaden your chest. Rest your hands in Jnana Mudra (see page 135). Hold for 30-60 seconds. Release the left leg with your hands, then the right. Repeat to the other side. Finish in Dandasana (see pages 14-15).

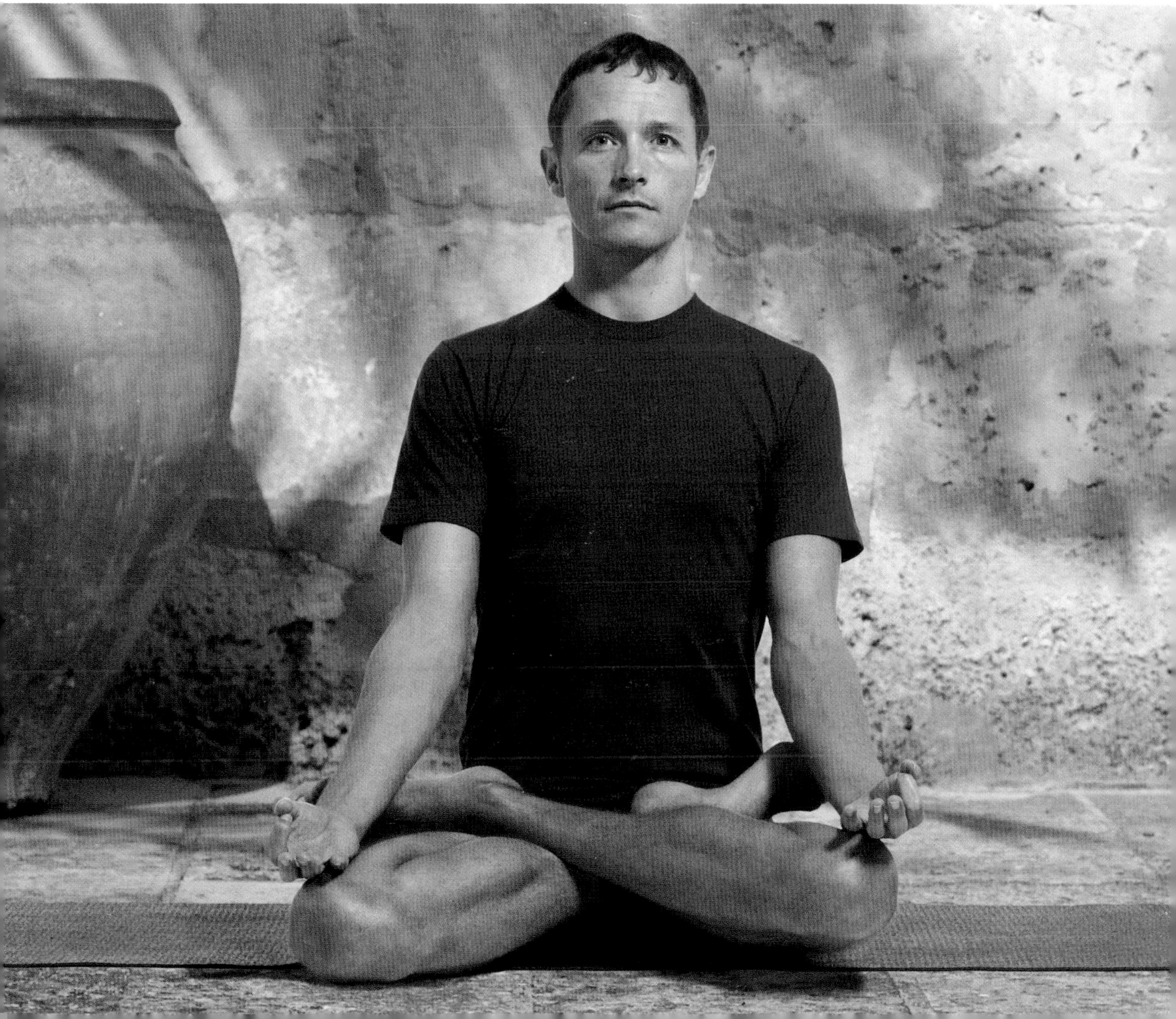

"Remember that the mantra is a seed, and ultimately you want to be seedless, or beyond the seed."

The Mantra Aum

Q. In the first chapter of the *Yoga Sūtra*, Patañjali mentions that one must repeat the mantra *Āuṁ* while meditating on its meaning. Do you personally chant or meditate with *Āuṁ* or some other mantra? If so, why don't you emphasize meditation more to your students?

"The word *āuṁ* is *akṣara*. It means imperishable, indestructible, undecaying. In the word *āuṁ,* three letters are involved. They are *ā*, *u*, and *ṁ*. *Ā* is the beginning of the alphabet. Creation begins from here. *U* is the continuity of the speech, and *ṁ* puts an end to communication. All the alphabets and words melt into these three alphabets. Out of the fifty phonemes in Sanskrit, all others melt and perish while the three (*Ā*, *U*, *Ṁ*) never fade or perish. These three are the principle cause not only for uttering the words, but also for communication and communion. Therefore, words being imperishable and eternal, the sages and yogis of India gave a divine touch to them. As *āuṁ* gets the supremacy over other letters, it is considered as the epithet of the Supreme – the God as well as the Self. *Āuṁ* being indestructible, the *ṛṣīs* saw this as *bīja mantra* or seed *mantra* on God.

Repetition of a *mantra* or sacred prayer like *āuṁ* is called *japa*. As I mentioned before, the mind tends to fluctuate and become distracted. By bringing it back to a single point like *āuṁ* or by looking at a candle or a rose or some other object, the *sādhaka* silences the thoughts and becomes one with body and mind. For me, focusing on the breath while in the *āsana* with total one-pointedness is meditation. It is with this steadiness of intelligence that one witnesses the presence of soul.

From the Indian point of view, *āuṁ* has a specific meaning. You open your mouth to say *ā*. To pronounce, you roll the tongue like *u*, *ṁ* stands for silence. In order to learn silence, you must close your mouth. These are the roots for speech, like the root mind or *mūla citta* for thinking, so they are considered as the divine sound. Patañjali wants you to do this with meaning and felt experience. Without experience, you cannot understand the meaning: you cannot experience just by knowing the meaning of it. Feeling must be there....

Patañjali wants, basically, the purification of body and restraint of *citta*. Therefore, my emphasis is on body and mind. For me, *āsana* is the *mantra*, the breath is the *mantra* and I have to understand the meaning of each *āsana* and feel the life force – the self – moving in with the rhythm of body and breath."

From "Iyengar talks about the Sutras", interview by Elise Miller in Pune, July 1983, Yoga Journal, July/August 1984.

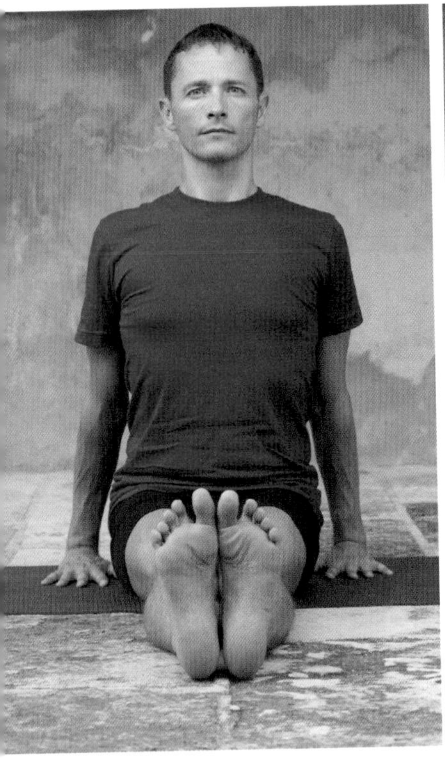

1 Sit in Dandasana (see pages 14–15). Have a wooden wedge or a rolled towel to hand if you need it in step 2.

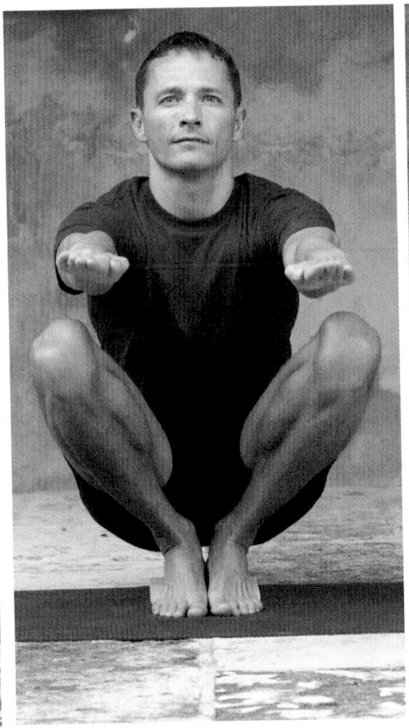

2 Squat on your haunches with heels and toes together and knees apart. If your heels do not touch the floor, place the support beneath them. Stretch your arms forwards, in line with your shoulders, palms down.

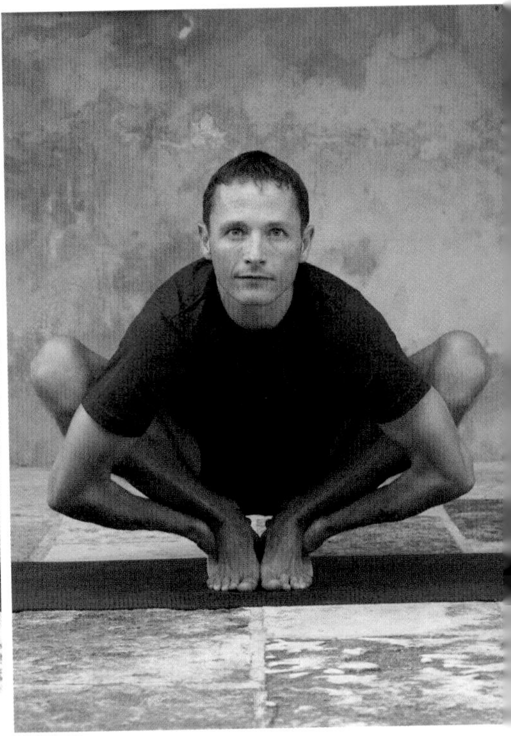

3 Widen your thighs and knees and move your trunk forwards until your armpits extend beyond your knees.

Malasana I

Garland Pose I

"The practice of *āsana* should be such that you not only find the centre of gravity on the physical body, but of your whole existence. The *āsana* has to be performed in such a way that the action, movement, adjustment, the energizing process of every bone, muscle, cell, is in touch with the core of the being."

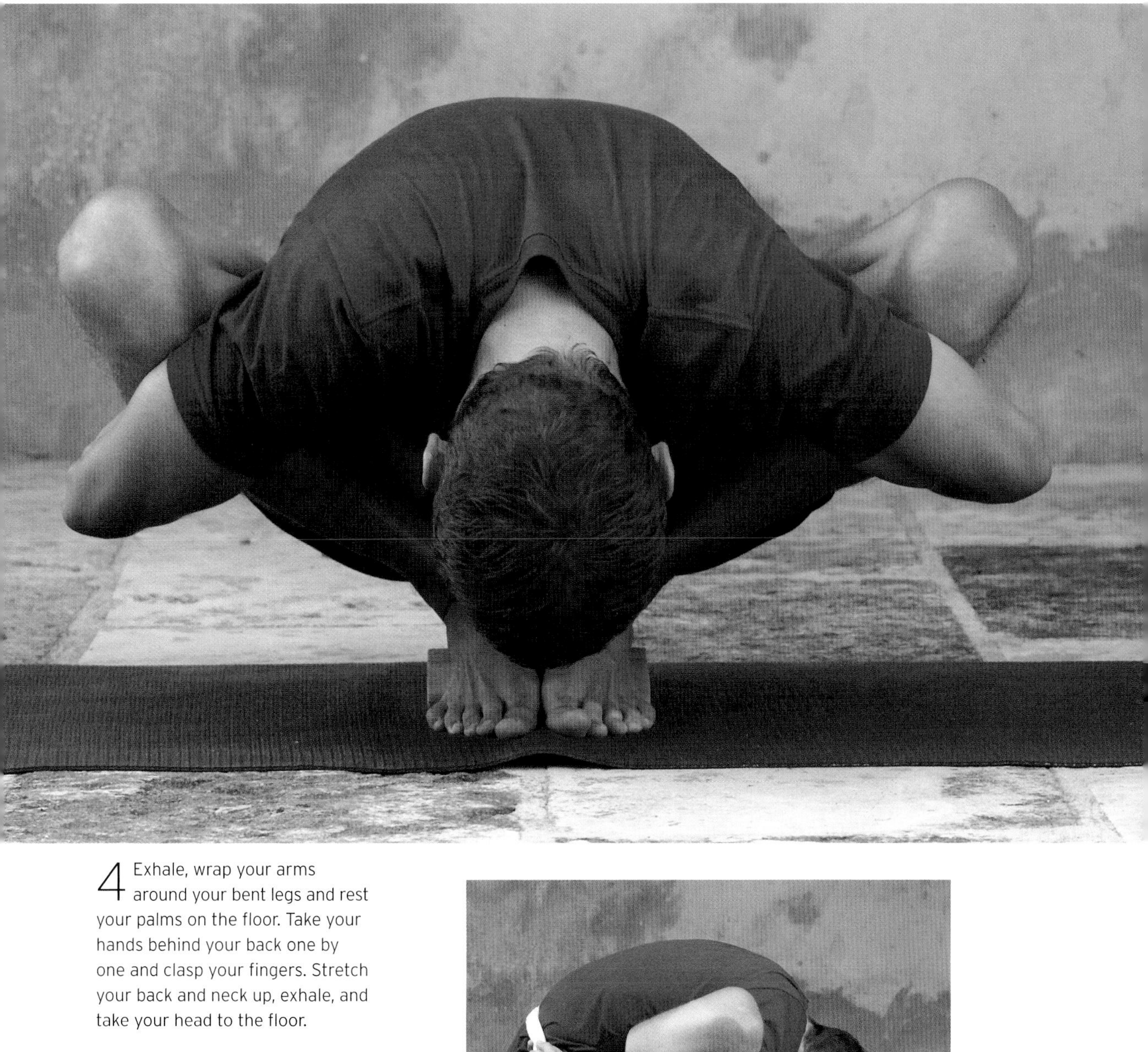

4 Exhale, wrap your arms around your bent legs and rest your palms on the floor. Take your hands behind your back one by one and clasp your fingers. Stretch your back and neck up, exhale, and take your head to the floor.

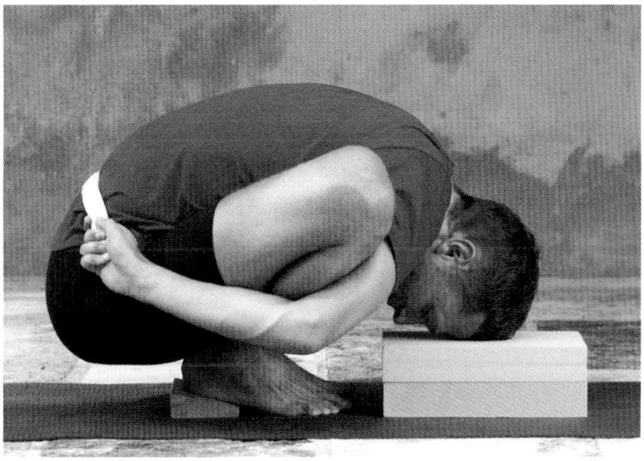

With props: If you cannot clasp fingers, hold a belt. If your head does not reach the floor, rest it on blocks.

"You never stop learning. I work constantly in my own practice and in my teaching."

Evolving as a Yogi

"*Haṭhayoga Pradīpikā* and *Śiva Saṃhitā* describe four evolutionary stages in the practice, starting from the gross and ending with the finest of the fine:

- *Ārambhāvasthā*: The beginning state, where one 'scratches the surface' (*Haṭhayoga Pradīpikā* IV. 70-71; *Śiva Samhitā* III. 28). This stage corresponds to *mṛdu* state of study in the *Yoga Sūtra* – that is the stage of anatomical analysis. After 'scratching' comes the second stage:

- *Ghaṭāvasthā*: *Ghaṭā* means a pot – the body is like a vessel or a pot (*H.Y.P.*, IV. 72-73; *Ś.S.*, III. 55-59). After scratching the first surface or layer of the body, comes the study of its inner functions, the circulation of blood, the function of the vital organs, the movement of breath, and so forth. This is *ghaṭāvasthā*. In modern scientific terms, *ghaṭāvasthā* is known as the physiological functioning of the human body. The *sādhaka* begins to feel how the internal anatomical action produces a physiological reaction. This state corresponds to *madhya* or average type of study. From this physiological reaction, a new awareness is developed in the mind, Suppose you think psychologically to flex the biceps more, or turn more; or extend the liver, strengthen the floor of the bladder and so on, you have to understand that the effect of *āsana* is not merely physical or physiological, but psychological also. *Āsana* practice strengthens the inner body. What is this inner body? The inner body is the mind – this is the third stage of growth in *āsana*. The mind feels; but cannot discriminate, so it takes and consults its friend, guide, and philosopher – the intelligence – and acquaints it with the body.

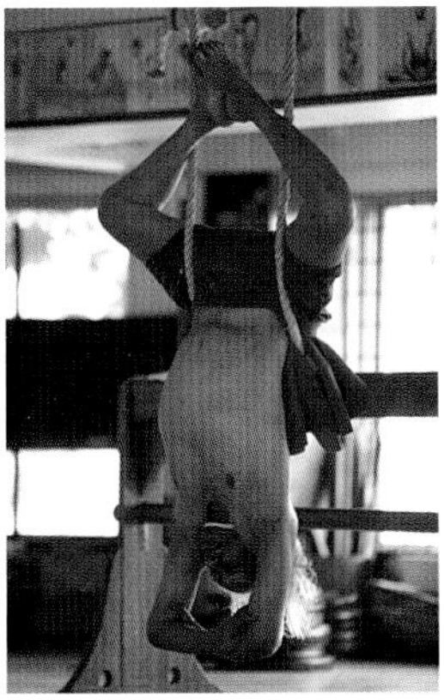

Guruji never misses his morning asana practice, which includes 20 minutes of inversions using a suspended sling.

- *Paricayāvasthā* (*H.Y.P.*, IV. 74-75; *Ś.S.*, III. 61-65): *Paricaya*, literally means 'acquaintance'. Here the intelligence is made to come closer in contact with the functioning of body, senses, and mind. This is the state of intimate knowledge, where the mind acts with the intelligence as a public relations officer between the physical and organic body.... Similarly, the mind takes the intelligence to the various parts of the body and introduces it to the anatomical body, physiological body, the physical organs, and senses of perception, by bringing the intelligence closer to the various systems of the body. Once this introduction is done, then the intelligence, the mind, the physiological organs, and the anatomical body function as a co-ordinated single unit. In this stage, the intelligence integrates the surface body and the inner body step by step to the core of the being, for the being to permeate. This state corresponds to the *adhimātrā* state of the *Yoga Sūtra*. Finally, comes the last evolutionary stage, that of emancipation.

- *Niṣpattiāvasthā* (*H.Y.P.*, IV. 76-77; *Ś.S.*, III. 66f): The state of accomplishment or consummation, where the consciousness and body (anatomically, physiologically, psychologically, and intellectually) become one. When they become one, dualities or differences between body, mind, intelligence, and consciousness disappear. ”

From "Yoga and Peace", talk in Barcelona, October 1986, first published in Dipika, *Iyengar Institute London, Winter 1986. Also published in* Victoria Yoga Centre Society Newsletter, *April 1988.*

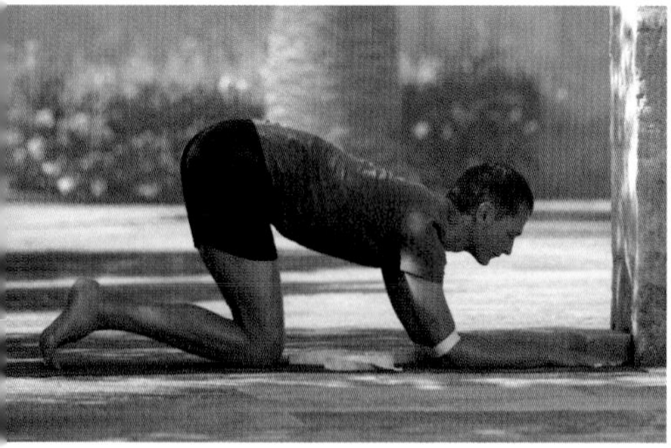

1 Place a mat and the long side of a brick against a wall. Secure a belt around your upper arms to keep them shoulder-width apart. Kneel on the mat, hands on either side of the brick. Position your thumbs and fingers so they make a right angle on each side of the brick.

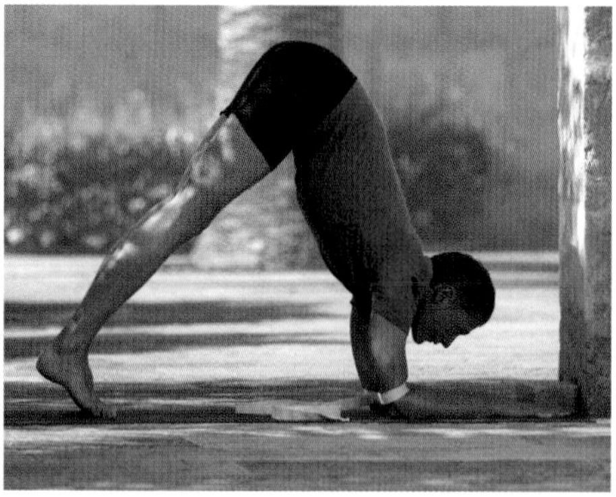

2 Keeping your forearms and hands parallel to each other, press your elbows, forearms, and palms into the floor. Straighten your legs, walk in a little, and come onto your toes. Stretch your neck and lift your head as high as possible.

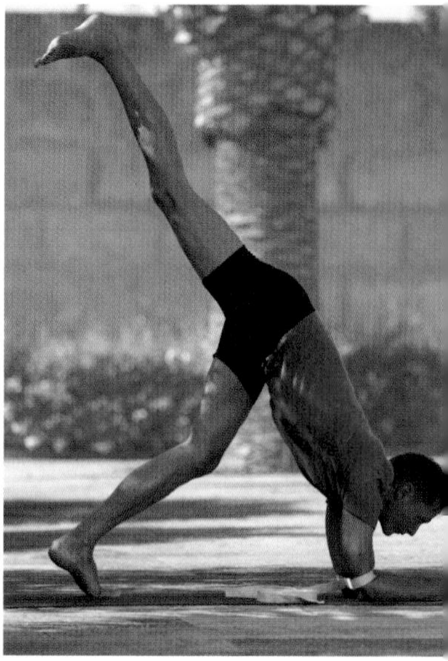

3 Bend your left leg slightly, exhale, and swing your right leg up, towards the wall. Follow immediately with your left leg.

Pincha Mayurasana

Peacock Tail Pose

"One will be surprised to know that he never touches the same corresponding back parts of the heels on the wall. He may be balancing but the sensations of the skin should tell him that the motor nerves extend on one leg while they are contracted on the other leg. While doing this *āsana* no one thinks this way, of touching the same spot and same parts as the other side of the body.... When such defects (*doṣa*) are dissolved, one has perfected the *āsana*."

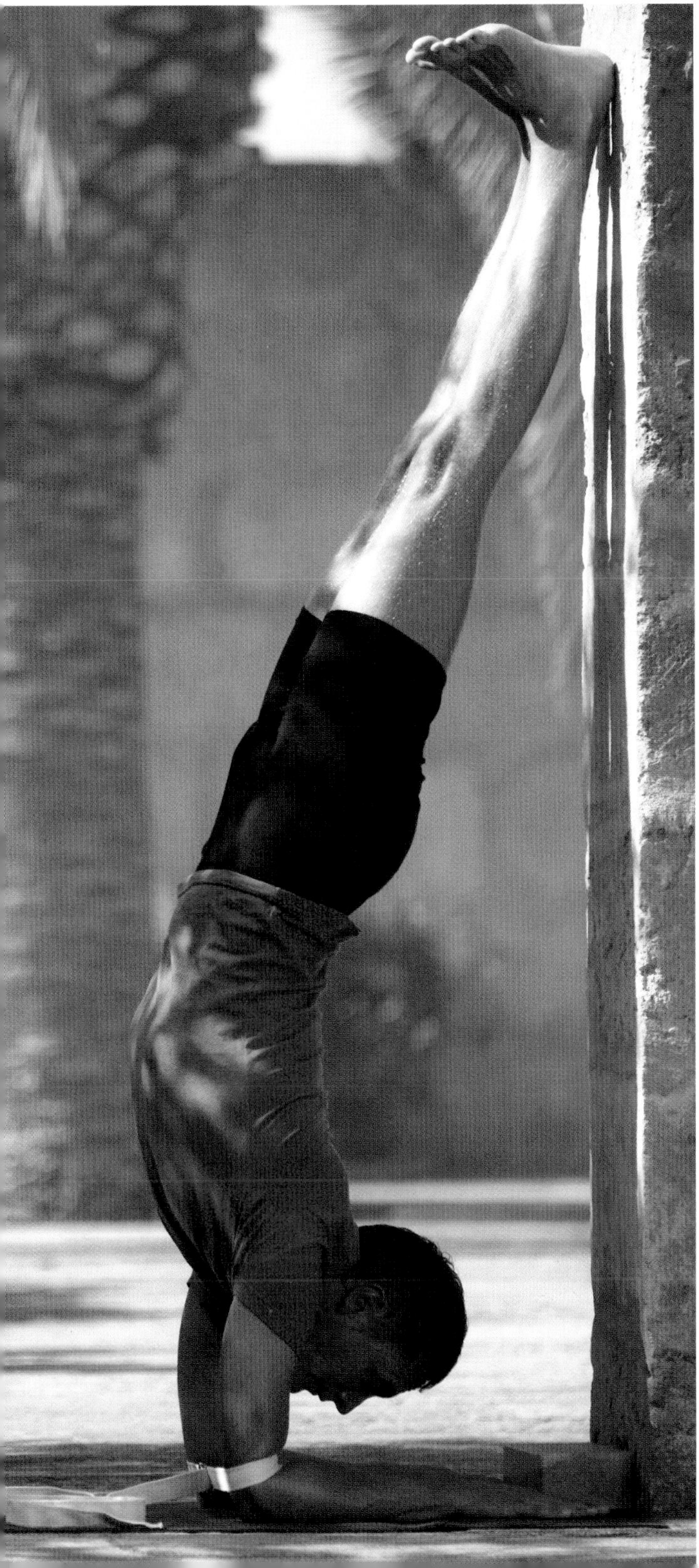

4 Rest your heels against the wall. Stretch your legs, knees, and ankles together, lift your shoulders and keep your head up. Hold for 20-30 seconds. Exhale and lower your legs one by one. Keep your head down for a few seconds before standing up. Next time, kick up the left leg first.

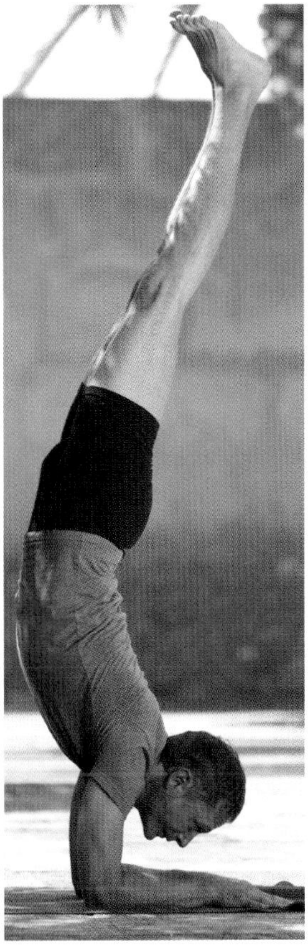

Free balancing: After practice, take your feet off the wall one by one and balance. Finally, work without the wall.

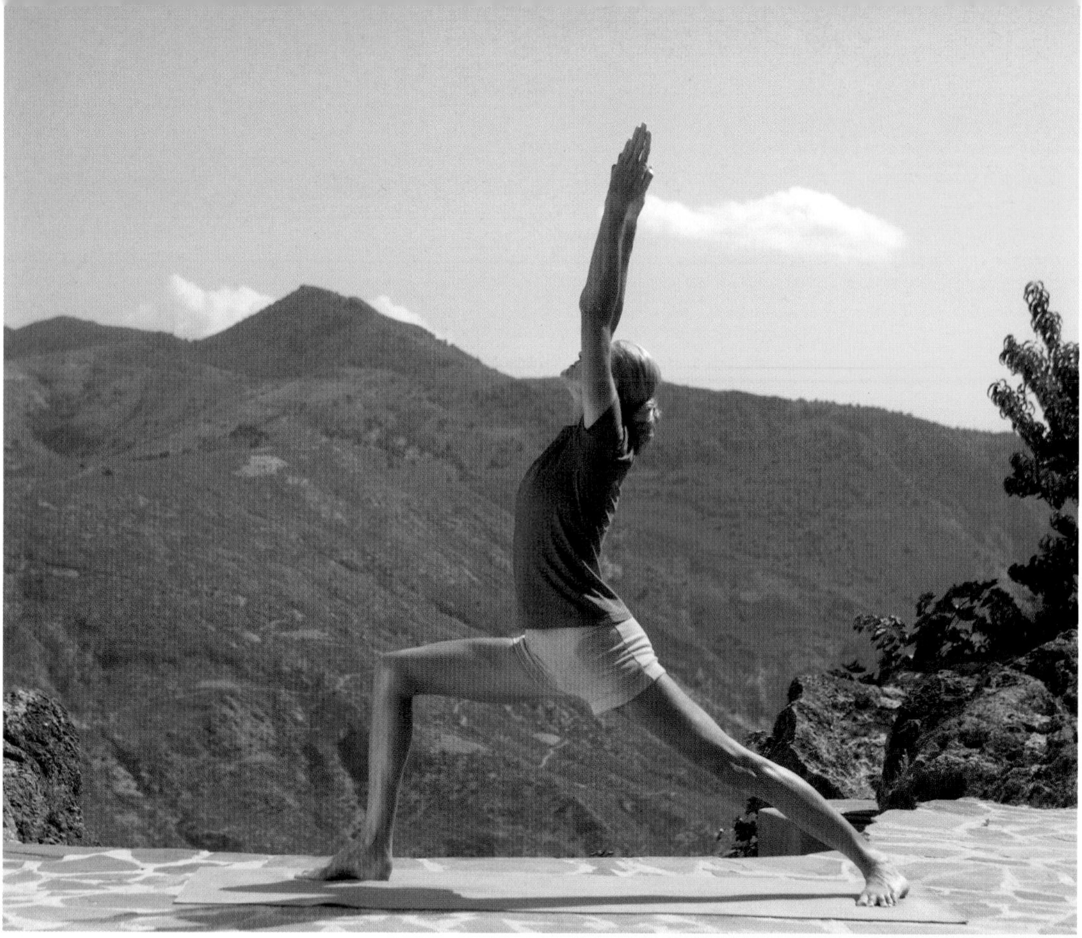

1 Begin in Virabhadrasana I (see pages 98–99) with your right leg bent and trunk facing right.

Virabhadrasana III

Warrior Pose III

"If the practice of *āsana* is a torture, who wants to do it? If you practise to learn and understand yourself, it is a joy and an eye-opener. It not only generates life-giving force, but acts as an inspiration to earn the nectar of knowledge. The cycle of evolution and involution continues and the intelligence does not stagnate. That is why you always find a newness in my practice and in my teachings."

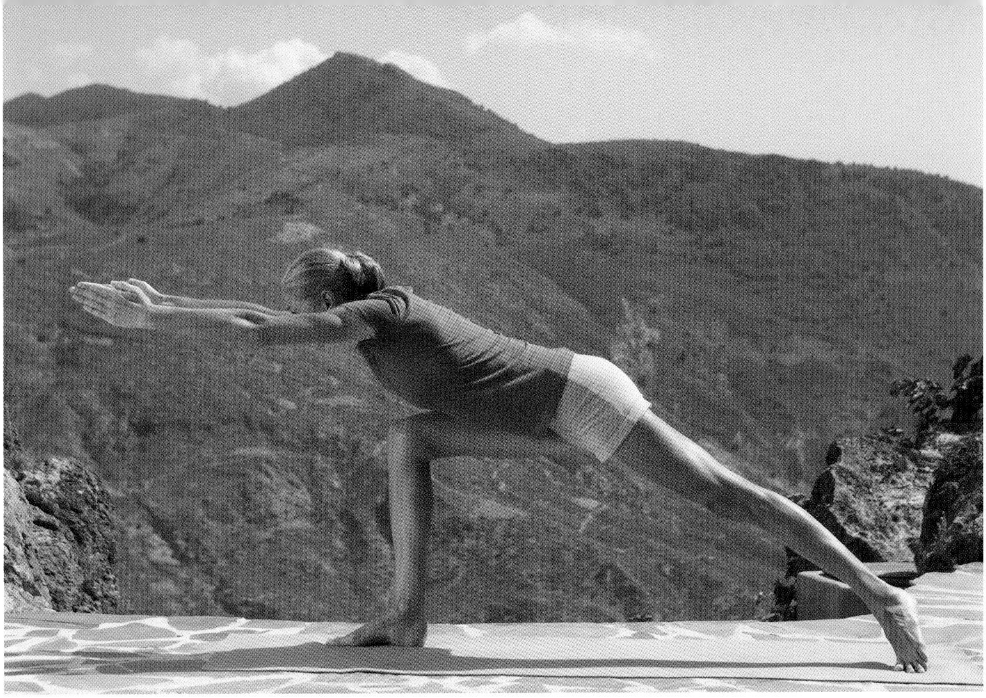

2 Exhale and extend your trunk over your right leg, resting your chest on the thigh. Stretch your trunk and arms forwards.

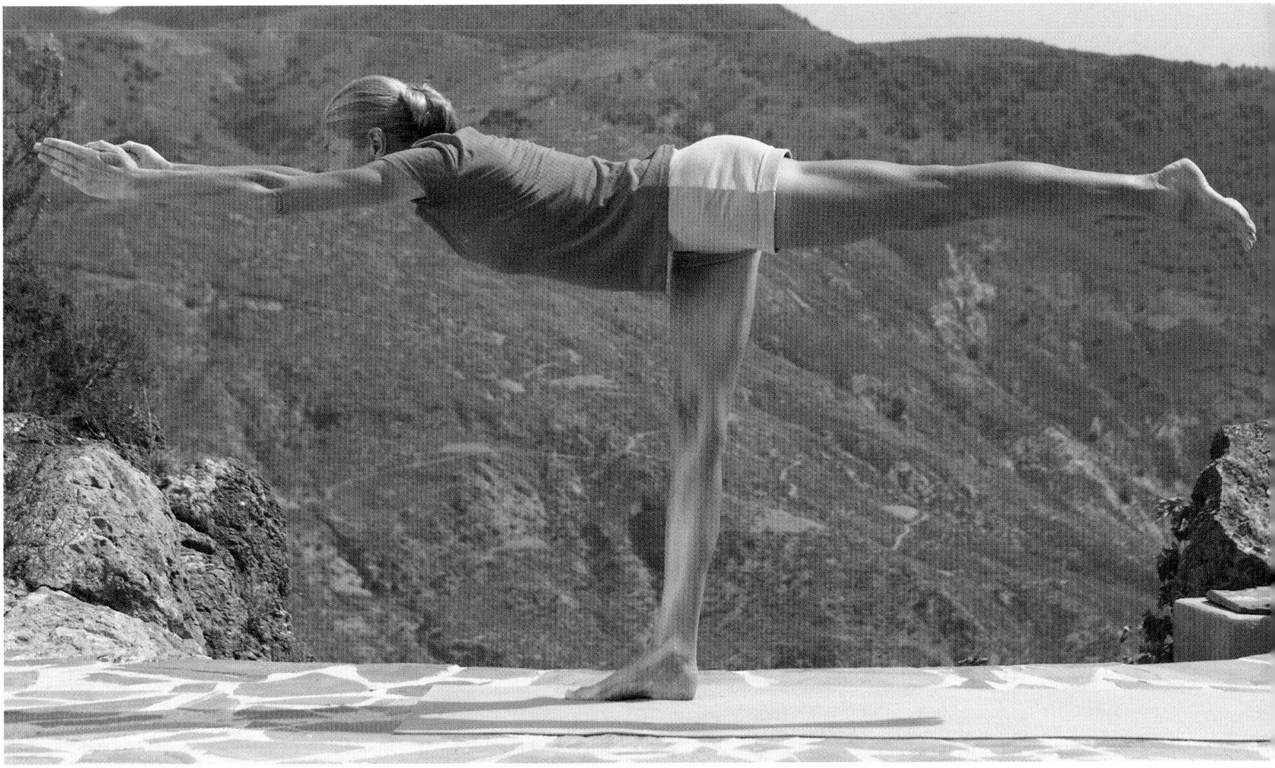

3 Exhale, raise your left leg, and straighten your right. Keep your hips level and chest, right leg and arms parallel to the floor. Look ahead. Hold for 20-30 seconds, breathing evenly. Exhale, bend your right leg, and lower your left into Virabhadrasana I. Straighten your leg, turn into Utthita Hasta Padasana (see pages 108-109), and repeat to the other side. Finish in Tadasana.

"Though he acts as a teacher, within himself, he should be a learner."

The Art of Teaching

"Teaching is learning, and re-learning is true teaching. Accept your pupils as a blessing from God for you to re-open your intelligence to re-think and re-act with wide open eyes. See the generosity of God who sends such students who pay for you to refine your *sādhanā* both in teaching and learning.

Each pupil who comes to you comes with some new problems. No two persons are alike. Therefore, teaching cannot be parrot-teaching. Each pupil has to be studied. The teacher has to go down to the understanding level of the pupils. The teacher has to get experience by thinking and learning adjustment processes as each different pupil opens new angles of thought.

Do not differentiate between yourself and the pupil. As the mother loves her children, the teacher should show affection in guiding them towards progression. If there is a gap between teacher and student, it creates egoism in the teacher and a communication gap between them. A teacher becomes a teacher because he knows and learns more to impart to his pupils. Teaching does not make one a master of the subject. There may be many unknown things to be known. Compassion, strictness, and discipline need to be utilized when necessary. Teaching needs love, compassion, firmness, and determination. There is nothing wrong with roaring like a lion on the outside but be a lamb inside.

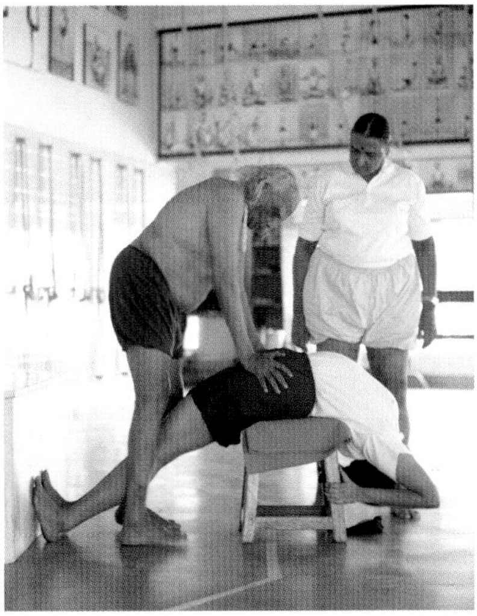

Guruji instructs his granddaughter Abhijata Sridhar in her morning practice, observed by his daughter Geeta Iyengar.

As a teacher I know one's responsibilities. I may assume a ferocious mantle in order to bring alertness and clarity in students as well as teachers while they are practising or teaching. As teachers when they come to learn from me, I make them forget that they are teachers but are pupils because I want them to learn and relearn, reflect and re-reflect on what they practise and teach.

When students come to me to learn, I treat them as God, as we are all children of God. From outside I treat them as pupils. As you see yourself in the mirror, I see also myself whether my teaching is correct by watching their faces which reflect their reaction fast. The teachers must be like this in order to develop the quality of right direction.

The teacher has to learn while teaching by blending his head and heart. He has to learn to weigh the intellect of the head and emotional intelligence of the heart in each student, which helps him to improve himself in the art of teaching. As a teacher, one must be a pupil within. As a teacher, some homework has to be done by investigating what was expressed and what was missing in teaching. Observation of errors helps to correct not only the students, but also oneself

continued

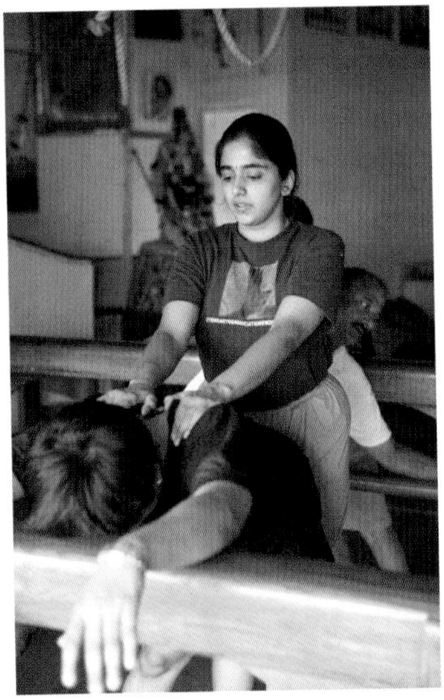

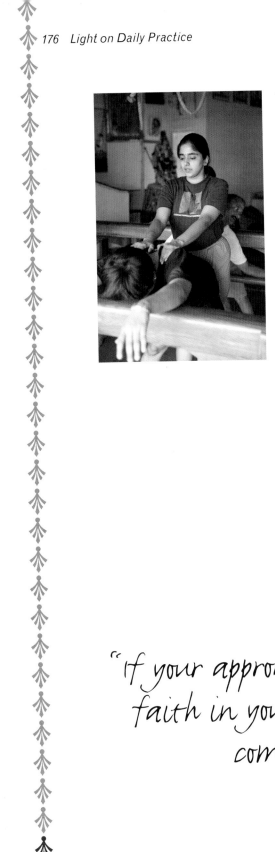

Guruji states that teachers must be guided by able teachers, but work at their discretion. Abhijata Sridhar learns from a family of distinguished teachers. Here, she passes on her observations during a medical class.

as a teacher. For this to develop, watchfulness and persistent effort are needed.

When pupils commit mistakes, the teacher has to think whether he too commits such mistakes. I did work like this before and I do this even now. This studentship in me has made me to be a good teacher.

So please do not practise yoga with the sole motive to become a teacher. If occasion arises, accept to teach. While learning, I never thought that I might have to teach. The circumstances forced me to become a teacher. If pupils did not come to me, I said that it was God's wish that I devote my time to more practice. And when pupils came, I would say to myself that it is God's wish to serve them. In both ways I took it as God's grace. ”

"If your approach is honest and you have faith in yourself, then the guidance comes from within."

Looking for a Guru

"When you go from one doctor to another for treatment, you need to explain in detail about your health history. A new doctor needs to know your past status of health, constitution, and your reactions to medicines and so forth. If he does not know that you are allergic to some medicines, both of you might end up in trouble. Similarly, a teacher keeps an eye on a pupil and watches his nature, constitution, mental set-up, physical ability, intellectual capacity, and accordingly, he imparts knowledge. In olden days the *guru* used to study the pupils who were asked to stay in the *āṣrama* or *gurukula* [residence] of a *guru*. They were called *antevāsin*. Now such life in *āṣrama* may not be possible, but we need a teacher who can judge and decide what is to be taught.

Moreover, when we go to several *gurus*, we neither learn nor get clarity. We land up in a confused state of mind. The mixing of methodology and confusion in the mind harms not only the *guru*, but also the pupil if ever one thinks of teaching. Take precautions before choosing a *guru*. In my early days, I used to read the name plates of lawyers on some bungalows, Bar at Law (England returned). Today, yoga teachers in the West are following the East on their advertisements, Yoga Teacher (India returned).

First, work steadfastly with one *guru*, learn, reflect, and assimilate. Then you become a *guru* to yourself. Your inner light begins to guide you. The matured intelligence leads you towards the exalted intelligence. That is what Patañjali calls *vivekaja jñānam*.

After assimilating, if one finds that his first *guru* is stuck without progress, then one can go to another *guru*. Your own consciousness then guides you whether the *guru* that you have chosen is the right one or not."

Extract on pages 174–76 from "A Real Teacher is a Pupil Within", Aṣṭadaḷa Yogamālā *Volume 8, pp100–103.*

Extract this page from "One Teacher or Several Teachers", Aṣṭadaḷa Yogamālā *Volume 8, pp94–95.*

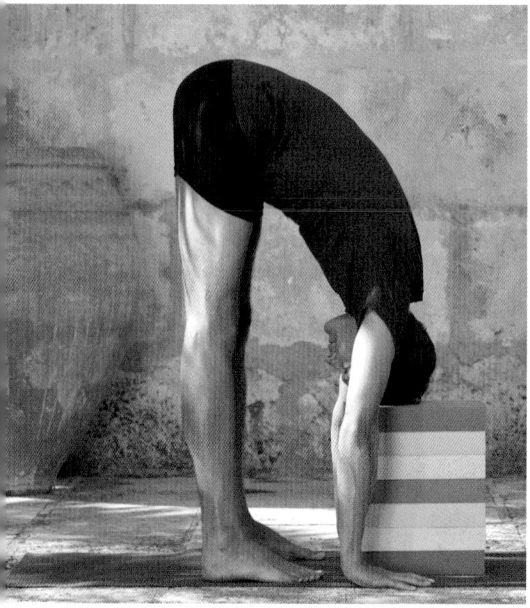

1 Begin in Uttanasana (see pages 114–15), feet hip-width apart. Rest the crown of your head on a stool or blocks (make the support high enough for comfort). Relax your arms. Hold for 30 seconds to 5 minutes.

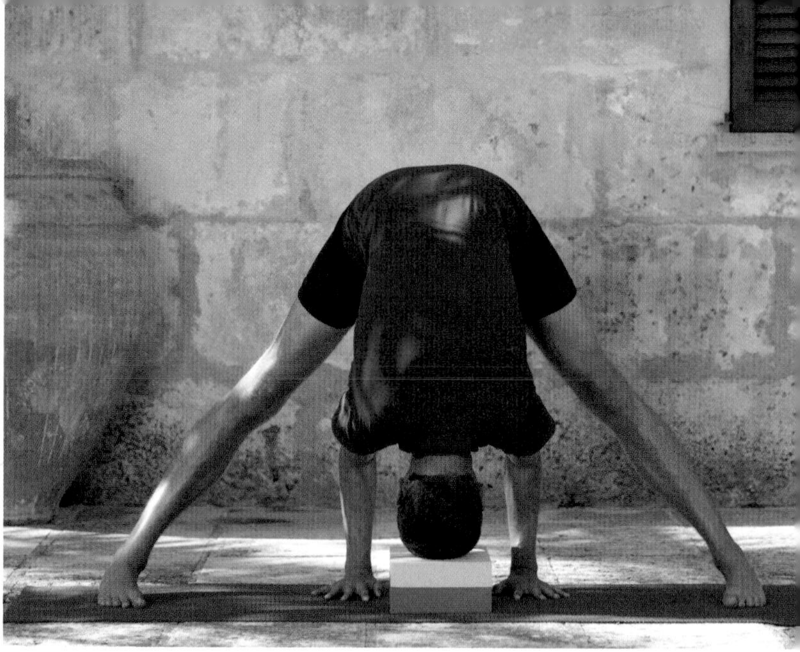

2 Step your feet 1.2m (4ft) apart, parallel to each other and facing forwards. Place your palms on the floor in line with your shoulders and rest your head on enough blocks for comfort. This is Prasarita Padottanasana. Hold for 30 seconds to 5 minutes.

Preparing for Salamba Sirsasana

Asana Sequence

"One has to begin by introducing the *āsana* where the flow of blood does not rush towards the brain cells but is made to percolate or seep through them, before attempting *Sālamba Śīrṣāsana*.... Give the sequence in such a way that it protects them from harm and injuries and builds up confidence physically, physiologically, and psychologically."

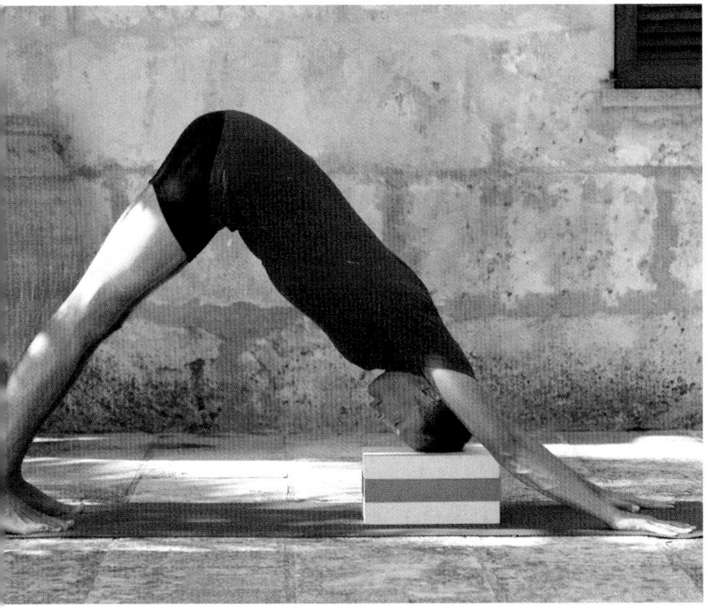

3 Come into Adho Mukha Svanasana (see pages 104–105), forehead resting on enough blocks for comfort. Hold for 30 seconds to 5 minutes.

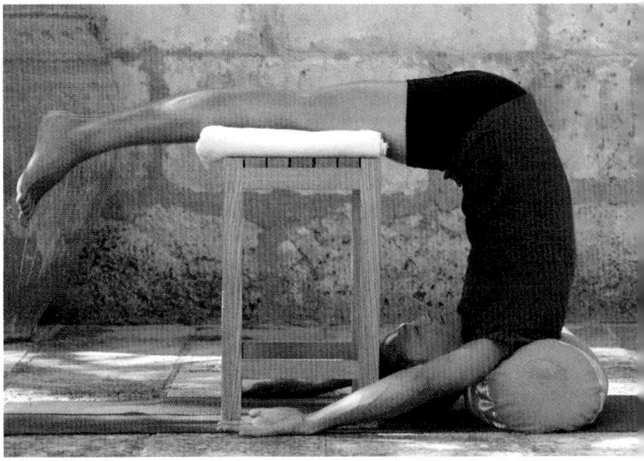

4 Come into Halasana with a chair or stool and bolster (see page 43), arms relaxed, and palms facing upwards. Hold for 30 seconds to 5 minutes.

5 Now place a folded blanket on your mat and learn to position your hands and arms correctly for Salamba Sirsasana (see page 72).

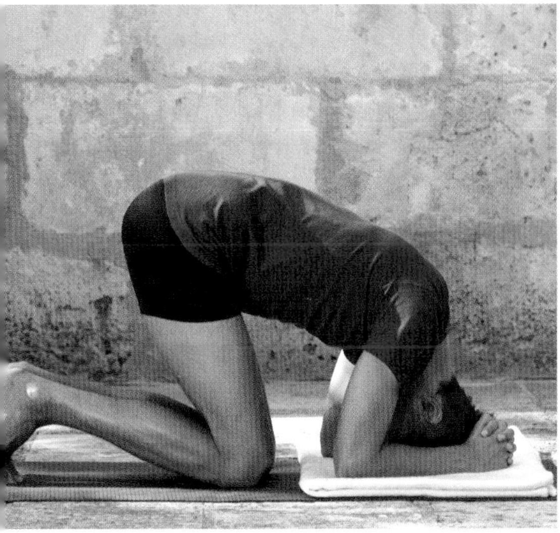

6 Straighten your legs, feet on the floor, to get used to the head-down position. When comfortable, ask a teacher to guide you up into Salamba Sirsasana (see pages 72–75).

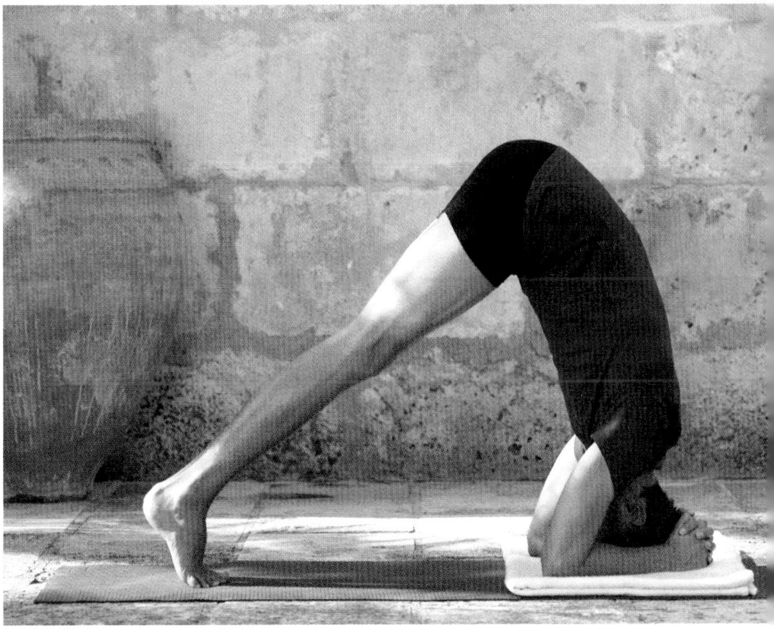

Bharadvajasana

Torso Twist (on a chair)

"Begin from simple twistings without creating hardness in the abdominal muscles for the spinal muscles to extend, without the stress. Train the abdominal muscles and organs to remain passive while performing lateral twists...it is advised to keep the abdominal muscles soft by rotating the torso instead of straining them."

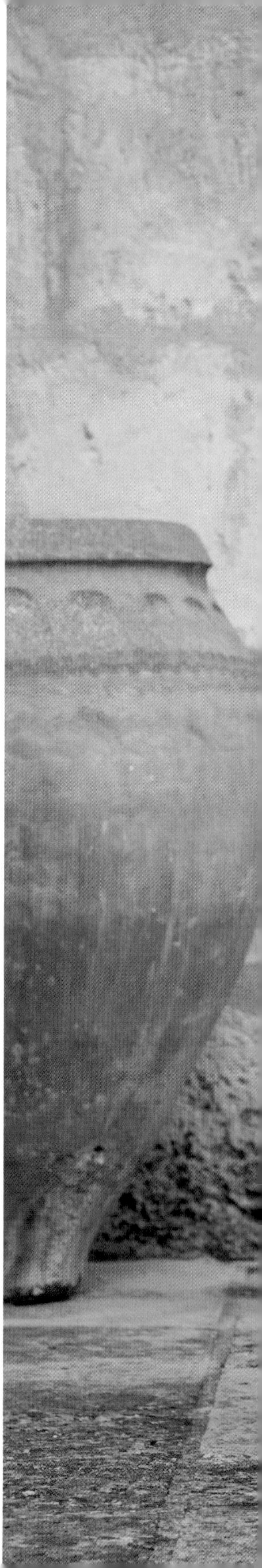

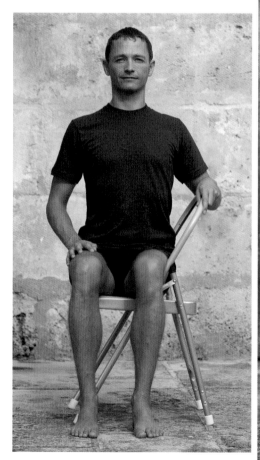

1 Sit on a chair sideways, with your left side next to the back. Keep your thighs and feet parallel and slightly apart. Sit erect and look ahead.

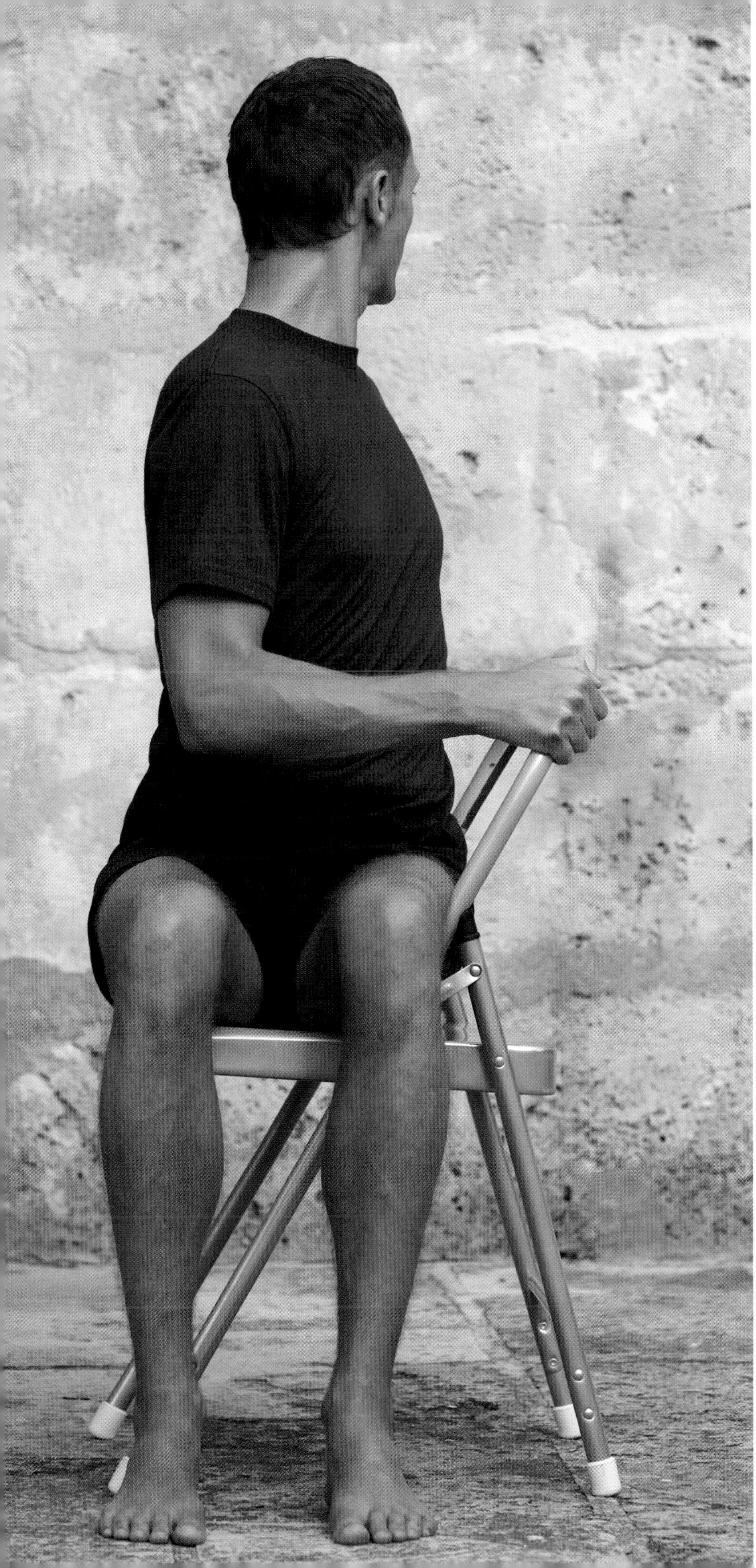

2 Inhale, raise your trunk, turn your chest left, and hold the chair back. Let your shoulderblades move in and shoulder bones roll back. Lift your spine, exhale and turn your head to look over your left shoulder. Hold for 20–30 seconds. Release your hands and turn forwards. Sit with the back of the chair against your right side and repeat to the right. Then relax.

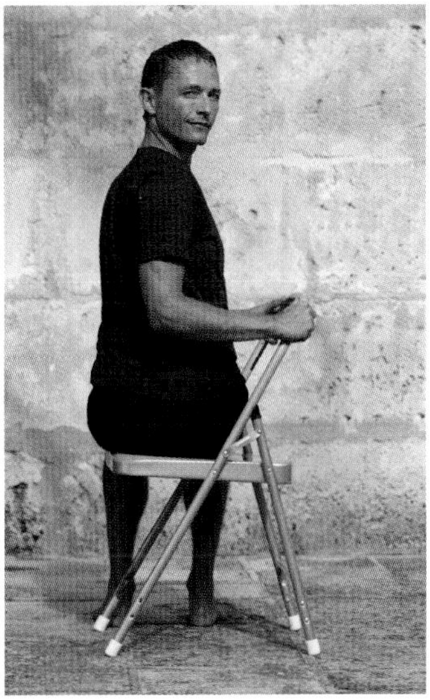

Bharadvajasana viewed from the back.

A Yogic Approach to Life

"If awareness has to flow in the right channel and spread everywhere, the asana has to be in a correct position."

Yoga and the Body

" We are wrapped and engulfed in five sheaths, namely *annamaya kośa*, *prāṇamaya kośa*, *manomaya kośa*, *vijñānamaya kośa*, and *ānandamaya kośa*. Let me give the gross translation. These sheaths are namely, the physical body of bones and muscles, the physiological or organic body of vital organs, the psychological body of the nervous system and mind, which includes the senses of perception, the intellectual body of the mental faculty, and the blissful body of the Self or *ātman*.

The practice of yoga has to interpenetrate these five sheaths known as *pañcakośa*. In order to simplify it further, let me tell you this. The nervous system is the bridge between the subtle body and the external body, called the physiological body. Or *manomaya kośa* is the bridge between *prāṇamaya* and *vijñānamaya kośa*. If the physical and physiological bodies are on one side, then intellectual and blissful bodies are on the other side. I address the nervous system as the psychological body or *manomaya kośa*. The nerves are like the bridge between the body and the mind. Therefore, for the practitioner it is very important to keep the nerves in a healthy condition. If the nerves are disturbed, they make the person completely dejected and depressed. The body, mind, and intellectual faculty, all get affected. That's why I consider the nerves as the bridge between the external body and the inner body. And these *āsana* are meant to develop strength in the nervous system. When this strength develops, then the physical body is forgotten, but the physiological body is taught to bring the body nearer to the mental body. Then, from the mental action you try to develop, as I said, the oneness of your intelligence. Suppose I am doing *Vṛśchikāsana*, the scorpion pose. I watch how my intelligence is flowing from the bottom of the feet and bottom of the toes, up to the bottom of the middle of the fingers of my hands. Is it flowing crookedly in one arm and straight in the other arm? We don't look at the pose then. We see how the inner body is working, how the inner awareness is working. We adjust not the body but the awareness. The moment the awareness is brought to function, then the body finds its right alignment and adjusts; as water finds its level, the awareness too finds its level. The intelligence flows according to the ways or paths we have created in our body. If the *āsana* is zigzag, the intelligence also flows zigzag. Awareness follows intelligence. Wherever you intelligize or energize, the awareness comes there.

Secondly, man is made of three layers. These are *kāraṇa śarīra* (cause body), *sūkṣma śarīra* (subtle body), and *sthūla śarīra* (gross body – the external body, which easily sees and cognizes). Practise of *āsana* takes the *sādhaka* from the external body to touch the subtle body and from there towards the causal body. Thus it connects and interweaves from the gross to the causal body and from the causal body to the gross body. This is how each *āsana* has to be done. ”

From "The Journey from Conative Action to All-Pervasive Awareness", Iyengar Yoga Institute Review, *San Francisco, Winter 1992.*

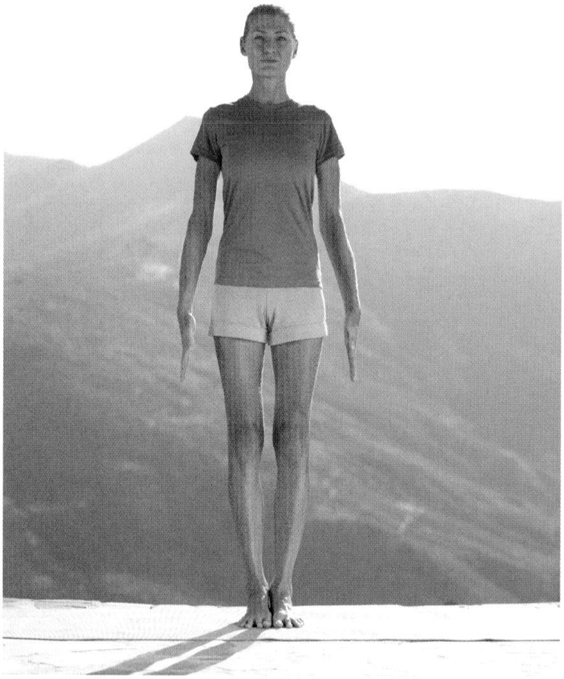

1 Stand in Tadasana (see pages 26–27).

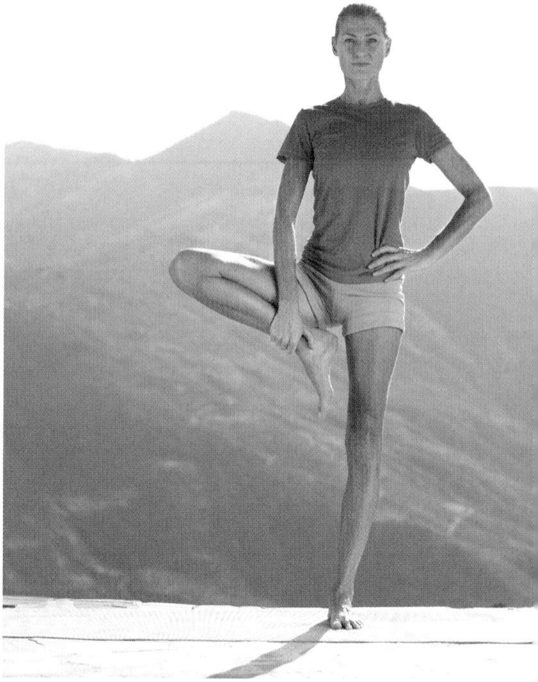

2 Place your left hand on your hip. Bend your right knee and catch the foot with your right hand. Lift your knee high and take it out to your right. Lift your chest.

Vrksasana

Tree Pose

"The Asvattha Tree is a giant banyan tree. Its roots extend deep and wide into the soil. Its trunk ascends, branching again and again carrying its leaves on its outer edge where they face the outer atmosphere, absorbing light, exchanging gases, and receiving the rain, directing its moistening fluid to bathe the entire organism.... We are the Tree. Our brain is the root, the trunk is our trunk with its spinal cord, and the branches are the limbs; arms and legs."

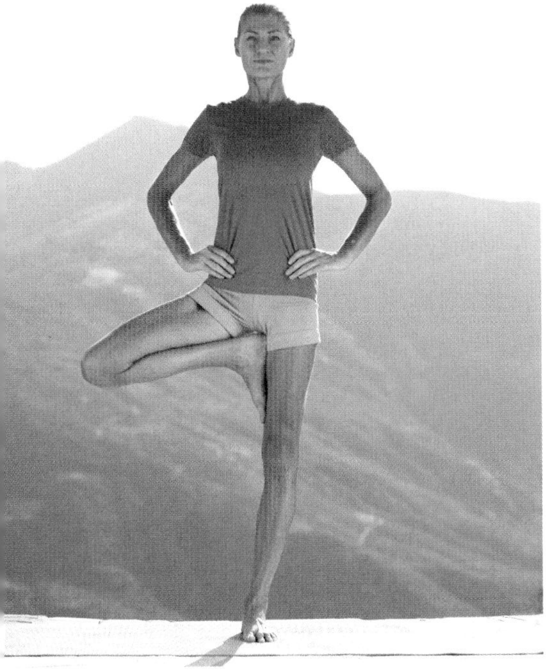

3 Place the sole of your right foot on your left inner thigh, heel pressing into the top of the thigh. Take both hands to your hips.

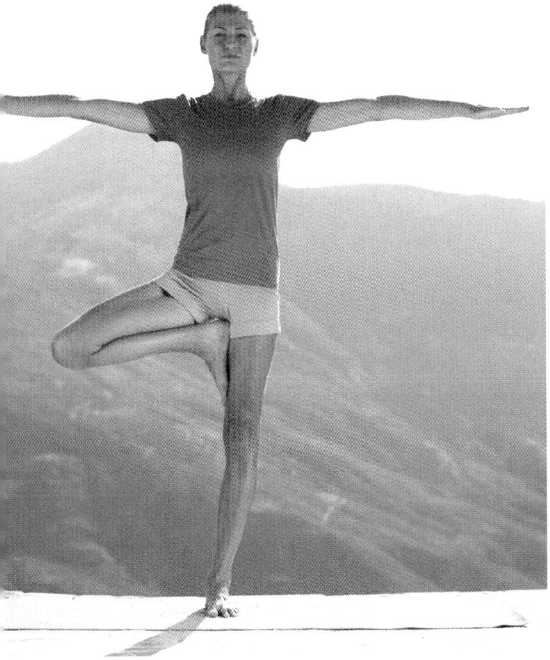

4 Keeping your standing leg straight and steady, press your right knee back. Extend your arms in line with your shoulders. Lift the sides of your trunk, open your chest, and look ahead.

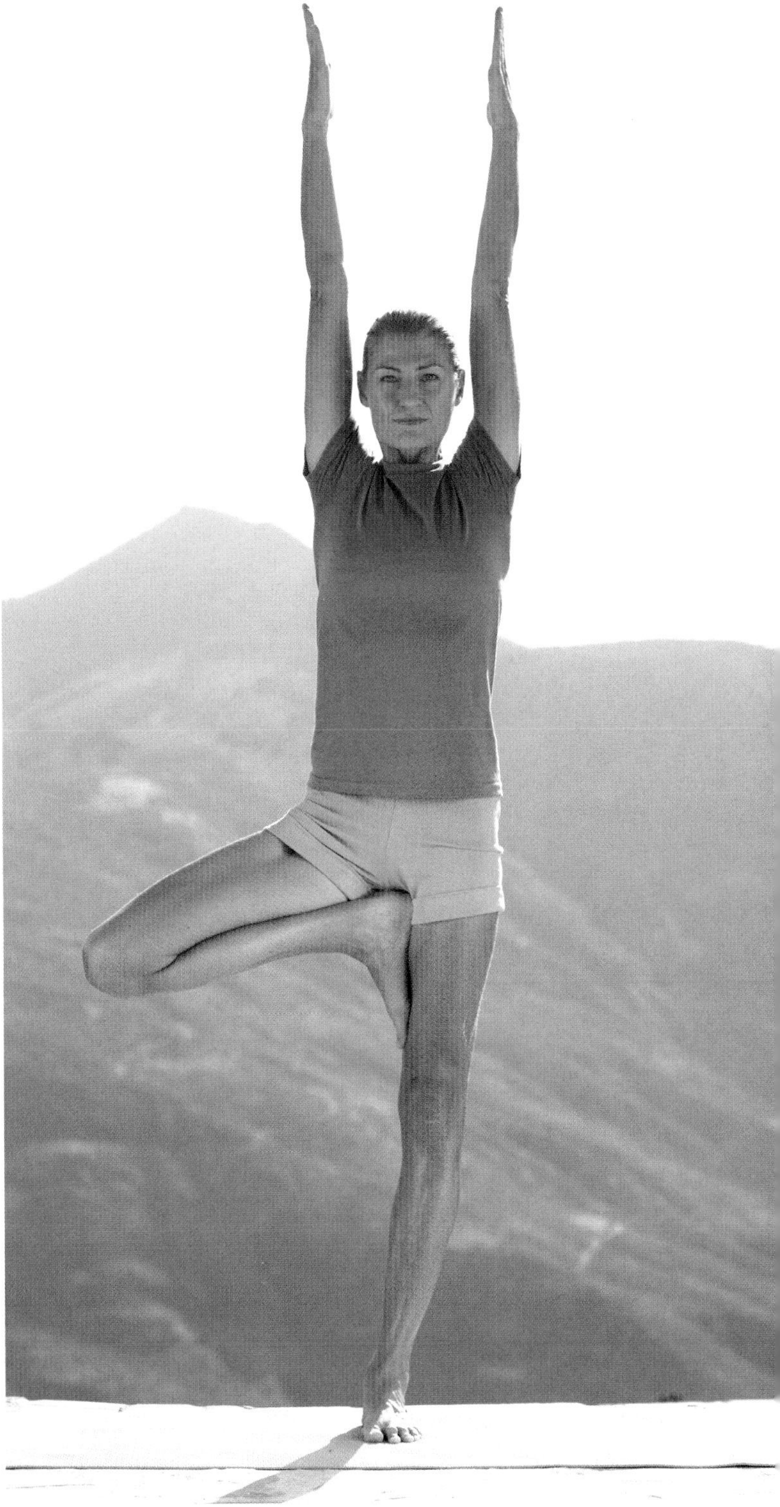

5 Turn your palms upwards, then extend your arms overhead. Hold for a few seconds. Lower your arms and raised leg and return to Tadasana. Repeat on the other side. Finish in Tadasana.

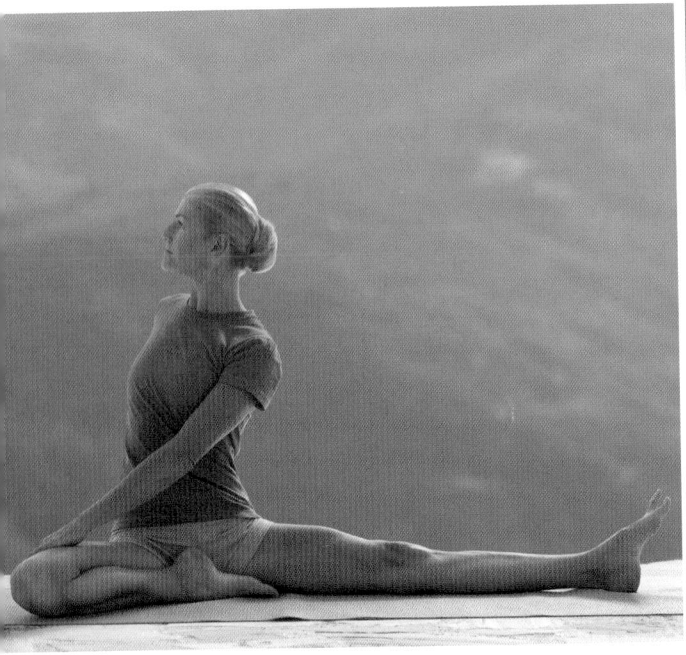

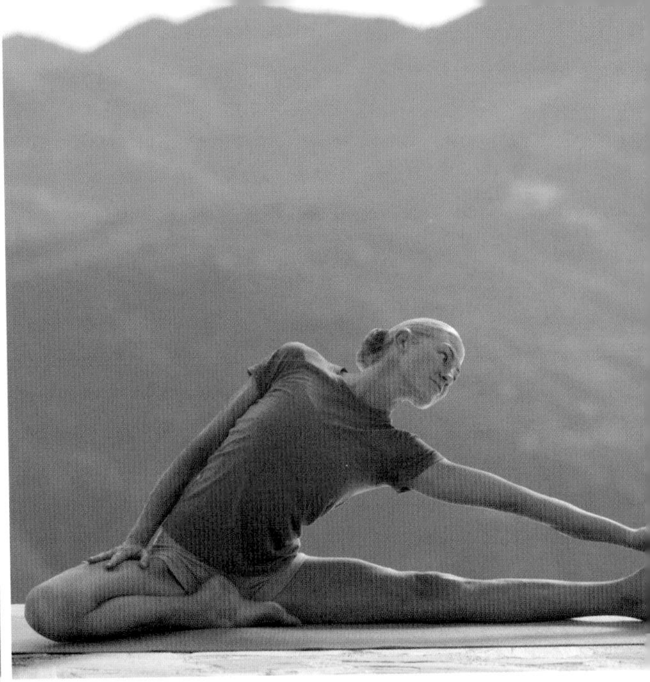

1 Sit in Dandasana (see pages 14–15). Bend your right knee and take the heel to the top of your right inner thigh, moving your leg back. Lift and turn your trunk to face your bent leg.

2 Extend your left arm over your left leg and rotate it, turning the palm up. Grasp your left big toe between the thumb, index, and middle fingers of your left hand. Look at your foot, turn your trunk to the right and lift your chest.

Parivrtta Janu Sirsasana

Revolved Head-on-knee Pose

"Yoga practice (*āsana*, *prāṇāyāma*, and *pratyāhāra*), gives us the tools for cleansing, toning, and ordering the organism into a harmonious whole, so that it may flower and fruit.... In [*Parivṛtta Janu Śirṣāsana*] there is a dynamic twisting action, which turns the core of the being, washing and cleansing the inner organic and nervous systems. Its vertical and horizontal aspects ensure the practitioner's intellect and emotions are balanced."

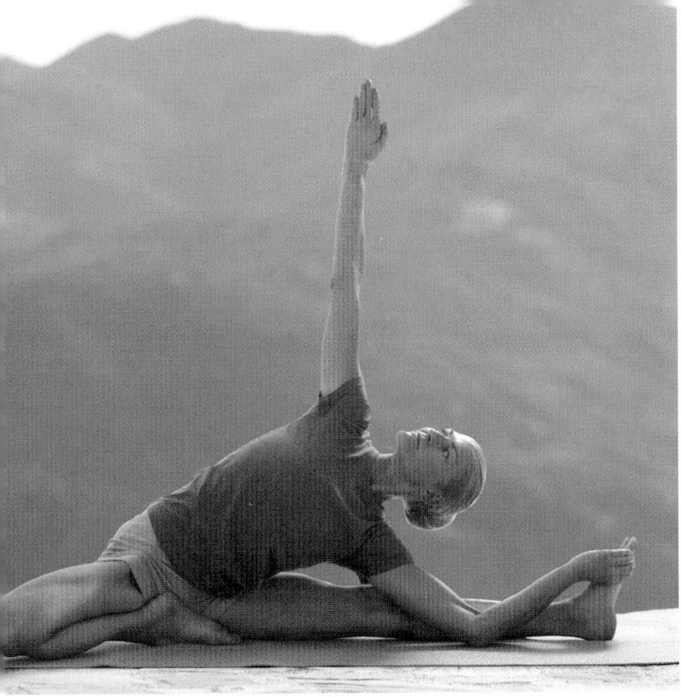

3 Bend your left elbow, drawing the left side of your trunk nearer your outstretched thigh. Extend your right arm upwards. Revolve your trunk to look up.

4 Extend your right arm overhead and catch your left foot. Widen your elbows, exhale, and rotate your trunk upwards. Try to bring the back of your left shoulder in front of your knee and turn more to rest the back of your left ribs on your knee. Hold for 20 seconds. Inhaling, release your hands, sit upright, and straighten your leg back to Dandasana. Repeat to the other side. Finish in Dandasana.

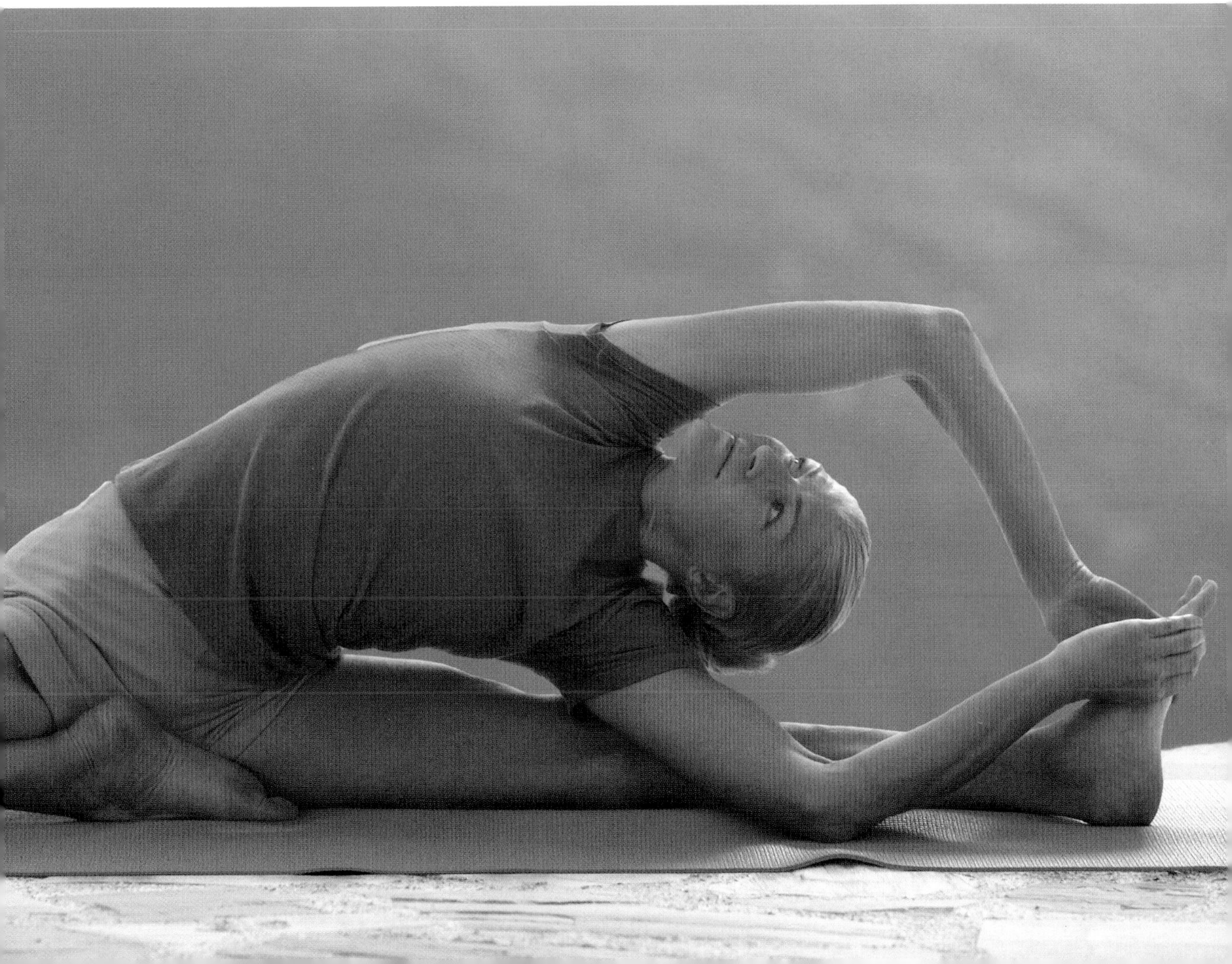

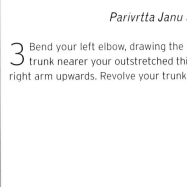

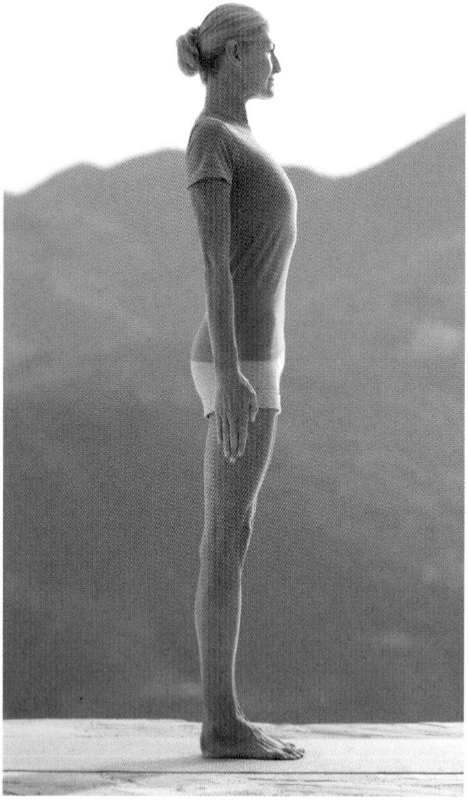

1 Stand in Tadasana (see pages 26–27).

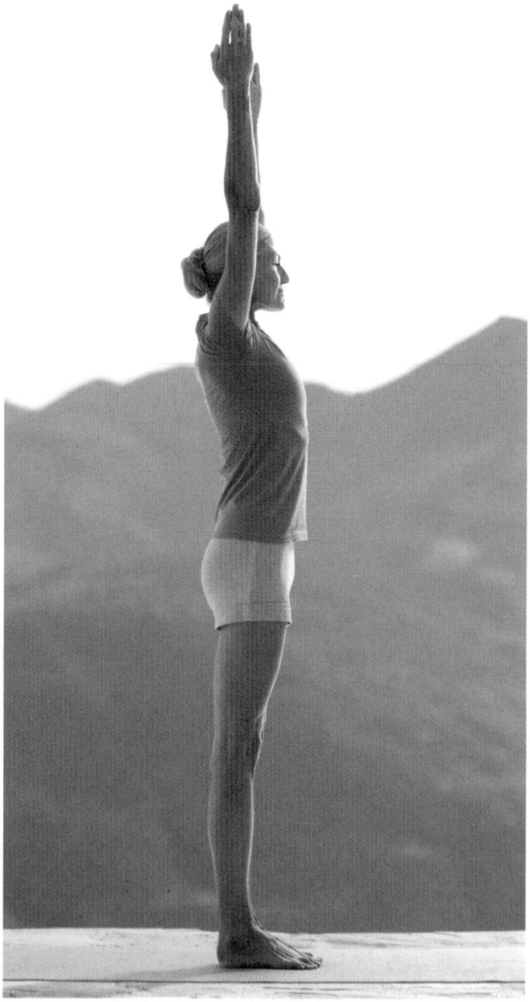

2 Extend your arms overhead, elbows straight, into Urdhva Hastasana (see pages 110–11). Keep your arms perpendicular to the floor and parallel to each other, and lift your sternum.

Utkatasana

Powerful Pose

"If you refine adjustments in the...skeleto-muscular body the physiological body co-operates while performing the *āsana*. In turn, they work effectively on nervous and glandular systems. The process of penetrating inwards makes us go from the grossest sheath towards the subtlest sheath of the body. Hence, the energy is made to reach not only the grossest but also the subtlest as well as the remote areas."

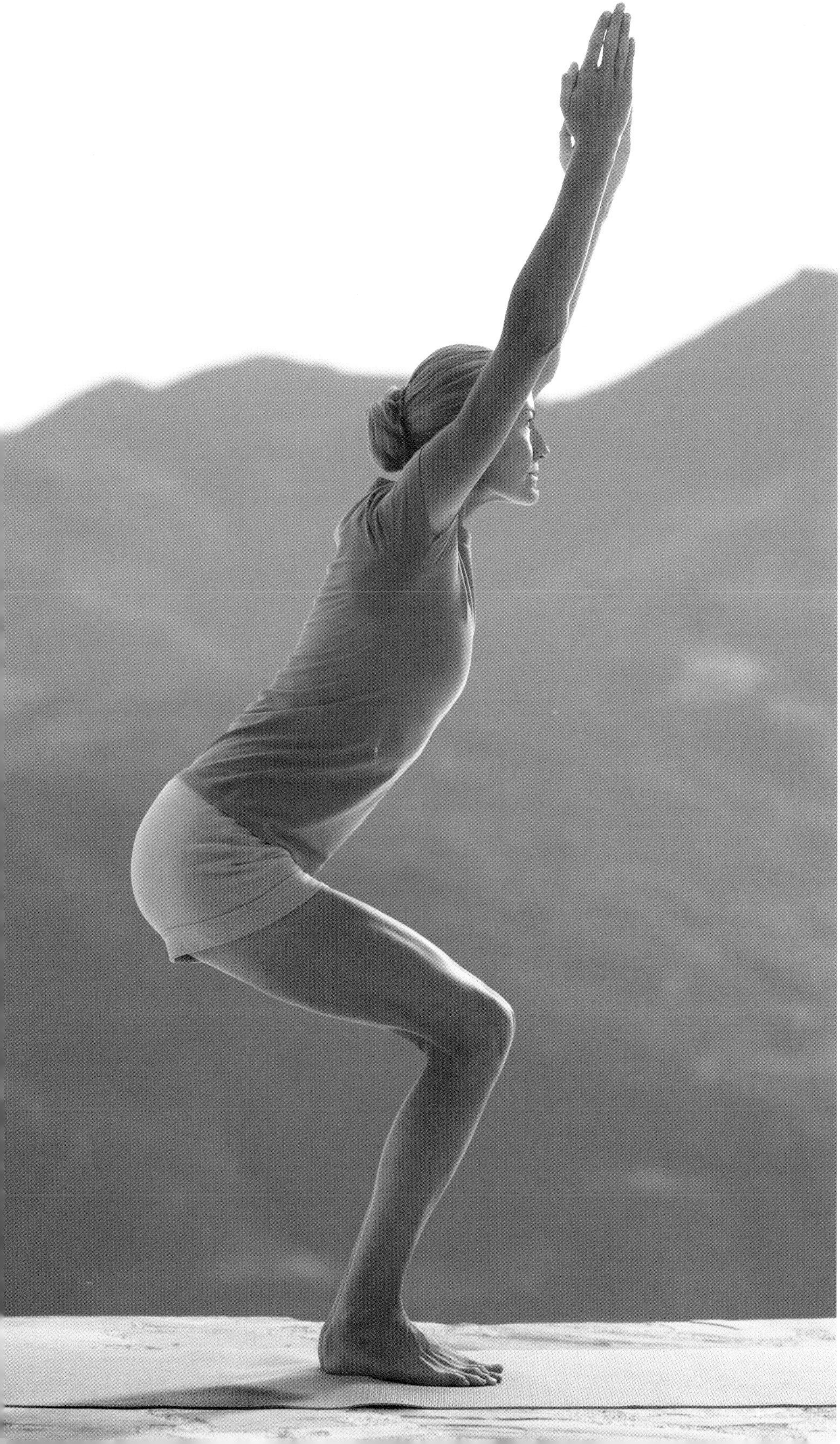

3 Exhale and bend your knees – try to bring your thighs parallel to the floor. Stretch your trunk upwards and keep your chest as far back as possible. Hold for up to 20 seconds, breathing evenly. Inhale, straighten your legs to return to Urdhva Hastasana, then lower your arms into Tadasana.

Yoga and Blood Circulation

“I have often emphasized the need to have fully potent respiratory and circulatory systems in order to maintain the health. All *āsana* as well as *prāṇāyāma,* directly and indirectly, work towards improving the quality and flow of this mighty stream of blood within us.

Our blood contains various components like plasma, immunoglobulins, fibrinogen, erythrocytes, haemoglobin, leucocytes, platelets, and other hormones and proteins. Every sixty seconds, 1,440 times a day, our blood travels through the 60,000-mile or 96,000-km system of the human body. These tidal waves of blood smash against the aorta, the body's largest artery, seventy times a minute, delivering their blows 2.5 billion times during the average life span. Rigid metal pipes could not withstand this battering for long. Yet, due to constant abuses, they take their toll.

Yogic practice does undo the damage that happens and puts the system back on track. Right from the standing *āsana* to the inverted and back bending *āsana*, the practitioner mobilizes the muscles, joints, bones, tendons, tissues, and fibres to squeeze, rinse, dilate, pulsate, and filter the blood through the immense network within the body. Sometimes wearing a ruby is said to help proper blood circulation for those who are anaemic. *Āsana* help first to have a healthy blood circulation in every nook and corner of the body....”

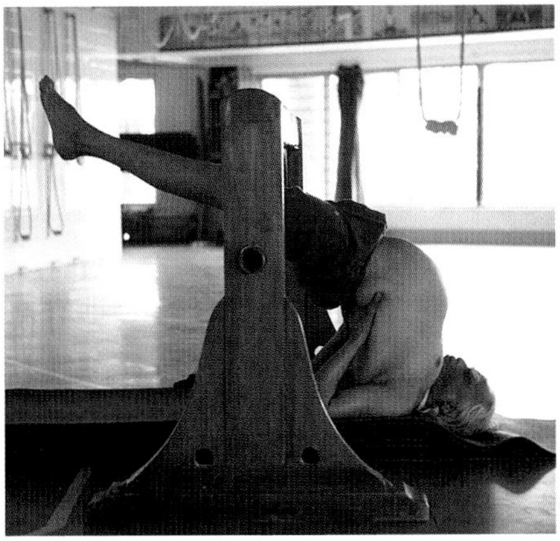

When the body is inverted, as in this variation of Salamba Sarvangasana, the venous blood flows to the heart without any strain due to the force of gravity. In addition, inverted asana exercise the liver, pancreas, and spleen, ensuring a generous supply of blood to these areas.

"The various types of pranayama help in enriching the blood circulation, nervous and glandular systems in a balanced state, keeping the mind clear and clean. The pure air channelled through pranayama enriches the blood."

From "Blood – a Gem", Aṣṭadaḷa Yogamālā *Volume 8, pp244–48.*

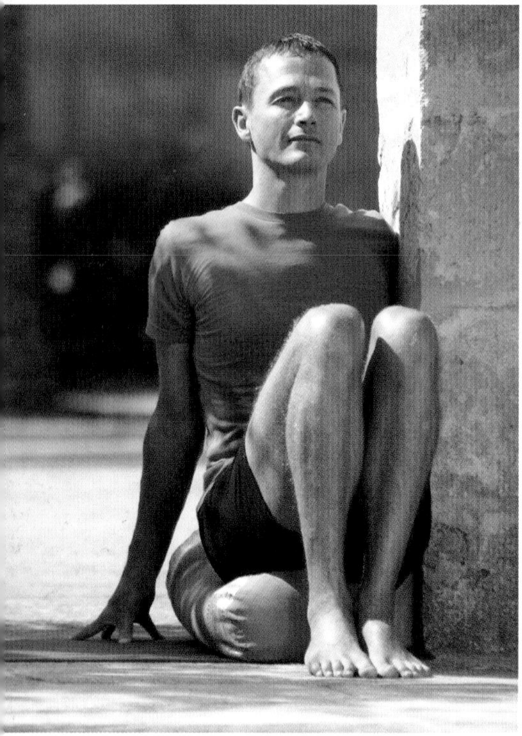

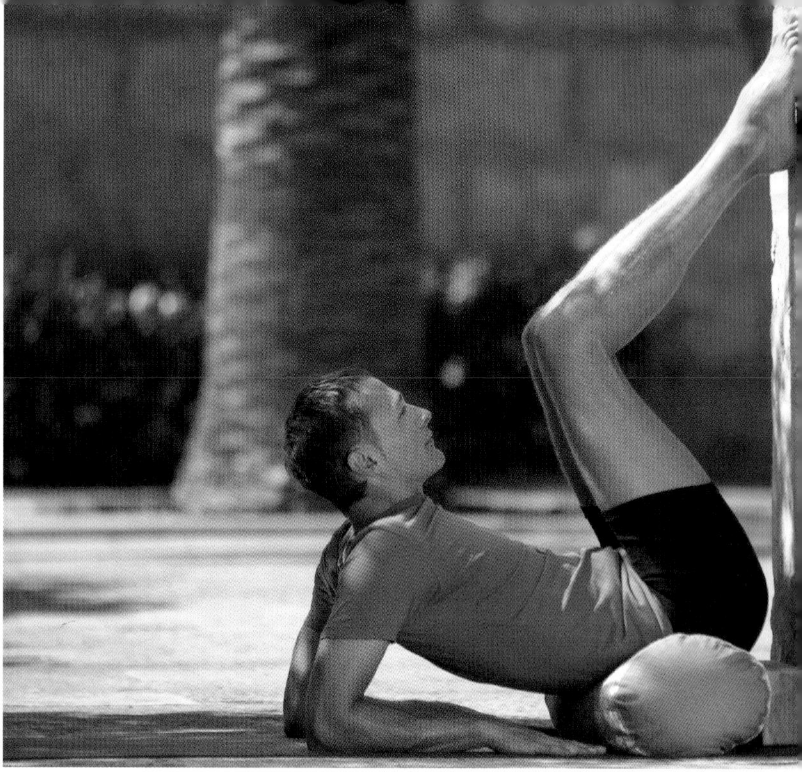

1 Place a brick with its long side touching a wall. Place a bolster parallel to the brick. Sit sideways to the wall on the bolster.

2 Swivel to face the wall, fingers behind you for support. Turn to the wall, lifting each leg up, knees bent. Push your palms down and move your buttocks nearer the wall.

3 Lower yourself until your shoulders are on the floor. Straighten your legs and rest your head and neck, chest lifted, and shoulders moving towards the bolster. Spread your arms to the sides, palms up, and close your eyes. Rest for 3-4 minutes. Cross your legs in Svastikasana (see page 134), pause, uncross your legs, push into the wall, and slide back to the mat.

Viparita Karani

Inverted Pose

"When [the protective muscles of the heart] are made to relax, then the direct muscles of the heart get relaxed. If one has to invigorate the cardio-vascular system in any other type of exercises, one needs to create tremendous movement in the body like jogging or running. This way one creates tremors made by vigorous movement, whereas in yogic *āsana*, one brings a good amount of blood circulation to heart muscles without irritating or making the heart to pump fast."

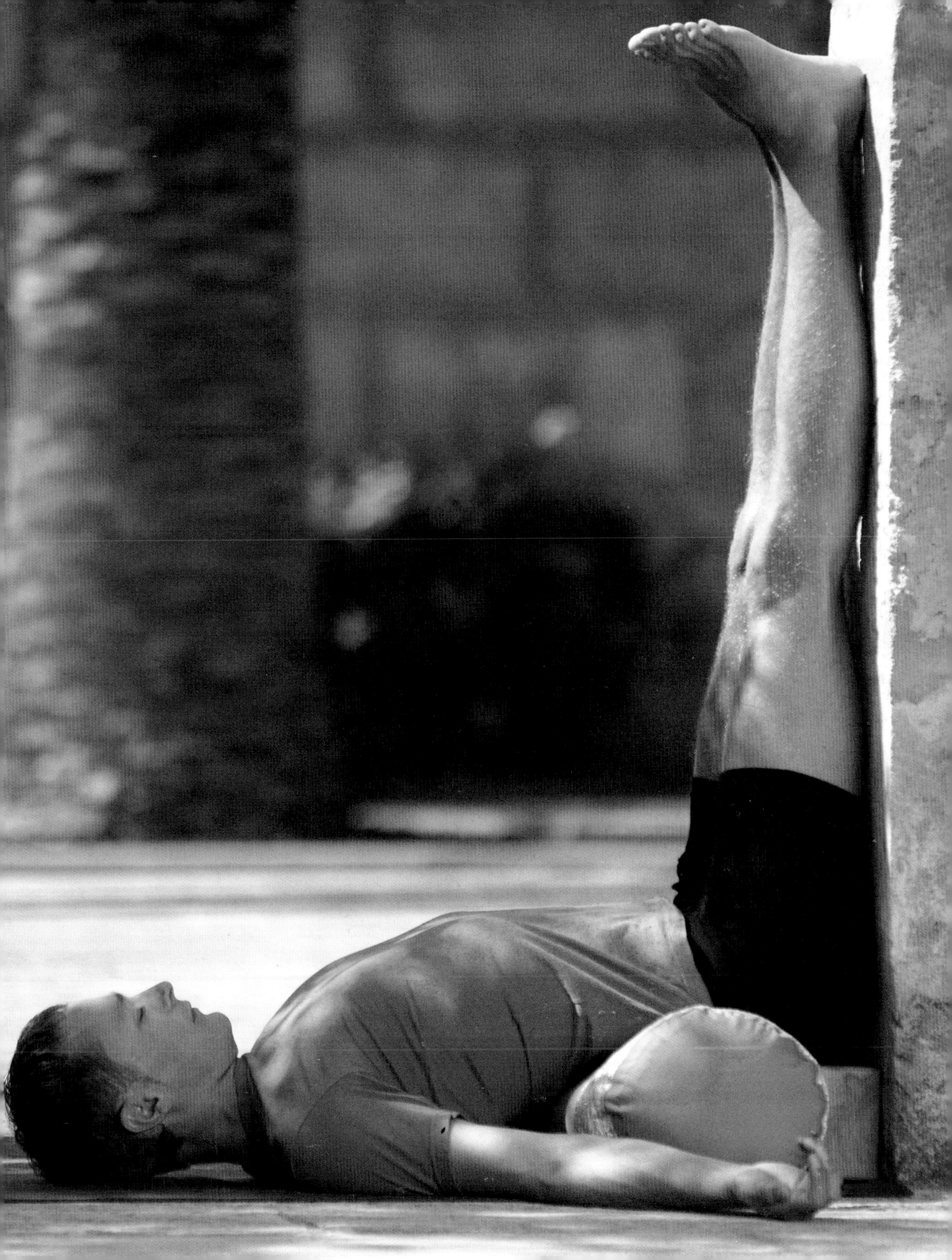

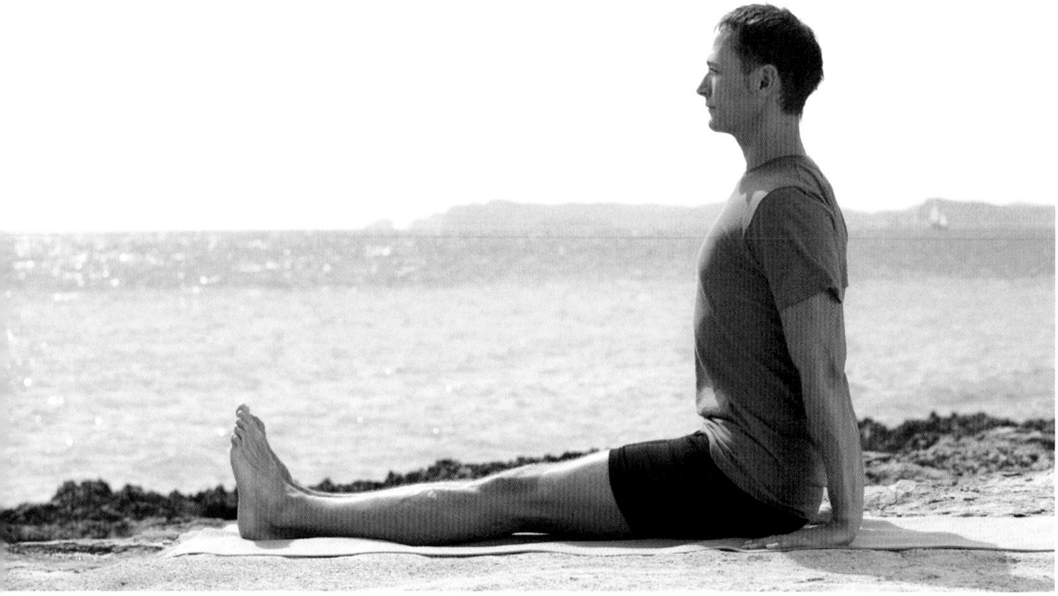

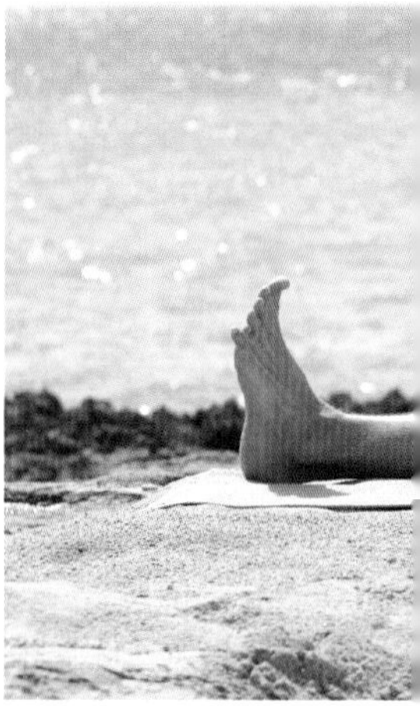

1 Sit in Dandasana (see pages 14–15).

2 Bend your right knee and pull the heel to the buttock. Press the foot down, exhale and lift your spine. Turn your torso 90° to the right. Bend your left arm and move the shoulder forward, over the bent knee, palm forwards.

Marichyasana III

Asana III Dedicated to the Sage Marichi

"With your conscious effort and attentiveness, the blood and the energy are supplied evenly throughout the body, and the cells are kept healthy. *Varāha Upaniṣad* speaks of *ratna pūrita dhātu* (the blood filled with jewels), a special constituent and essential ingredient of the blood in the body.... It conveys that the quality of the blood should be brought to the level of a jewel. That is the effect of the *āsanas*, which build up the cellular system as jewels".

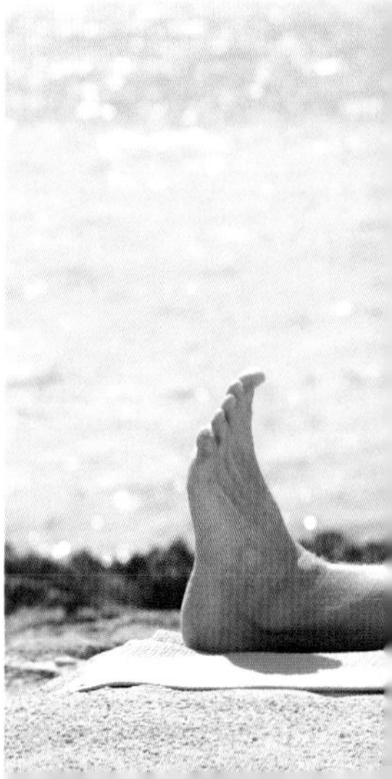

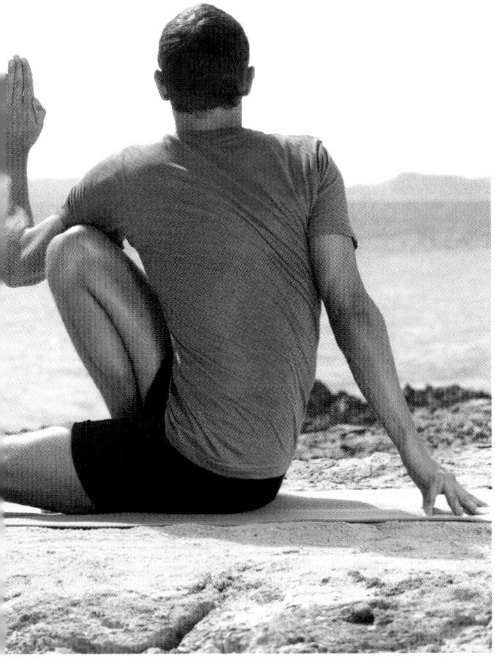

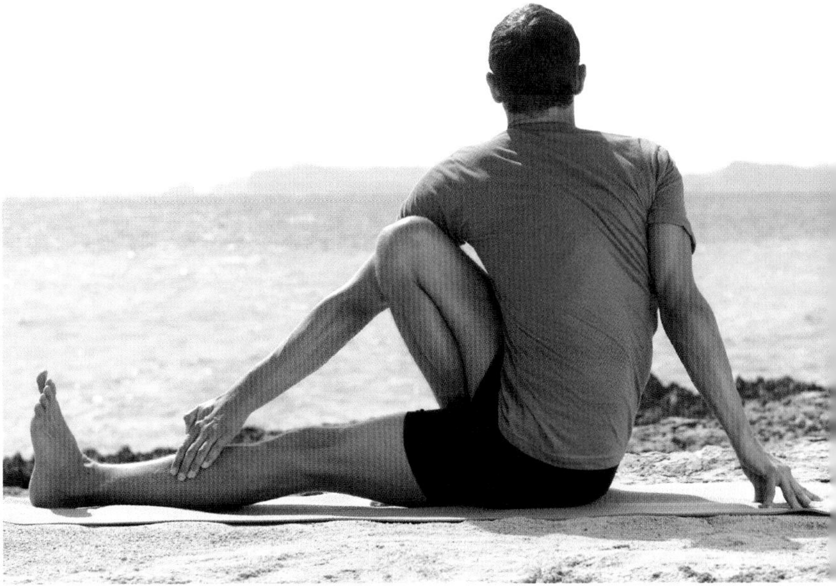

3 Extend your left arm from armpit to elbow. Press your right foot down and turn further, pushing the armpit against your outer knee.

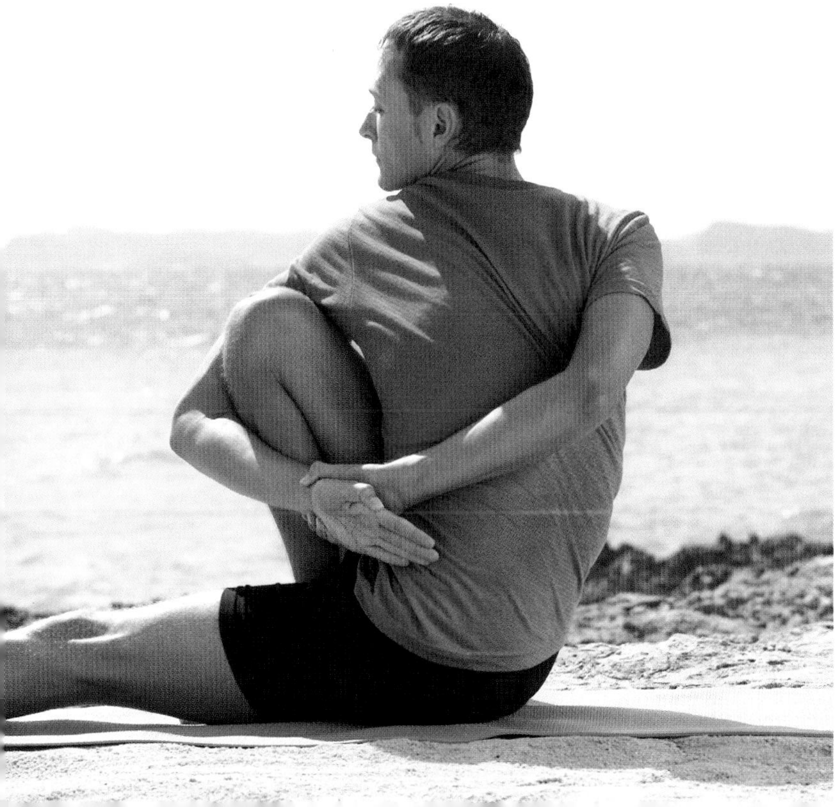

4 Exhale, wrap your left arm around your bent shin and thigh, reaching towards your waist. Clasp your left wrist with your right hand, or vice versa, palm facing outwards. Extend the outstretched leg and turn your head to look towards it. Hold for 20-30 seconds. Release your hands and rotate back to centre. Lower your bent leg into Dandasana. Repeat to the other side. Finish in Dandasana.

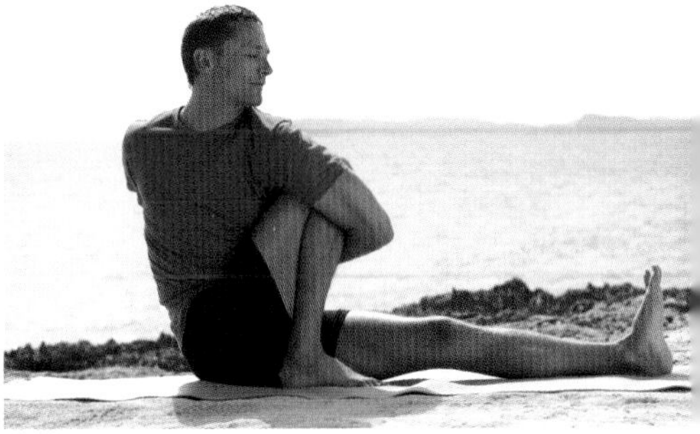

Marichyasana III viewed from the front.

Pasasana

Noose Pose

"As doctors tighten the tourniquet at certain areas to control the blood circulation, *āsana* work in the same manner. When you do *Marichyāsana*, or *Paśāsana*, what do you do? You do not allow the blood to circulate in certain parts and you change the blood flow from these areas to move where the gates are opened for circulation to take place or saturation to take place. When you release the pose, the blood spreads and is supplied to the dried area. This is the way in which the energy is produced by the *āsana*."

Note: As this is an advanced pose, no instructions are given. To compare Guruji in the final pose, see **Light on Yoga**.
"Does the *āsana* evolve or do we evolve? *Āsana* are adopted by us. As we involve ourselves more in their practice, we evolve. Obviously the quality of presentation of *āsana* improves as we proceed. Though we often use the word 'perfection', it is not easy to reach."

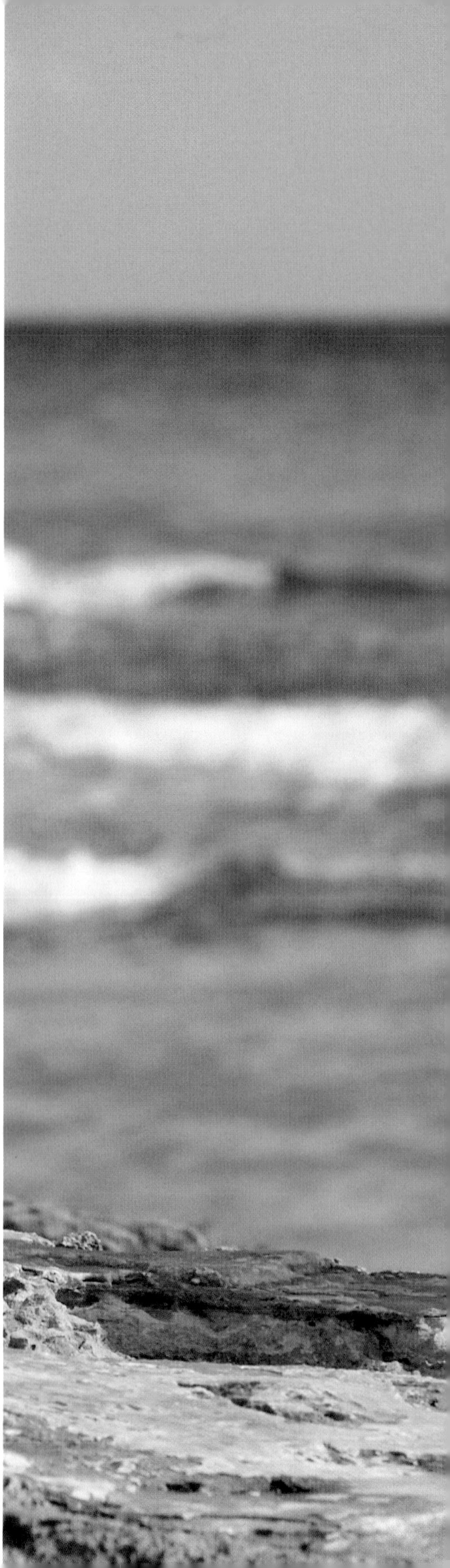

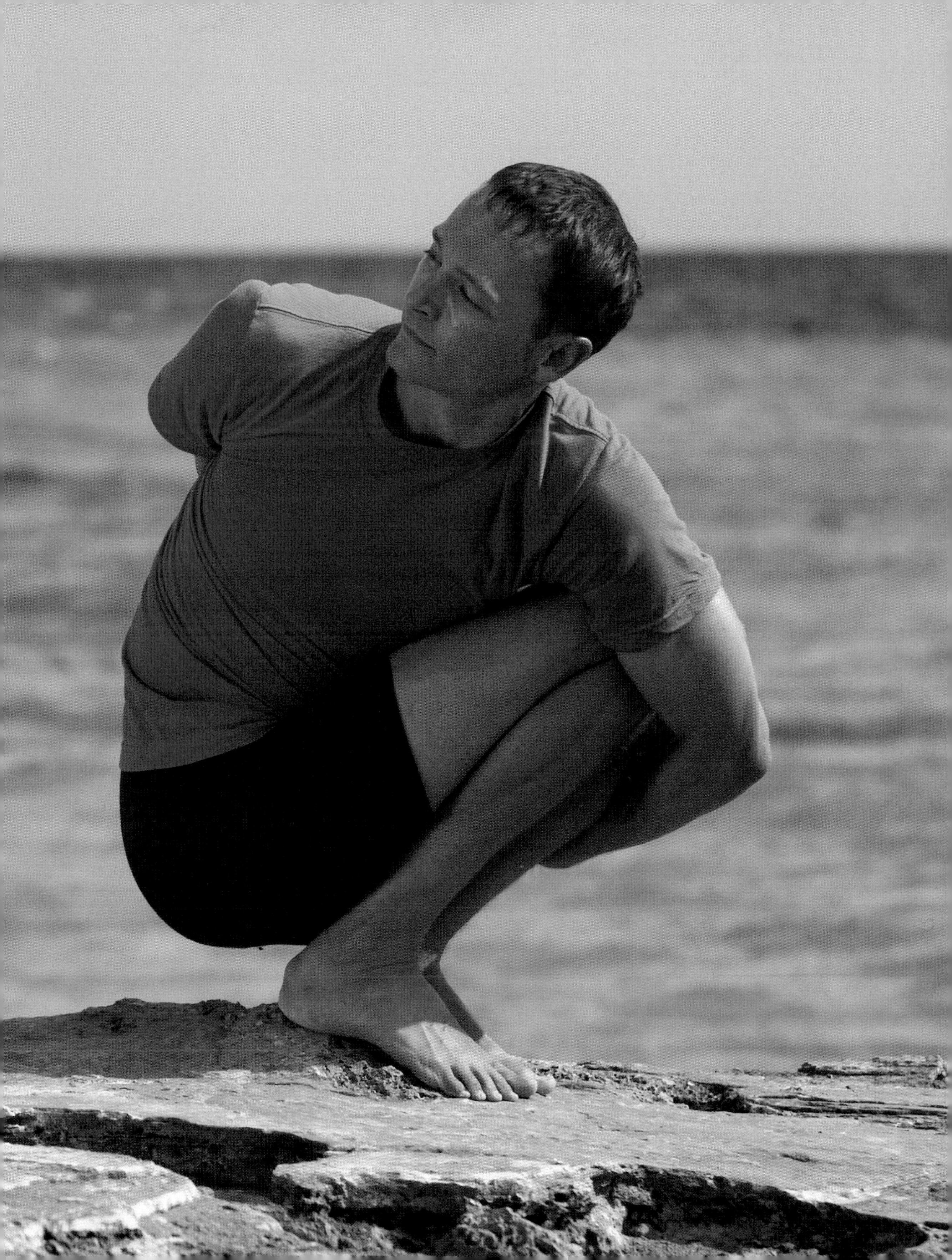

The Spinal Column

"We are made up of the respiratory, circulatory, digestive, nervous, glandular, and genito-excretory systems. Each one is dependent upon the other for healthy rhythmic functions. The secretions of the hormonal system are considered to be an essential factor for the tranquillity of the mind. The house of all these various systems is the spinal column (*merudaṇḍa*). The spine, its muscles, its nerves, and its fluid keep all these systems functioning in concord. The science of yoga was aptly discovered by yogis in order to culture the *merudaṇḍa* or *viṇādaṇda* so that the shoots of the spine like the fibres, sinews, cells, nerves, senses, mind intelligence, ego, and consciousness are kept healthy.

The spinal column has different parts such as the coccyx, sacral, lumbar, dorsal, and cervical regions. Networks of plexuses and ductless glands are situated in contact with the various parts of the spinal column, and they can either cause disturbances in health and poise or help to build up good physical health and mental poise. Yogis studied the human body in their own ways, particularly the spinal column. Through their intuitive capacity they studied the energy centres within the spinal cord and named them *cakra*.

Cakra means a wheel, a diagram, a cycle, or a circle. As the wheel of a gigantic machine is connected to a flywheel, around which the entire machine moves like a chain, similarly the rhythmic discharge of the *cakra* affects the functioning of physical, physiological, mental, mystical and spiritual depressions or elations. *Cakra* is the store house of power; they are seven in number.... Because of the location of various *cakra* as explained in yoga texts, many authors hold them to represent the plexuses or ductless glands. The *cakra* may or may not be these, though their situation corresponds very closely. If plexuses and glands work on psycho-physiological levels, *cakra* work at the level of spiritual enlightenment.... In order to know the functions of the plexuses, glands, or *cakra*, one should

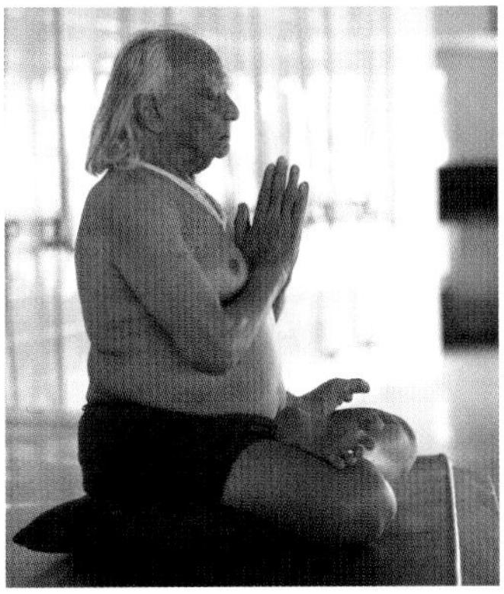

Practice of yoga keeps the fluid of the spine in a steady state, without fluctuations, says Guruji. The observant practitioner may feel the fluid rising while sitting erect, as here in Padmasana.

know something about the nervous system. This system in the human body has three tiers. They are the peripheral nervous system, autonomous nervous system and central nervous system. The peripheral nervous system gets its feedback from the senses of perception and organs of action. The autonomous nervous system is semi-voluntary, as it functions on its own as well as through the volition of the mind. The central nervous system is electrifying, dynamic, and functions with the help of judicial intelligence.

The *cakra* are hidden in the core of the spinal canal, which is said to be thinner than a hair, and have access to the entire functioning of the body.... The cord being exactly in the centre of the body, the yogis named it *madhyama nāḍī* or middle nerves. Thus, the middle nerves represent the central nervous system of modern medicine. We are all aware that with all of the modern scientific equipments, very little is known about this central nervous system. According to the yogis, the energy discharged from the *cakra* is known as life force (*prāṇa śakti* or *jīva śakti*), while the autonomous nervous system is said to be on the right and left sides of the spinal column as an inner part of the nerves (*antaraṅga bhāga*); the peripheral nerves are external part of the nerves (*bahiraṅga bhāga*). Though the functioning of the central nervous system still eludes modern science, it was known and understood by the yogis through their intuition and deep study. ”

From "Physiology and Cakra", talk by B.K.S. Iyengar on his 70th birthday.

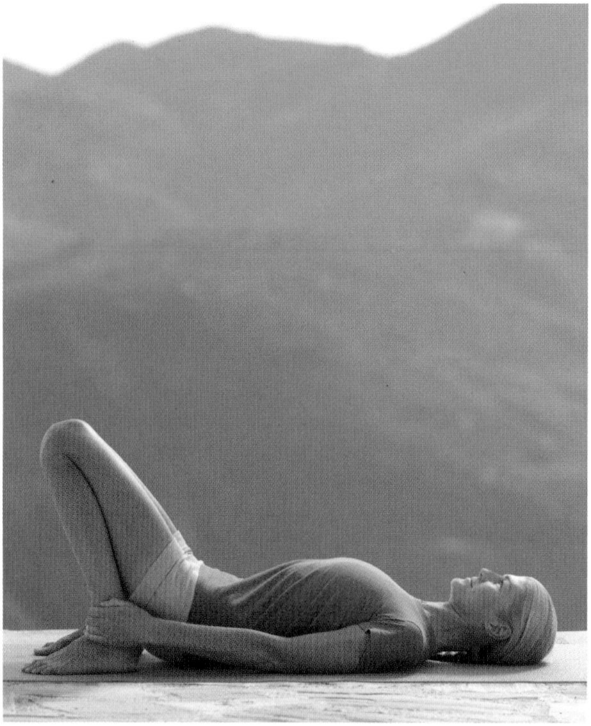

1 Lie on your back with your knees bent and feet hip-width apart. Draw your heels close to your buttocks.

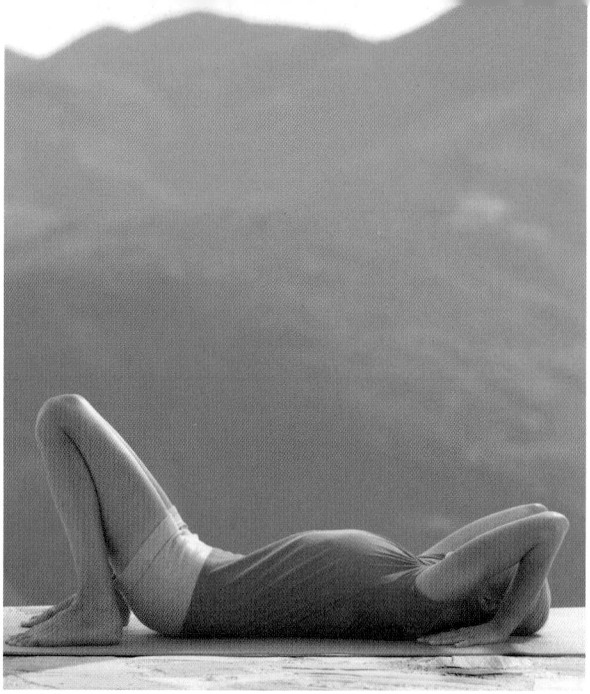

2 Bend your elbows and place your palms on the floor beside your ears, fingers pointing towards your shoulders.

Urdhva Dhanurasana

Upward-facing Bow Pose

"In *Ūrdhva Dhanurāsana* one expresses the stretch by extending the body and expanding the chest. The most interesting thing that happens in this *āsana* is that though the body extends and expands, the mind moves inside the body. Watch this inward movement, which is the same as it happens in *dhāraṇā*. Such experiences do not come from books but through direct observation and reflection. When attentive stability is built up, naturally it makes one move towards *dhyāna*."

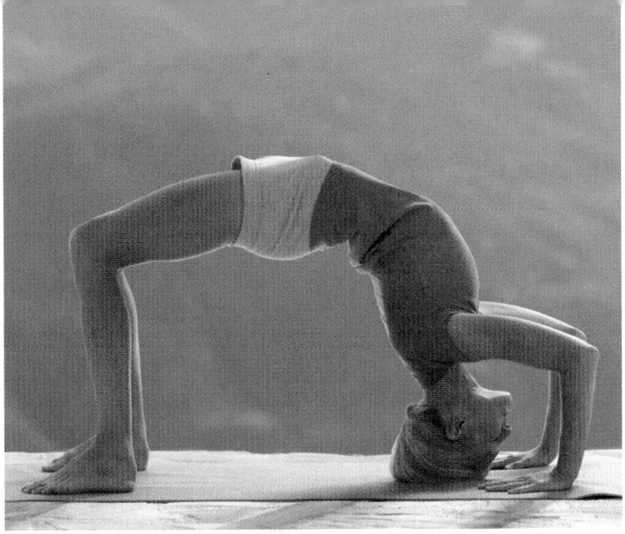

3 Exhale, press your feet down, and lift your buttocks. Keep your feet parallel. Press your palms down, raise your trunk, and rest the crown of your head on the floor. Maintain the lift of your tailbone, buttocks, shoulders, and the back of your chest, and align your elbows and knees.

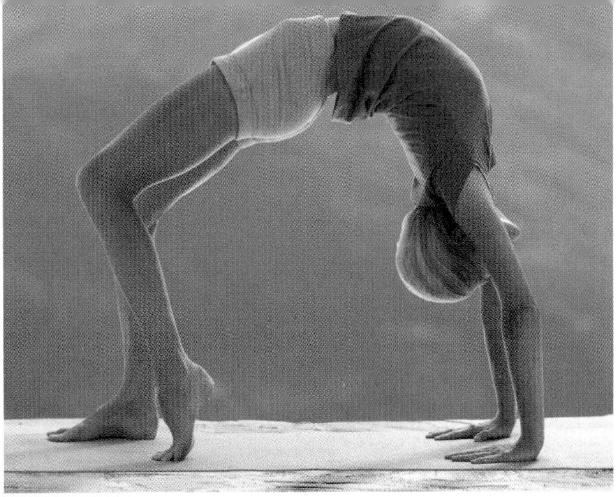

4 Exhale, press into your hands and feet and lift your trunk and head. Straighten your arms, pull up your thighs, and arch your back. Take your head back without straining your throat. There should be no pain in your lumbar. Lift your heels (walk your feet in) and sacrum, lengthening your lower spine towards your legs and your chest towards your head.

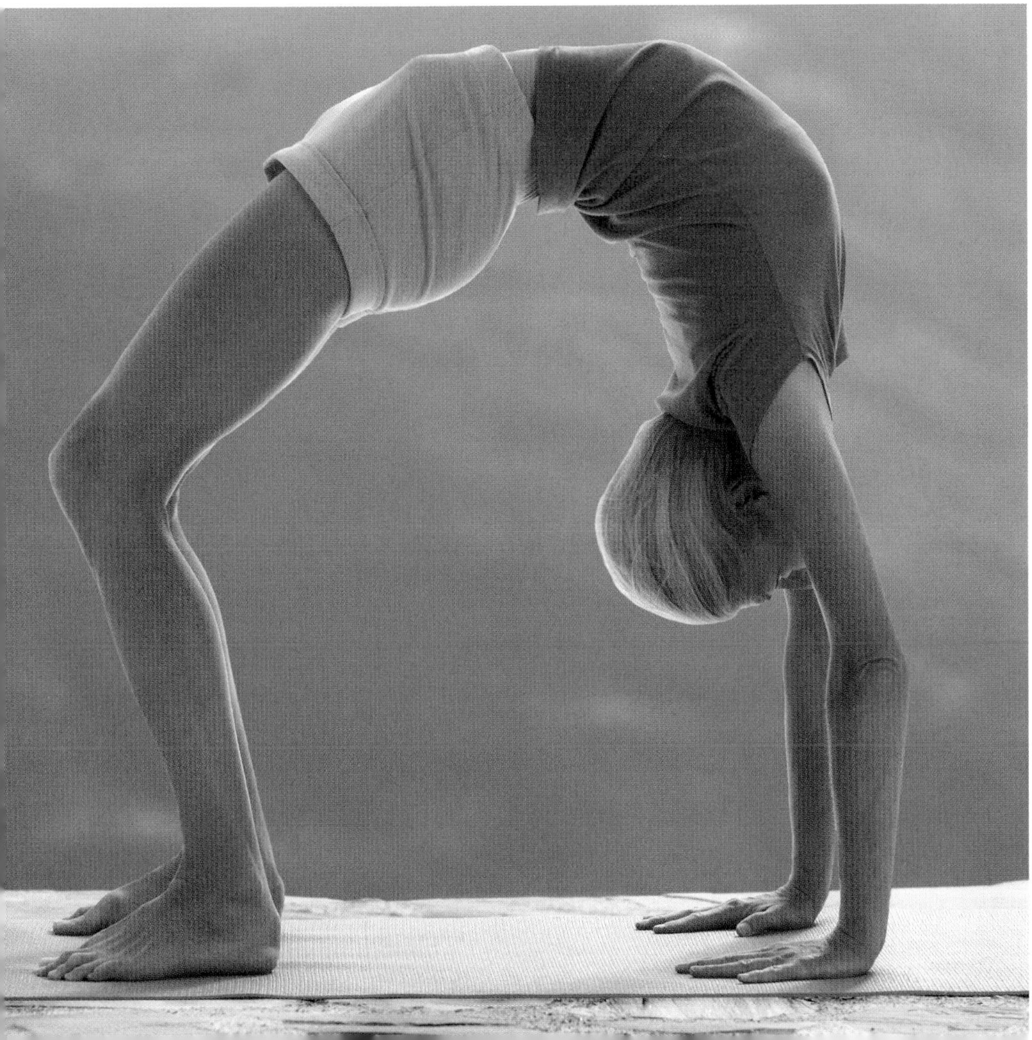

5 Maintaining the extension of your spine, lower your heels. Hold for 30–60 seconds. Exhale, bend your elbows and knees, and lower the crown of your head to the floor. Lower your back and buttocks to the floor, then rest.

"In order to unite the mind with the soul, the body, which is the foundation, has to be kept healthy."

Yoga for Overall Health

"By nature, the body is inert, dull, and sluggish; the mind, vibrant, active, and dynamic, and self, luminous and illuminative. Practice of yoga destroys the sluggishness of the body and builds it up to become equal to that of the active and sensitive mind. Then both the body and the mind are made to transcend to the level of the illuminative self with perfect health in body, stability in mind and clarity in intelligence.

The body is one of the finest precise instruments on earth. It has about three hundred odd joints, seven hundred odd muscles. We do not know how many minor muscles and link muscles are in this machine. If the nervous system were stretched as a single thread, it would reach from Mumbai to London. If arteries, veins and capillaries are connected together, they run to 100,000 kilometres [62,137 miles]. The lungs are as broad as a tennis court, supplying about 250 millitres [9 fluid ounces] of oxygen to the blood. The heart rhythmically beats about seventy times per minute pumping about 5 litres [10½ pints] of blood per minute. This is enough to know how much one has to be vigilant to shape the body in order to possess good health.

Nature fortunately provides this precise instrument – the body – with the means to adjust its rhythm to the turmoils of day-to-day pressures and environmental stress. It is also astonishing that in spite of imbalances created by the possessors of the body, it maintains its balance in spite of

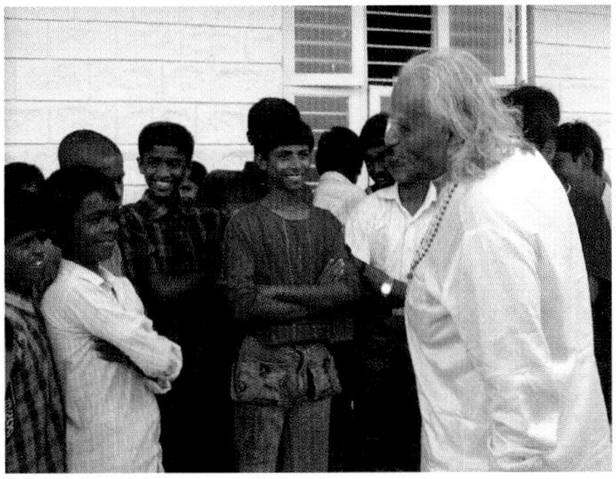

Asana and pranayama are just two aspects of yoga's eight-fold path. Here, Guruji engages with the ethical dimension of practice, meeting a group of teenagers at a charity project.

human over-indulgence in satisfying their greedy wants. When the limits are overstepped, physical, physiological, and psychological diseases set in.

Yoga has eight aspects known as *yama*, *niyama*, *āsana*, *prāṇāyāma*, *pratyāhāra*, *dhāraṇā*, *dhyān,* and *samādhi*, forming ethical, physical, mental, intellectual, and spiritual disciplines. The first two aspects of yoga are from time immemorial, known as do's and don'ts or *rīti* and *nīti*. The next three are for progressive evolution of the practitioner and the last three are the wealth of yoga which comes by following the first five principles.

Yoga not only works and triggers the whole body, but also develops and illumines the intelligence for the sight of the Self. It connects the anatomical and physiological bodies, as well as the mind and the soul of man. It deals with the structure of the body and proper functioning of the muscles with perfect flow of blood current in the blood vessels. It provides even distribution of bio-energy or life force, the very *prāṇa śakti,* and channels the mind to a state of calmness to face life without becoming a victim of circumstance and environment but as a master of them. Yoga starts from the health of the body and makes one climb the Everest of spiritual contentment, poise and peace. ”

From "Yoga for Overall Health", Courtesy of All India Radio, Pune.

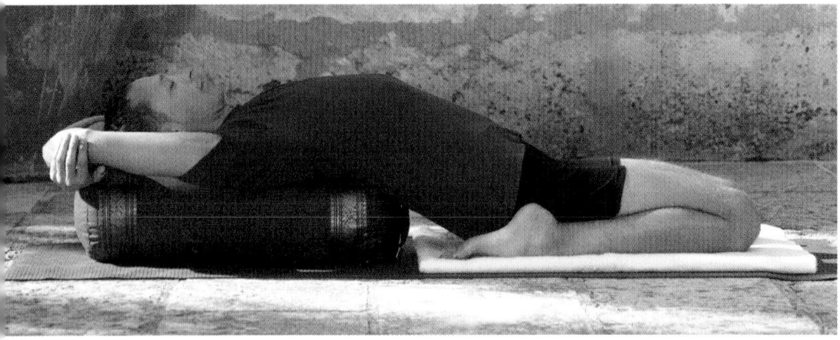

1 Place a folded blanket over the lower half of a mat and a bolster vertically along the centre of the upper half. Recline over the bolster in Supta Virasana (see pages 238–39) for 5 minutes, if possible, before sitting up.

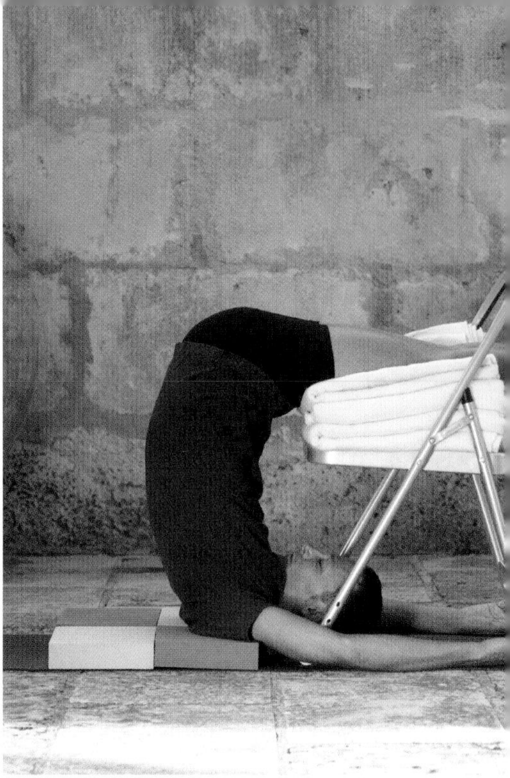

2 Place a chair on a mat with 2–3 folded blankets on the seat. Align four blocks in front of the chair. Recline over the blocks, tops of your shoulders at the edge nearest the chair. Lift your hips and legs into Halasana (see page 124), thighs on the blankets. Extend your arms overhead and hold the chair for 5 minutes, if possible. Reverse the actions to come down.

Encouraging Relaxation

Asana Sequence

"The practice of certain groups of *āsana* and *prāṇāyāma* sequenced properly creates space inside the body and flushes out the impediments which block the blood from flowing in the blood vessels and clears the energy blocks in the nervous system, thus preparing man to bear the load with ease in the neuro-endocrine and immune system. Besides these, the eyes, the windows of the brain, and the ears, the windows of the mind, are made to relax...."

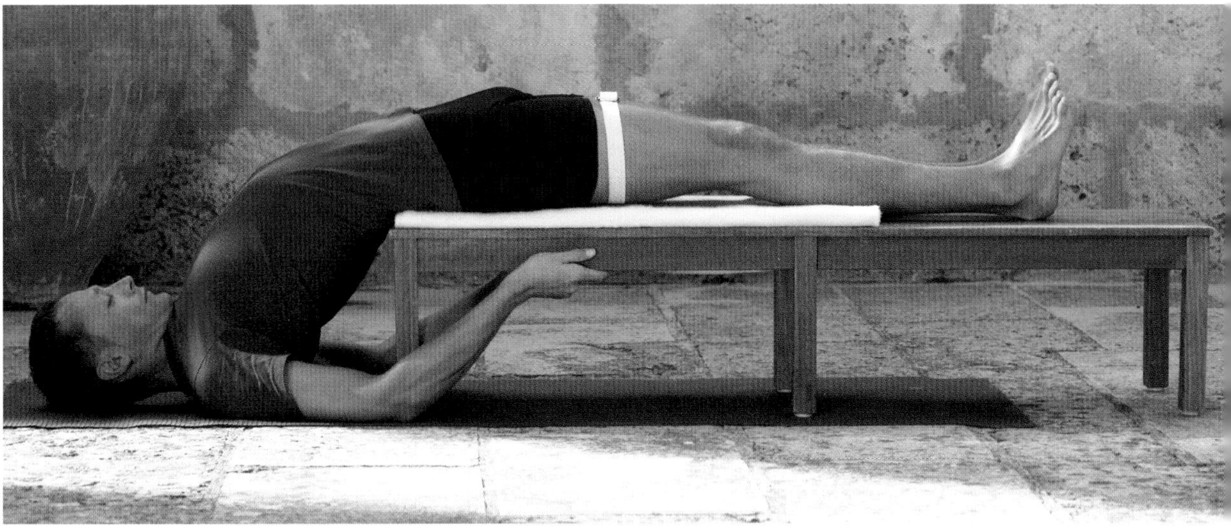

3 Place a low bench on a mat, with a folded blanket on the end. Sit on the blanket with a belt around your upper thighs to secure them together. Bend your knees, hold the bench, and slide back until your head and shoulders rest on the mat. Straighten your legs into Setubandha Sarvangasana (see pages 230–31). Try to hold for 5 minutes. Slide down to the mat.

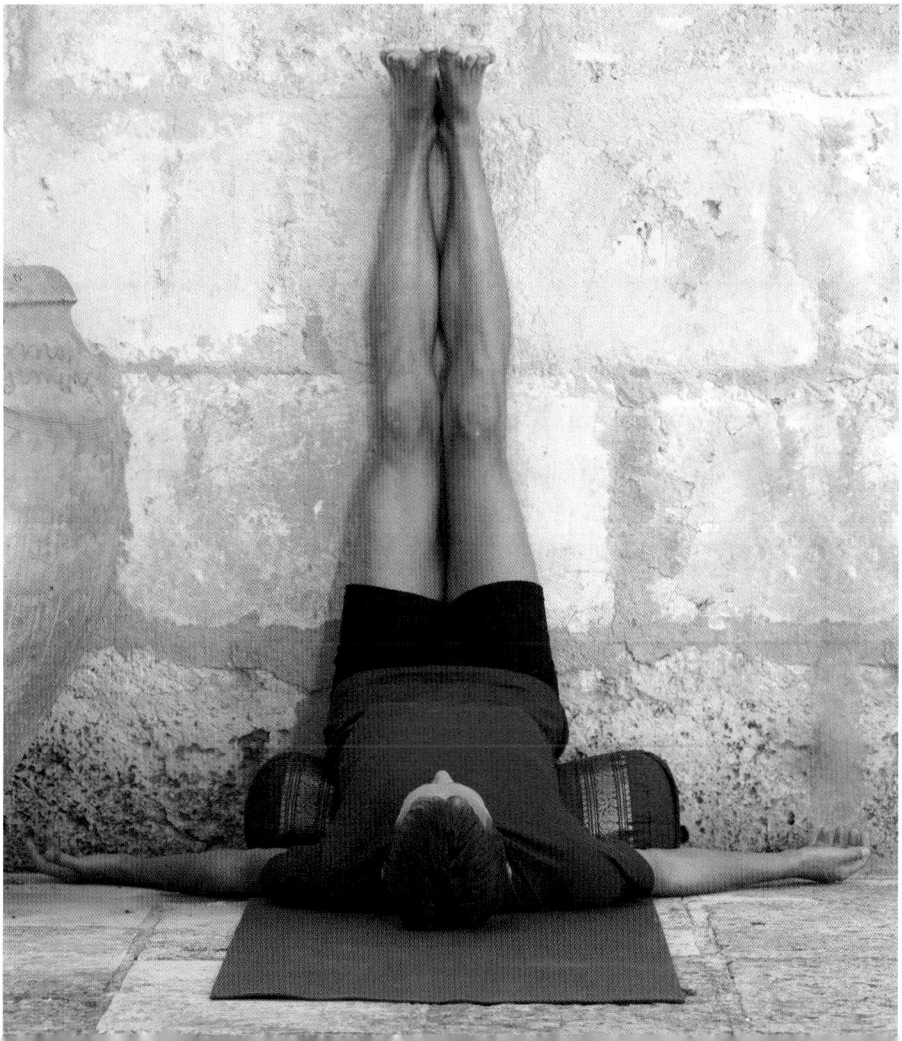

4 Place a mat and bolster against a wall. Sit on the bolster with one shoulder, hip, and thigh against the wall. Swivel around and recline over the bolster, legs up the wall in Viparita Karani (see pages 194–95). Try to hold for 5 minutes. Bend your knees and push into the wall to slide out of the pose.

Yoga for a Stress-free Life

“Industrial development and urbanization have no doubt triggered a fast life. Science and technology have given us the boons of physical comfort and leisure. But we do not allow our mind to pause and think. We throw ourselves mindlessly from one endeavour to another, believing that speed and movement is all in life.

Where is the time to think or ponder, to contemplate or introspect on the process of life? In the East, we are a shade better. In the West, there is the paradox of a communication upsurge going hand in hand with disastrous communication gaps. Husbands and wives have no time to talk to each other, parents have no time to communicate with their children. The result is alienation from our near and dear ones and from the whole of society. This has built up violence in petty matters with all kinds of perversions and tensions bottling up which result in an escalating crime rate. Here to our rescue comes the *sūtra* of Pātañjala Yoga, *yogaḥ citta vṛtti nirodhaḥ* – the art of restraining the consciousness and of keeping in a state of restful motionlessness.

The way out

Ancient sages, *ṛṣis*, and seers, literature and scriptures set a great emphasis on what man does in this world in accordance with his past chain of *karma* and previous births. Their guidance is on how to construct ways and means for better living. For this they take us towards the yogic way of living. The approaches of the western psychotherapeutics and that of the East with its 'wisdom' are fundamentally different. Western techniques provide physical relaxation and superficial quietness.

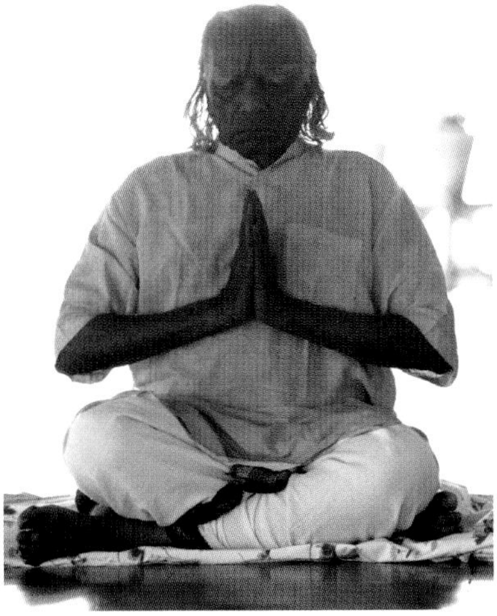

Guruji begins each day with an hour of pranayama practice; pranayama helps to control and calm the mind and recharge one's energy.

This yogic approach is control of the movements of the mind. The mind is a great culprit. Self control will save many a situation, if the individual can retain his poise of mind, stay cool, and be able to do the *sādhanā* without getting unduly perturbed or agitated. Having done what could be done, one is then prepared to await patiently the outcome or consequences of the action.... Yoga believes in developing a strong fabric which will withstand the onslaughts of the fluctuations, the ups and downs, the pleasure and pain, or a mixed product of despair, hope, frustration, failure, triumph and so forth.

Yoga is a natural tranquillizer for the urges from within which we call 'likes and dislikes'. The discontent, frustration, disappointment, hopes, success, greed, ambition, sex and neediness in love veer round our expectations. All these situations are a part of normal daily life with its inevitable conflicts, oppositions, clash of interests and ideas, collision of mutual ego, limited or little understanding of the points of view of others. In the midst of hurry, and at times of stress or emergency, basic human values alter, latent impulses become more urgent. The conflict within the individual snowballs and gives rise to psychosomatic diseases.

continued

Yoga comes to the rescue

The first limb of yoga (*yama*) is a social virtue to observe in life while in contact with others. The second (*niyama*) is the individual discipline by which to improve oneself for the betterment of life. The third (*āsana*) is for the maintenance of health and steadiness of mind. Health is a perfect balance of body, mind and soul, free from disease and at the same time protecting, sustaining, and supporting the living cells to lead a positive, constructive, and creative life. Life is a combination of consciousness, intelligence, mind, senses of perception, and action. The mind is like a mirror, receiving the aspirations of the self and acting through the senses for enjoyment and attainment. It has a dual role to play at both ends. It receives and acts for the impressions from the self to the senses, or from the senses to the self. If the mind acts without discriminative power, the body and the self become the abode of suffering. Hence, the practice of yoga purges the impurities of the body, bringing beauty, strength, firmness, calmness and clarity, revealing a happy disposition without creating any dualities between body, mind, and self.

The fourth limb (*prāṇāyāma*) is the extension, expansion, prolongation, requisition, and distribution of vital energy and consciousness to spread well in its field, the body and mind. It is said that where breath is, there the consciousness is. So correct *prāṇāyāmic* practices regulate man's habits, desires, and actions, and act as a bridge in unifying the body, the mind, and the self.

The fifth limb (*pratyāhāra*) brings the senses and mind under control and stops the dual functioning of the mind by diverting it from the enjoyment of pleasures towards the union of the self. The last three limbs (*dhāraṇā*, *dhyāna* and *samādhi*) are collectively termed as *saṁyama*, meaning integration. ”

Q. You say that the diaphragm is the window of the soul.

"No! I said that the diaphragm is the medium between the physico-physiological and psycho-spiritual bodies. What I said was that if the eyes are the windows of the head – brain – the ears are the windows of the heart – mind. If any emotional or intellectual upheavals take place, the first reaction is on the diaphragm."

– Why? –

"Why? Suppose you are suddenly frightened, then what happens to your diaphragm? What shape does it take? It shrinks. Suppose you are full of delight, how does the diaphragm move? You lift your chest. Don't you lift your diaphragm also? Don't you feel the exhilarating sensation, while in sorrow, depression is felt?

When one is afraid, often one says that the solar plexus gets gripped due to the fear complex. But it is not the solar plexus that gets gripped. It is the diaphragm that suddenly contracts, thereby applying pressure on the solar plexus when you are nervous or get frightened.

Why do yogis have a calm mind? Because they don't allow the diaphragm to become tight or to become hard, or to expand excessively; they do in such a way that the elasticity of the diaphragm is maintained permanently.

(*Gurujī* pretends to strike the journalist lady in the abdomen.) Look, I just pretended to strike her; what happened to the diaphragm? Instinctively, she got scared, she gripped her diaphragm.

Though the diaphragm is a physical organ, it is in direct contact with the mind, consciousness, and the self. If it is balanced and stabilized, it brings a sort of freedom to the mind, intelligence, and self. So *prāṇāyāma* is mentioned by Patañjali so that, through the control of the breath and energy, control of the diaphragm too takes place. As you win over the diaphragm, control of your mind too sets in."

Extract on pages 208–210 from "Yoga for Stress-Free Life", Aṣṭadaḷa Yogamālā *Volume 3, pp107–10.*

Question from "The Strength of Yoga", interview by Roger Raziel in Paris, April 1984, first published in Le Monde Inconnu *July 1984, and in* Victoria Newsletter, *May 1991.*

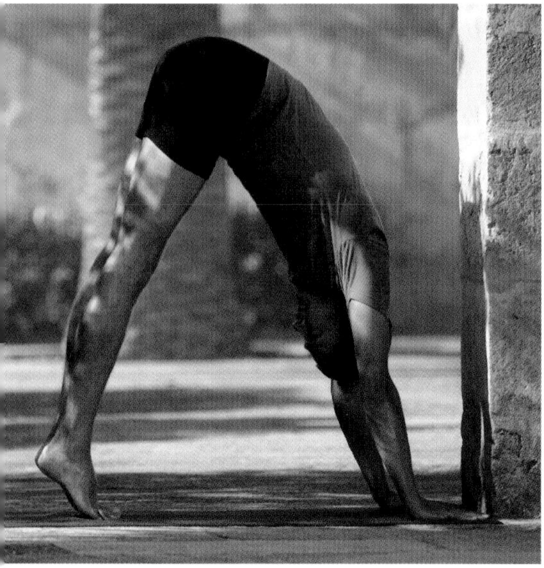

1 Place your mat with the short end by a wall. Stand in Tadasana (see pages 26–27) 90cm (3ft) from the wall. Place your palms by the wall, shoulder-width apart.

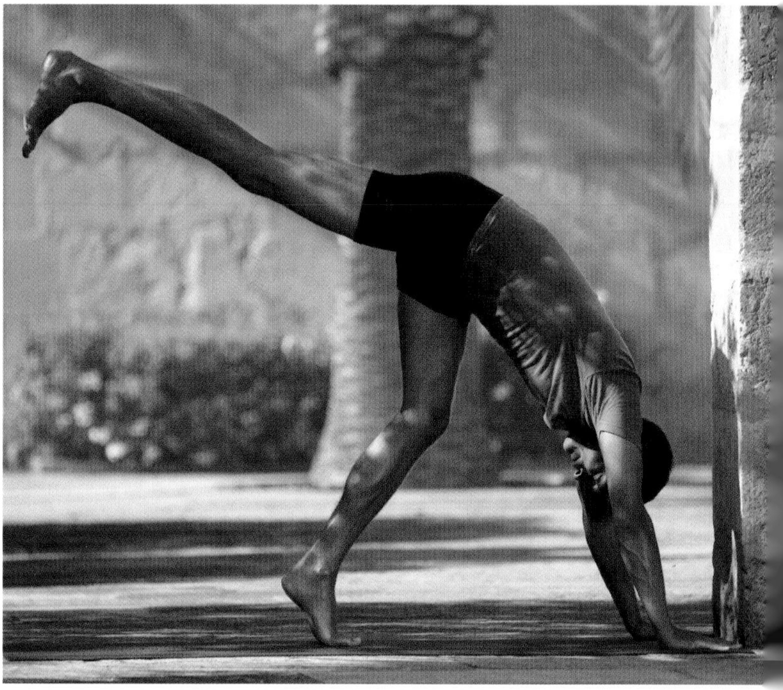

2 Keeping your arms fully stretched, bend your knees, exhale and swing your right leg up, towards the wall.

Adho Mukha Vrksasana

Downward Tree Pose

"The supersonic speed in thinking and action drains the physical frame, tenses the nerves, and taunts the intellect. If one cannot release these tensions and relax, one develops sleepless nights, which in turn affect the thinking faculty.... To focus his attention with his body, senses, and mind, he is made to perform *āsana* like [*Adho Mukha Vṛkṣāsana*] to flush and irrigate the brain."

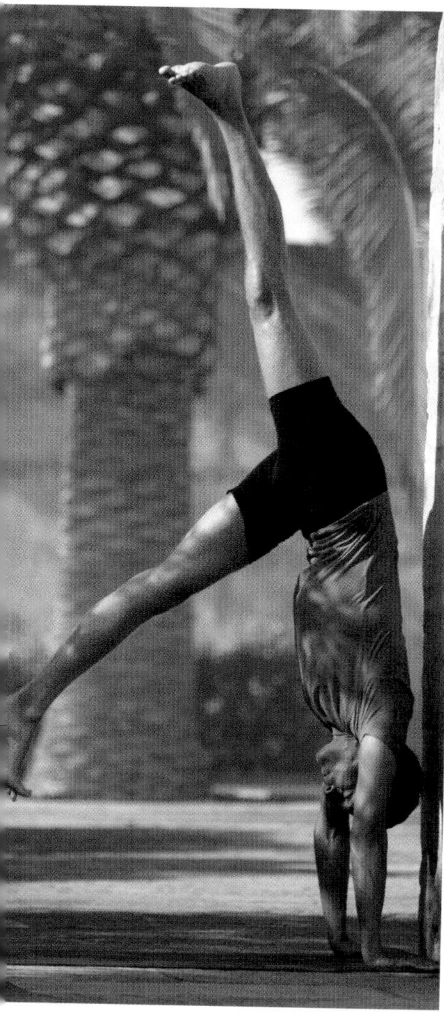

3 Immediately follow on with your left leg.

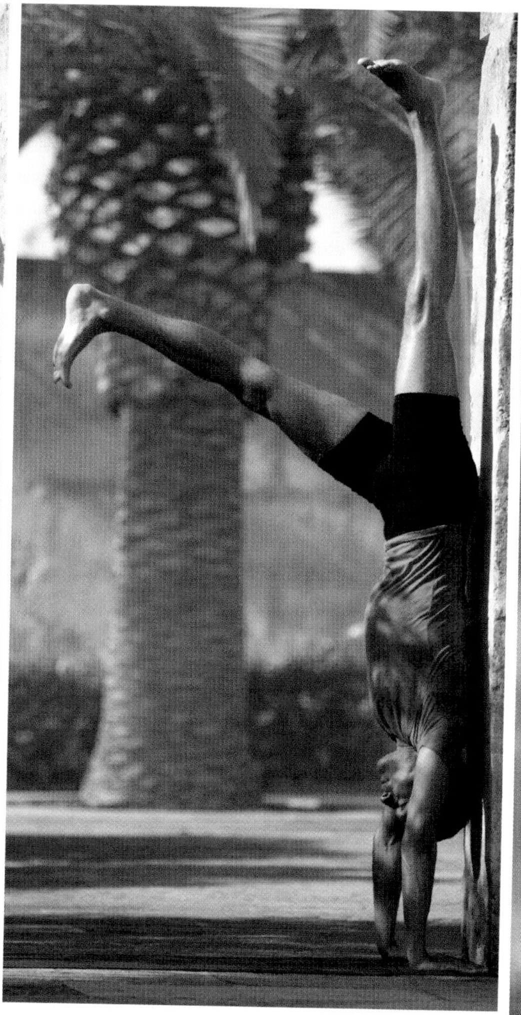

4 Bring your heels to rest on the wall and stretch both legs up.

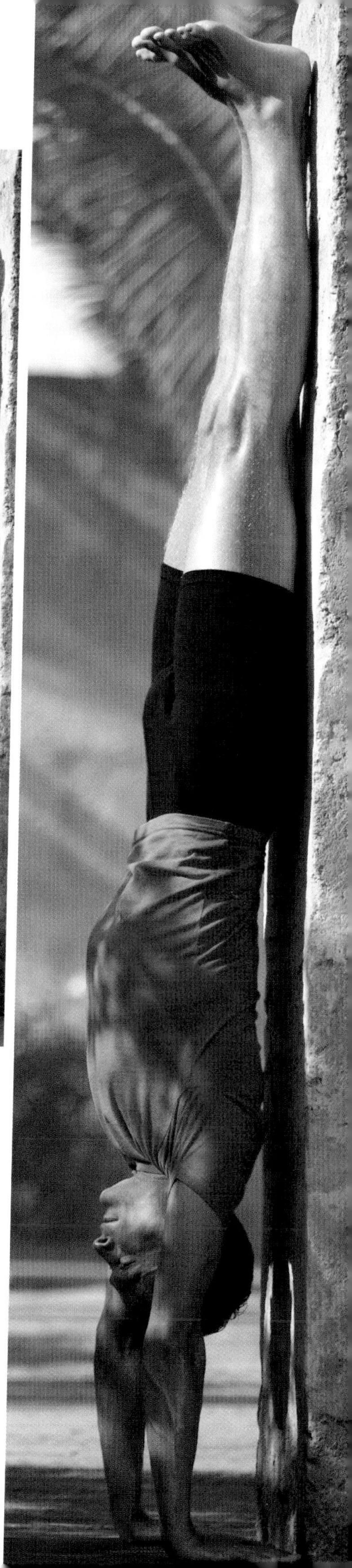

5 Hold for 20-30 seconds. Exhale and bring your legs down one by one. Keep your head down for a few seconds before standing up. Next time, kick up first with the left leg.

Salamba Sirsasana

Headstand (with brick and straps)

"Yesterday in *Śīrṣāsana* I kept a brick between the legs and the tailbone went in. At that time wasn't your ego auspicious? When the brick was not there you disturbed the tailbone with your egoistic intelligence. This is how you have to understand the functioning of the ego, which expresses through your action, through your posture and gesture as well."

Note: You will need help in the pose from an Iyengar yoga teacher.

1 Fold a mat in four and place it beside a wall with a brick and two belts nearby. Come into Salamba Sirsasana (see pages 72–73) and extend your heels up the wall.

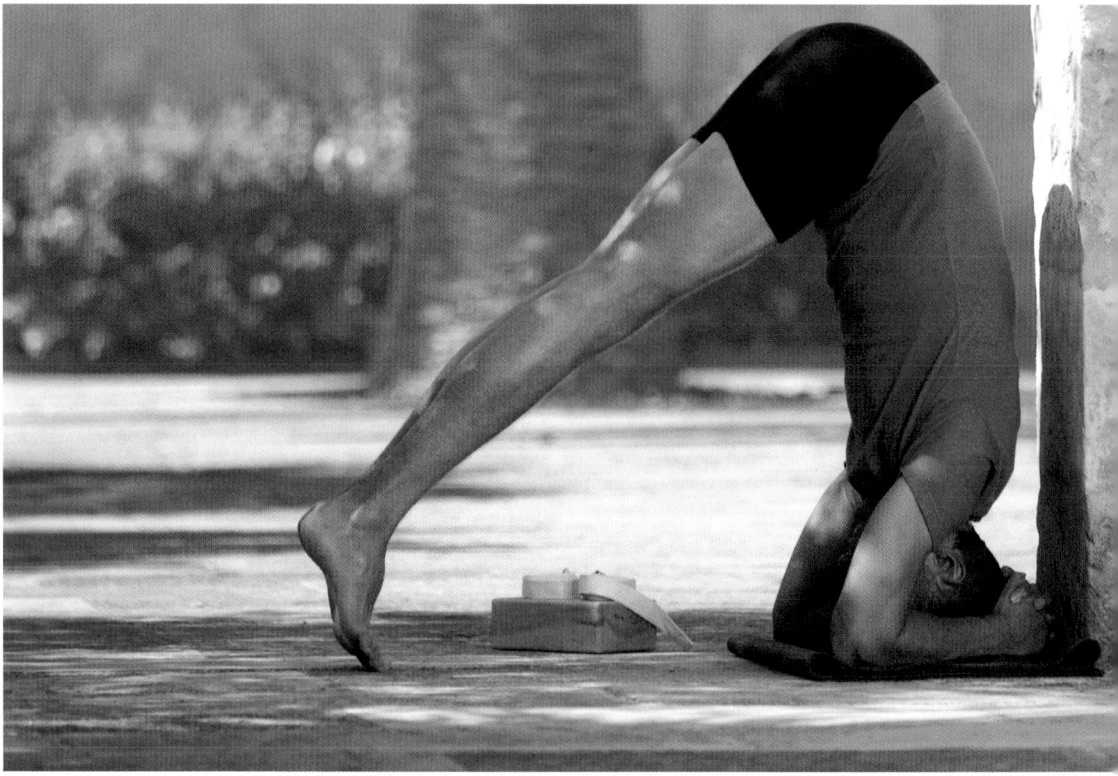

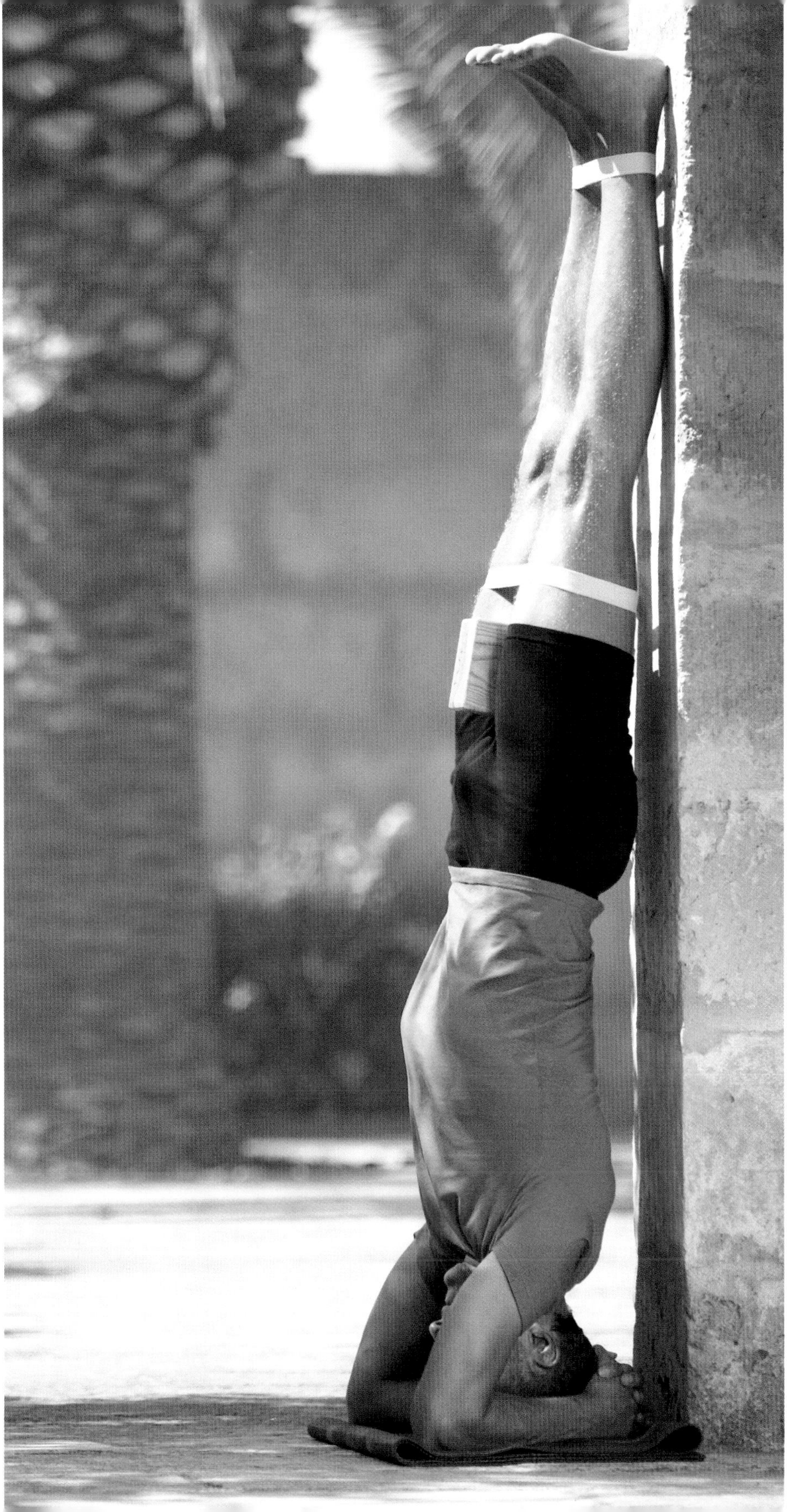

2 Ask the teacher to position the brick horizontally between your thighs, touching your perineum, then to fasten the belts around your thighs and ankles to keep your legs together. Hold for 3–8 minutes. Ask the teacher to remove the props before you lower your legs. Rest your forehead on the floor for a few seconds before sitting up.

Yoga and Ethical Living

"Ethics and spiritual discipline are like two eyes of an individual. They cannot be separated."

Q. Can you talk about the importance of ethics in terms of practice and relationship to yoga?

"Ethics is a way of life. Moment to moment, in each movement or action one has to observe the ethical pattern, as ethics are the base for spiritual growth. As such, the ethical disciplines explained in the *Yoga Sūtra* of *yama* and *niyama* are the foundation to be followed. For example, while in *āsana*, if my one right toe is turning out and left toe is turning in, there are no ethics involved and it becomes an undisciplined practice. If it is incorrect on one side and right on the other side, the readjustment of a wrong placing in the right direction is ethics.

As I said the other day when you were doing the *āsana*, if you are stretching more on the right side and less on the left you are doing *hiṁsā* to one part, *ahiṁsā* to the other. One part is moving in purity, the other part is moving in impurity. This is known as ethics.

If you remember, I told you today, when you were doing *Paśchimottānāsana,* if the right eye is moving forward and the left eye is not moving, one is in ethical

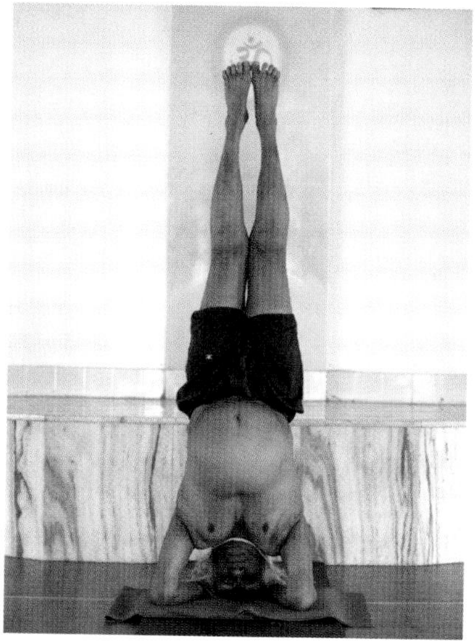

Whoever engages in spiritual practices has to have ethical discipline, says Guruji, and this begins with the perfect alignment of each asana, as here in Salamba Sirsasana.

discipline and the other is not. Ethics is not a way of just thinking, but a way of doing with thinking. It is the process of re-alignment of the body, senses, mind, intelligence, and consciousness, which have to be put together.

You cannot separate ethics from physical or mental discipline. You cannot discipline physically without ethical means. Even the breath that you take has a certain regulated flow. That regulated flow is ethics. You sit for meditation and close your eyes; but how the eyes are to be closed is ethics."

"It is impossible for anyone to experience salvation or reach God without ethical discipline."

From "Paths are Many, But the Goal is One and the Same", interview by Norman Mackenzie, December 1982, Yoga Center of Victoria Newsletter, *March and April 1983.*

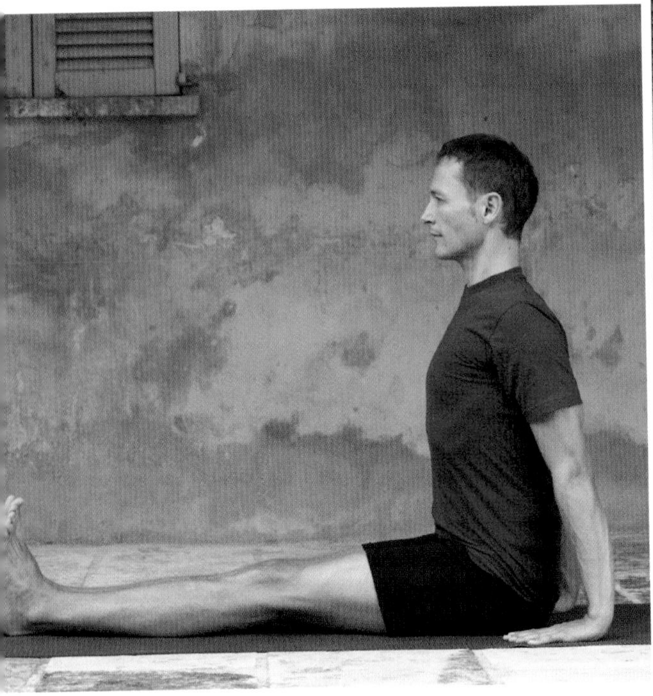

1 Sit in Dandasana (see pages 14–15).

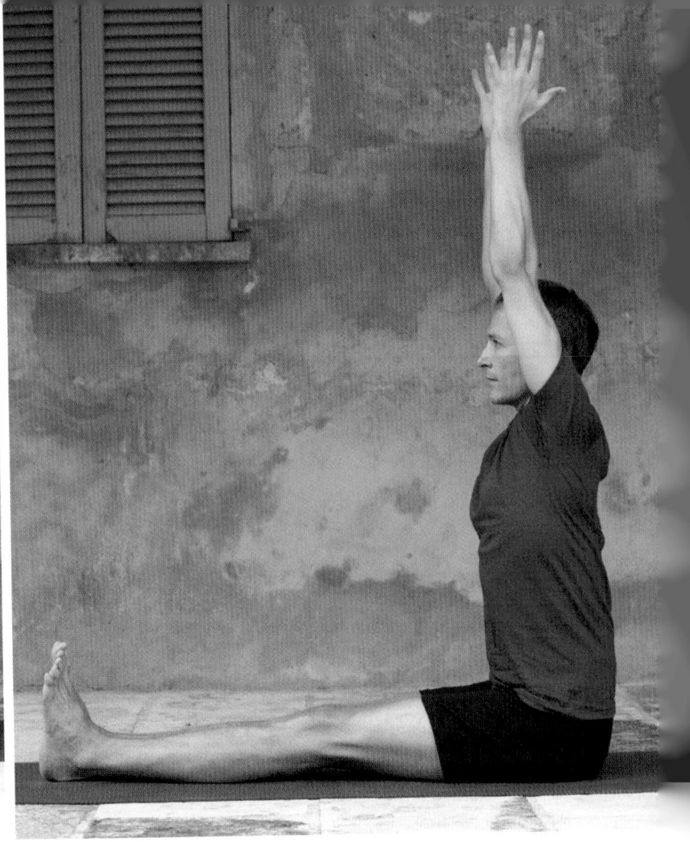

2 Extend both arms overhead until they are perpendicular to the floor and parallel to each other, palms facing. Stretch your spine up.

Paschimottanasana

Intense Back Stretch

"If your right leg is stretching and your left leg is not, you believe that the left leg is in *ahiṁsā* and the right leg in *hiṁsā*... You think that the stretching is *hiṁsā* and non-stretching is *ahiṁsā*. In both cases, you are creating *hiṁsā*. If one is a deliberate aggression, the other is a non-deliberate one. The moment when both legs are equally stretched or equally relaxed, there is neither violence nor non-violence. This is how you have to study the ethics in *āsana*."

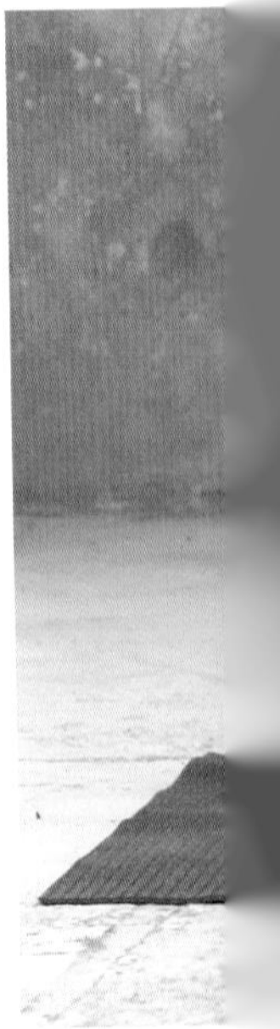

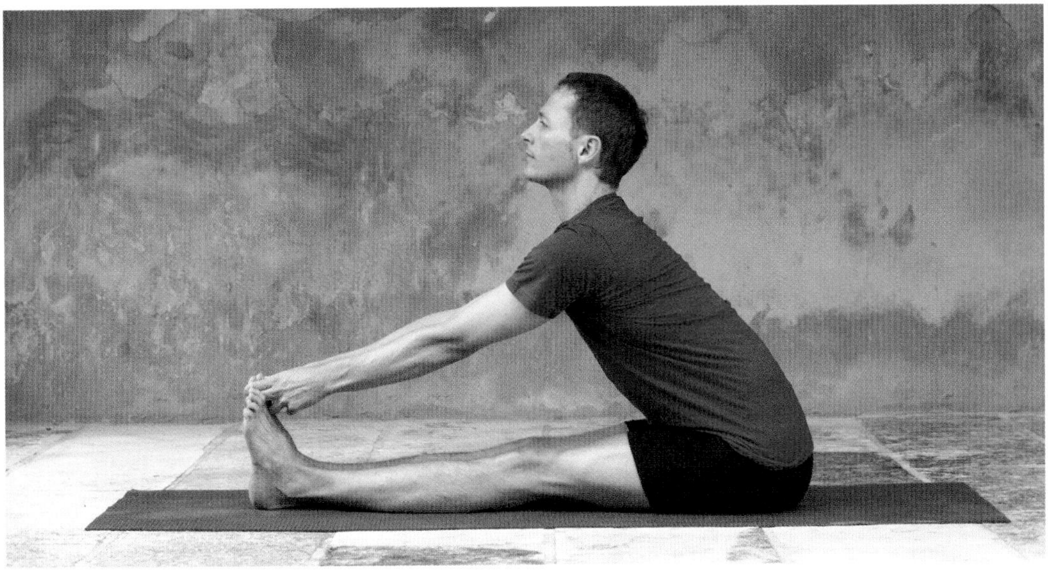

3 Exhale, stretch your arms forwards, and grasp your big toes between your thumbs and your first and second fingers. Look up.

4 Exhale, extend forwards from your lower back and both sides of your waist. Stretch your hands beyond your feet, if possible, clasping your right wrist with your left hand or vice versa. Hold for 30 seconds. Inhaling, release your hands, and lift back to Dandasana with the spine concave.

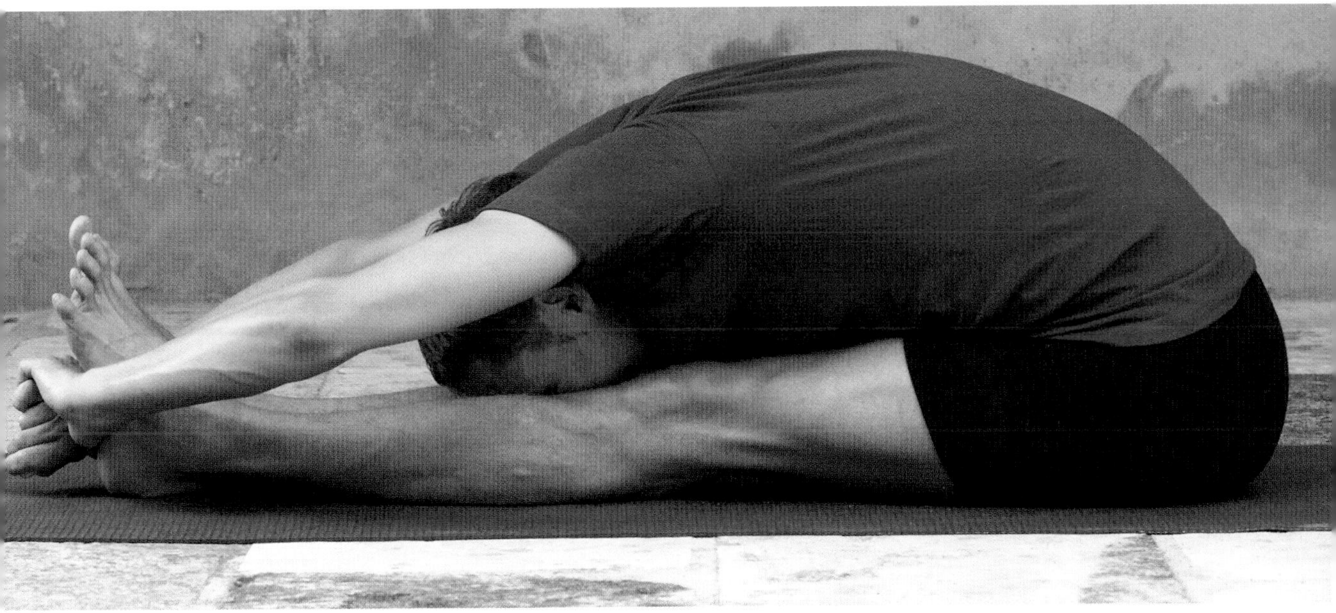

"If one wants to have sharpness and alertness while practising yoga, then one has to change his food habits."

Yoga and Diet

"Plenty of literature is available on food and diet for yogic practice. For them food comes first and then yoga. For me, it is yoga first, then food. Practice of yoga is important to me and I live on whatever suits my *sādhanā*.

Lord Krishna says, in the *Bhagavad Gītā*, that the suitable food for *sāttvic* growth is that which is delicious, soft, sweet, substantial, agreeable, and promotes long life, vitality, energy, health, happiness, and cheerfulness. *Tāmasic* food is that which has no taste and flavour, but is stinky, unclean, remnants and leftover. In my childhood, I did not know what is *sāttvic* or *rājasic* or *tāmasic* food. Whatever food the circumstances were providing me, I ate for survival. But my yogic practices nourished me and kept me healthy and alive with the stale and tasteless food.

My diet depends upon what type of practice I plan to do. I avoid that food which affects my practice. In case I need to attend family problems the next day, I may perform the *āsana* of tomorrow or the day after or the day before and adjust my diet in such a manner that practice won't suffer the next day. My system cannot take hot, savoury, spicy food. Even among the so-called good food, I choose what is congenial to my system and my practices.

If one remains on light food or on a diet and one type of food each day, this may make one feel weak. *Āsana* practice guides one in having sensitivity for eating what the body needs each day. Sometimes the system demands liquid food and sometimes sweet or salty food which all comes from the dictates of the body's needs.

My food is what an average Indian eats. I am a vegetarian. My main food is a bit of rice, one vegetable and yogurt with honey in the day and milk with chapatti and vegetable at night. But as far as solid food is concerned I don't think my system needs much. It is the discipline of yoga which has disciplined my food. That is why I am not fussy regarding food.

There cannot be a single type of food congenial to yogic practice. *Haṭhayoga Pradīpikā* says avoid too much food (*atyāhāra*). Eat only when hungry, or when saliva oozes from the mouth as one sees the food. Only eat what the system demands. Some say that the moment they smell something good, their mouths begin to water. But this cannot happen to one who is practising yoga. One can experiment oneself. Regular, disciplined, and genuine practice of *āsana* and *prāṇāyāma* for some months makes one indifferent to one's favourite dishes even if they are placed in front of him. Stop practice for eight days, then indiscipline sets in, and old habits return. When practised regularly, the digestive system gets stimulated and one eats less than what one normally consumes. After yoga, the system needs less fuel. Even metabolism turns into *sāttvic* quality in yoga *sādhanā*. By yogic practice, one enjoys food but does not indulge in it. ”

From "On Diet and Nutrition", Aṣṭadaḷa Yogamālā *Volume 8, pp51–59.*

Yoga as a Nature Cure

“ Our body is a combination and co-ordination of five elements: earth, water, fire, air, and ether, with five qualities namely odour, taste, form, touch, and sound. You can call these the atomic structures of the above five elements. All these elements with their qualities are in our body. Through the organs of action and the senses of perception, we can feel these elements and the qualities of the elements.

While practicing *āsana,* you begin to control the elements so that they function in unison, and through the practice of *prāṇāyāma,* you do the same with the atomic structures of the elements. This means that through *āsana* and *prāṇāyāma* practices, you learn to recognize and control the ten elements and qualities of nature in you. At the next level comes *citta*, comprised of mind, intelligence, and ego, which are to be co-ordinated attentively with the organs of action and senses of perception in order to make all facets of nature function healthily....

The practice of *āsana* and *prāṇāyāma* controls these elements not for remedial purposes but in order to earn permanent health. In *āsana*, the body is placed in various positions. The act of positioning the body is done by *pṛthvi tattva* (earth element). After positioning, we reflect on what we have done. This act of reflection is an interaction of *āp tattva* (water element). As a reaction, we readjust and repose. This is *teja tattva* (fire element). Then we check whether our consciousness and intelligence are touching everywhere evenly and whether we are aware of each part. This act of reasoning comes from *vāyu tattva* (air element). Extension, expansion, or contraction caused by the diffusion of intelligence are movements within the body and they belong to *ākāśa tattva* (ether element)....

In *āsana*, when one uses one's power or weight on certain parts, it is done by the earth element. This element works on stability and firmness. The element of water is purification of blood current through sterilization. The element of fire reacts and shapes each part of the body in that particular *āsana*. The element of air mobilizes and brings movement as per requirement. The element of ether creates space for expansion or contraction according to the movement.

The inner energy is *prāṇa* and the consciousness is *prajñā*. *Prāṇa* and *prajñā* are twins. Energy and awareness go together. Wherever energy moves, awareness flows; and wherever awareness reaches, the energy moves. While performing an *āsana*, *prāṇa* and *prajñā* – the main instruments – are used to adjust the five elements. For instance, when one suffers from acidity, one may do *Paśchimottānāsana* and other forward extensions to overcome the burning and vomiting sensation; but at the same time, one has to exhale in such a way that the energy is moved in the abdominal region and the abdomen is pacified consciously so that fire and air in that region are pacified.

One should know while doing the *āsana* where the power should be, where one should harden and where one should let loose, where one should have stability and where mobility. One should watch what sort of vibration is felt within the body. Why is there sensitivity at one place and insensitivity at another? One has to see whether the extension is away from the body or towards the body. With proper understanding, the elements are adjusted to remain in a balanced state.

The elasticity of the body is often considered the criterion for performing *āsana*. The parameter of elasticity does not provide the right way of judgement. Rather, it should be an adjustment of the elements. ”

From "Is Yoga a Nature Cure?" speech at a conference held by the Karnataka Prakrtika Parisad, Bangalore.

Can Yoga be a Therapy?

“Therapy is a healing art, used not only to combat disease but also to rehabilitate those who are afflicted with physical, organic, mental, and social problems. Can yoga help therapeutically to relieve and cure their sufferings so that they live with a healthy body and a happy disposition of mind?

The ancient healing art of yoga has stood and will stand as an unrivalled form of therapy for centuries. Basically, yoga is not therapy though healing is its sideline; it is mainly a spiritual healing science and an art of uniting body, mind, and soul as a single entity to merge finally in the Universal Soul.

According to *haṭha* yoga, diseases are man-made, man-invited, as well as environmental and affected by natural imbalances. According to *Sāṁkhya*, *āyurveda*, and yoga, imbalances take place and diseases set in when the soul conjuncts with nature. These imbalances are in the form of disease, weakness, sloth, indecision, carelessness, idleness, incontinence, illusion, disappointments, instability, distress, despair, body-infirmity, and laboured breathing. Due to present day stress, strain and speed, these obstacles get aggravated in one's physico-mental health. Hence, Patañjali puts forward *aṣṭāṅga yoga* in order to live in the joy of health and tranquillity.

As science has advanced, and is still advancing, diseases multiply too. As modern comforts have facilitated life, the result has been that our body has become lazy; joints and muscles have lost movement, power and growth; and various systems like the respiratory, circulatory, digestive, glandular, urinary, and eliminatory systems are rendered inefficient, these being but the vehicles of health of mind and harmony of the self.

Āsana plough the inner body and stimulate the necessary supply of bio-energy and blood to irrigate each area of the body for efficient

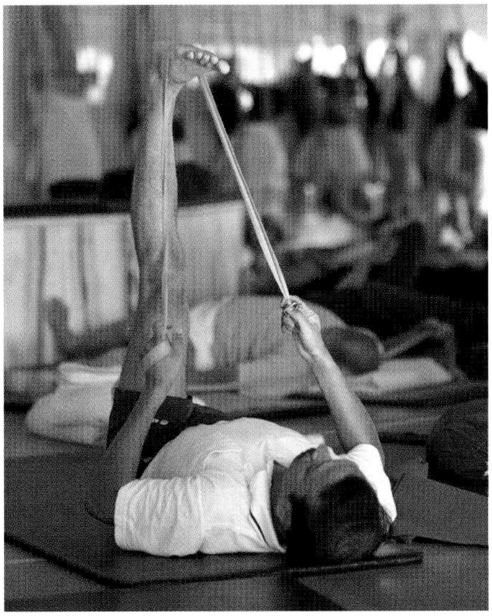

Each asana animates the bio-chemistry of the body, and props enable all to reap the benefits.

functioning. They also stimulate the diseased and affected parts by making each cell fulfil its function before it dies. *Prāṇāyāma* helps to store much vital energy as a reserve force to act when necessary. *Dhāraṇā* and *dhyāna* keep the mind calm and serene.

Thus, yoga not only acts as curative therapy but also as a preventive art in keeping the body healthy and firm, mind clear and clean with emotional stability so that the *sādhaka* is healthy both inside and outside. Patañjali has not forgotten social health too. He says that friendliness, compassion, delight, indifference towards happiness and sorrow, virtue and vice are the ingredients of social health.

Hence, yoga covers the inner field as well as the outer for a better, healthy, happy, long life though its aim is freedom and beatitude (*mokṣa*). ”

From "Can Yoga be a Therapy?", Aṣṭadaḷa Yogamālā *Volume 3, pp125–26.*

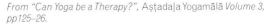

Sarapanjarasana

Bed of Arrows Pose

"When [Bhīśmācārya] was totally injured in *Kurukṣetra*, he kept himself alive with sheer will power. He lay on a bed of arrows, known as *śarapañjara*.... But was it not a strain for him to lie on a bed of arrows? He preferred to lie in the same position. Why? Because he was supported by arrows at the cardiac nerve. The ventricle of the heart was supported and that brought him a restful state.... In the Institute, those who suffer from cardiac problems are asked to do this *āsana*."

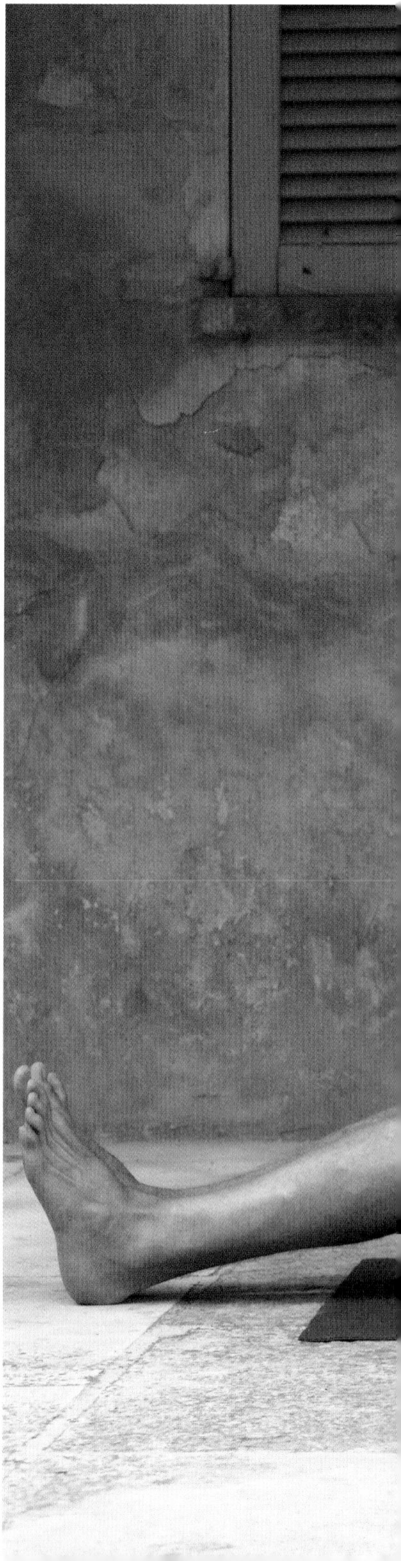

Note: Practise with an experienced Iyengar yoga teacher. Place a stool at the end of a mat, with a folded blanket on top. Position 4-5 blocks, depending on your height, in front of the stool, to support your dorsal spine when your head rests on the stool. Place two blocks to support your tailbone. Balance upended bricks on the blocks. Position two further bricks between the blocks, one on each side, to support your hands. Sit on the lowest blocks (remove the brick) and rest your dorsal spine on the higher brick. Position your head on the stool and support your tailbone with the brick. Extend your legs (rest your soles on a sandbag for increased recuperation). Place the backs of your hands on the side bricks. Hold for 5 minutes, building up to 10. Bend your knees, lift your buttocks, and remove the brick. Finally, raise your head and back.

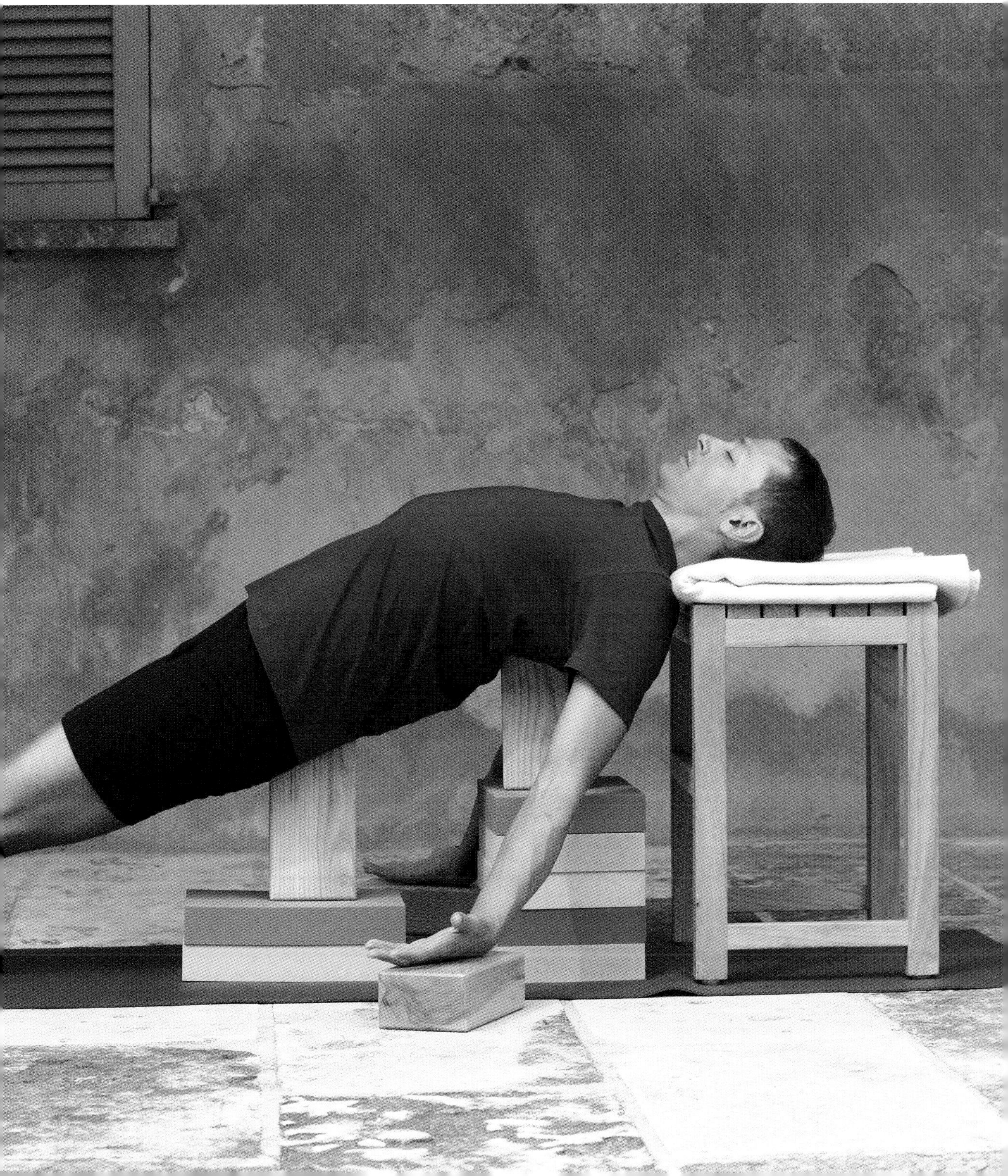

Yoga for Mental Equilibrium

“As body and mind are naturally integrated, they influence one another. Hence, *āsana* practice not only affects the body but affects the mind and in turn both affect the self. The mind, being very mercurial, gets caught in sorrows, pleasures, emotions, and moods. *Āsana* has the power to work in such a manner that they can change the attitude of our body, mind, intelligence, and ego confidently to undergo a stream of change by making them ecstatically happy and exultant so that they move together in unison and meet the soul.

The varieties of *āsana* help our musculo-skeletal body to undergo changes with the help of our mind. For example, if the shoulder blades are out, one will have a hunch back, the slight structural defect is enough to change our mood and attitude. A caved in chest does not allow one to breathe correctly. A protruding abdomen restricts movements and makes one lazy. Therefore, varieties of *āsana* are necessary if needed to change the structure of the body.

Similarly, if one of our inner organs suffers with some problem, it affects our mind. For instance, take glandular system. If the thyroid has less iodine, there will be more secretion of hormones, and on account of this obviously one suffers from mental imbalances. Hypo- and hyper-thyroidism affects both body and mind. Adrenals change the personality of man. High blood pressure causes anxiety and fear. For this reason, innumerable *āsana* were discovered and propounded by ancient yogis, in order to gain permanent over-all physical and mental health and harmony....

Mental health needs both intellectual as well as emotional stability. The intelligence in a person has two branches. One branch moves towards the

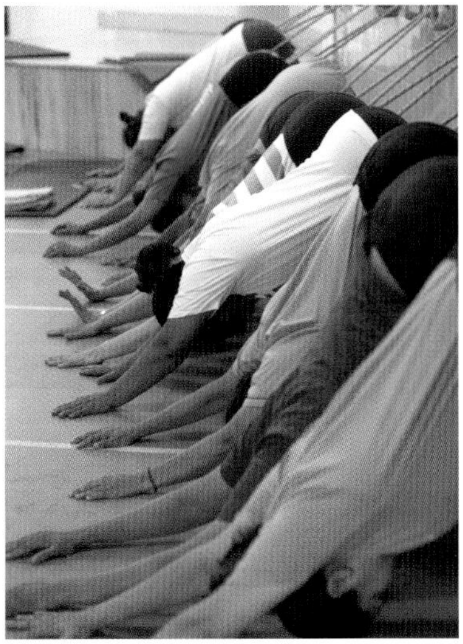

In Adho Mukha Svanasana supported with ropes, the brain becomes quieter and the emotions more stable.

brain while the other towards the heart. When one is depressed, the upward flow of energy facing the brain gets retarded. The retarded energy makes one brood and sinks the mental heart. Some *āsana* work on emotional quietness by stabilizing the emotional centre. Some *āsana* help one in developing intellectual sharpness, alertness, smartness, and power to endure any type of physical load whereas some other *āsana* help the mind move inwards to penetrate the interior mind. Particularly, the inverted *āsana* not only bring intellectual clarity but also emotional stability. In these inverted *āsana,* the head is subdued and heart is energized. The life-energy flows in these regions creating joy without any disturbances.

The practice of *āsana* stimulates deep bio-chemical changes. The brain and the glandular system undergo a transformation. The metabolism of the body is adjusted and corrected according to the requirements. One understands where to activate the body and where not to activate, what one has to do and what one should not do. Discriminative way of thinking and presentation brings change and affects the doer for the good to gain mental equilibrium. ”

From "On Aṣṭāṅga Yoga – Asana", Aṣṭadaḷa Yogamālā *Volume 7, pp110–12.*

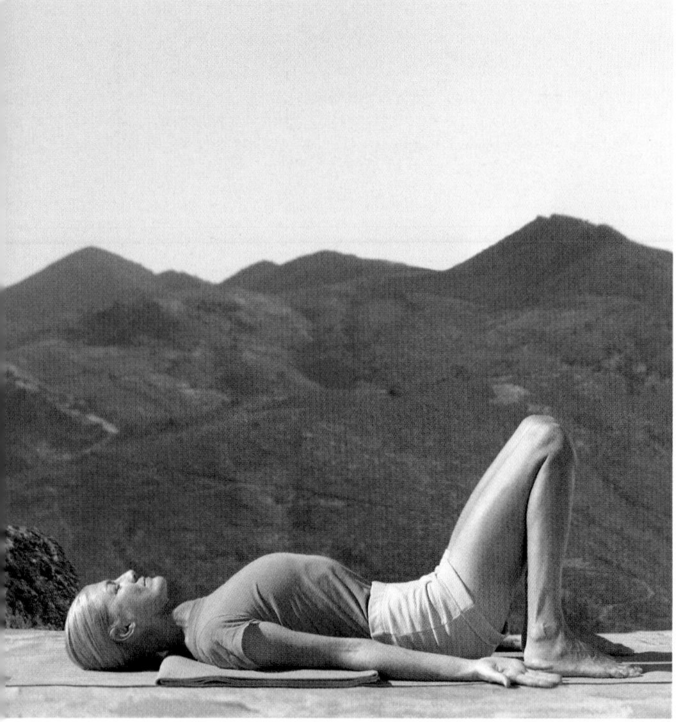

1 Place a folded mat beneath your shoulders. Bend your knees, place your feet hip-width apart and your arms by your side, palms facing up.

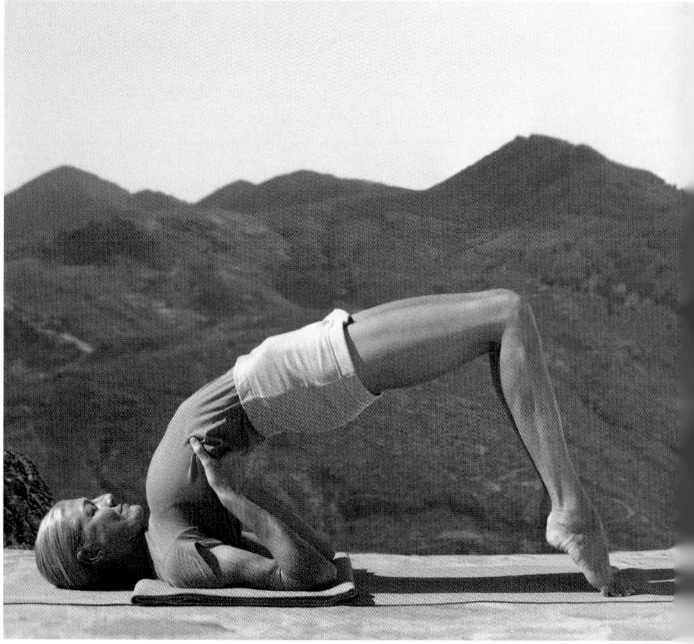

2 Exhale, press your arms and feet down to help lift your buttocks and hips, then place your palms on either side of your spine. Lift onto your toes, raising your sacrum to increase the height of your pelvis, the extension of your spine and the lift of your chest.

Setubandha Sarvangasana

Bridge Pose

"The gateways for human health are the respiratory and circulatory systems. When you do *Setubandha Sarvāṅgāsana* the lungs expand automatically. In this *āsana*, the breathing process increases indirectly even without the knowledge of *prāṇāyāma*. That is why patients find relief as there is no strain. The chemicals of the blood change, which gives them health."

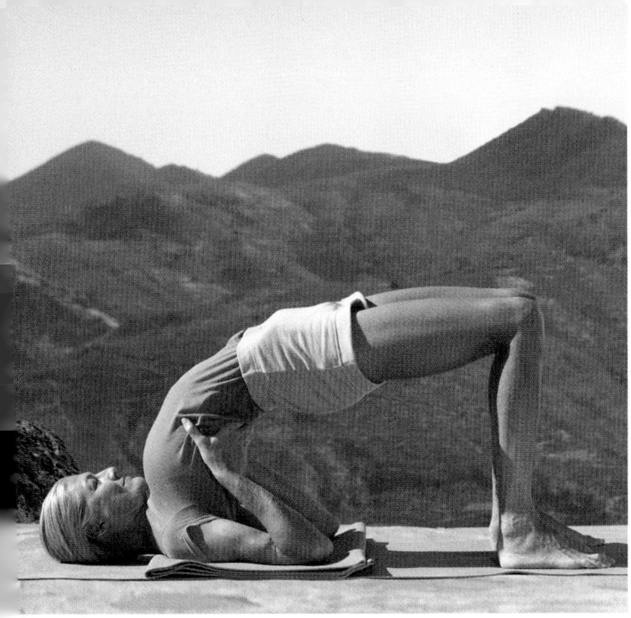

3 Press your shoulders and upper arms down and forearms up to maintain the lift of your chest and pelvis, then lower your heels. Hold for 30–60 seconds. If you are a beginner, lower yourself to the floor and rest.

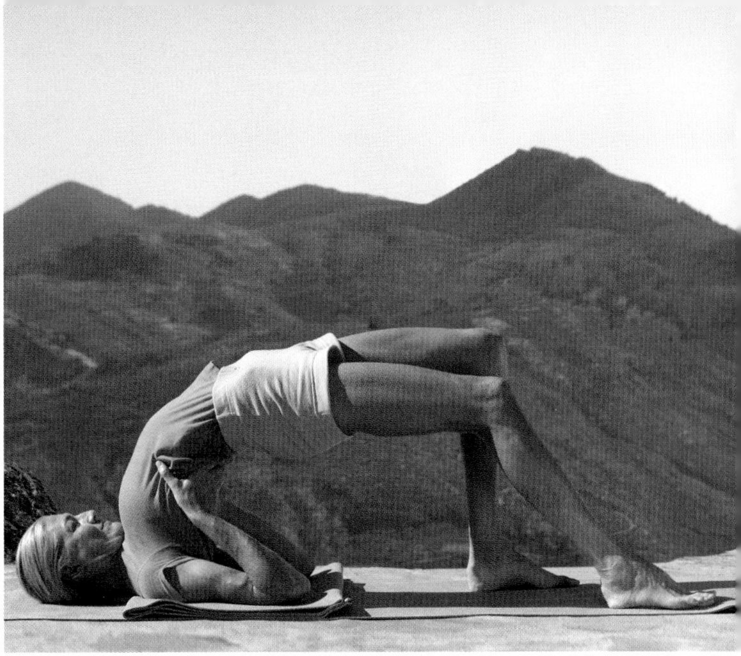

4 Now stretch out one leg, maintaining the lift of your chest and the extension of your body.

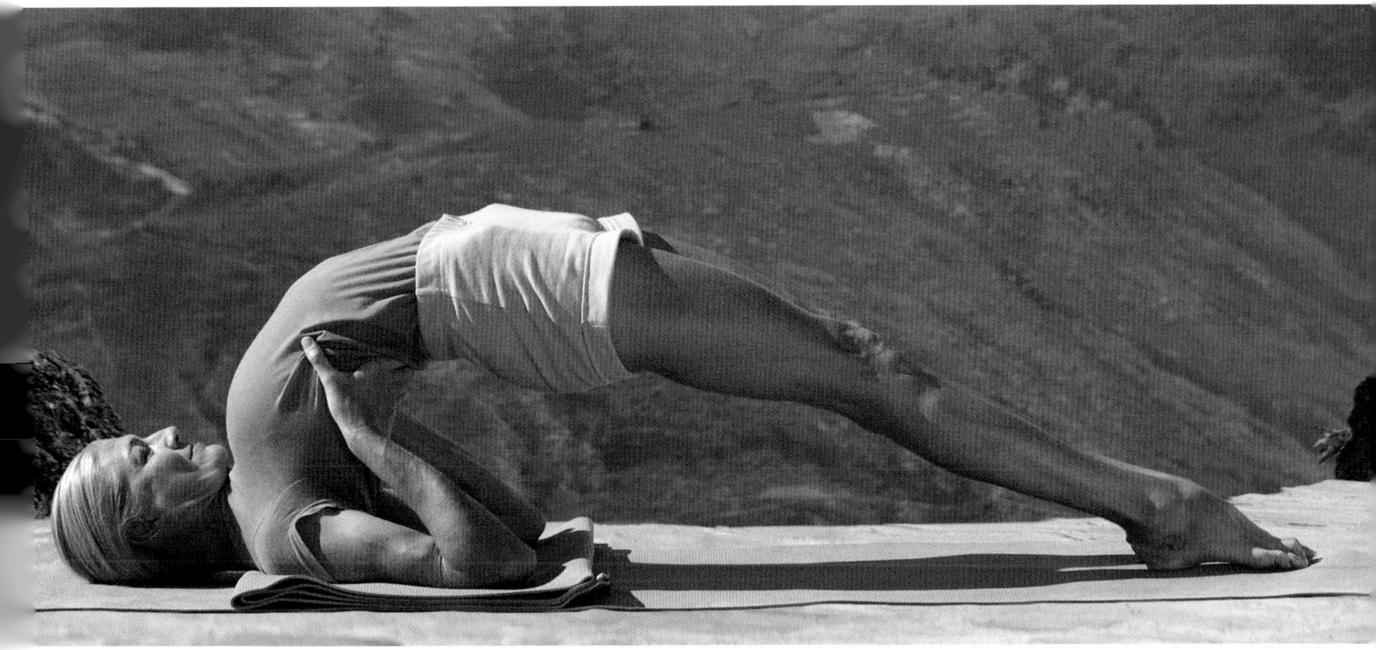

5 Extend your other leg, then straighten both legs. Keep lifting your hips and chest. Hold for 30–60 seconds. Bend your knees and walk your feet towards your buttocks, then lower yourself to the floor and rest.

"A friendly approach is needed to develop constructive ideas."

Yoga for a Better Life

Q. Can you give some idea of your experiences with drug addicts and prisoners?

"I have to think about what *āsana* would help to remove the vacuum in them. As they go silent, empty and dull within, I have to be with them moment to moment to fill the awareness and attention in their way of living while practising. I have to make them work on *āsana* to live in the present that creates exhilaration. I have to show them that nature abounds with exhilarating principles through which yogic *āsana* tickle and trigger their nerves. This sensation in them has made many to be free from smoking, alcohol, and drug addictions and transforms them for better living and high thinking.

Regarding prisoners, they are aggressive and destructive, yet soft in their hearts. Their intelligence is limited in understanding moral behaviour. In prison they do repent their crimes and like to find solace. Mild practice does not convince them. They love the speedy sequences of doing *āsana*, which exhilarate the brain, and difficult *āsana*, which attract them. So we teach what they ask and slowly change them for the better. At San Francisco, seeing a few hard core prisoners was a delight for me. They all embraced me and kissed me when I talked to them and showed what they can do in their cells to keep lively. They liked it and are as humane as we are, but circumstances make them choose that path. With compassion, firmness, and a friendly approach to *āsana*, they come to smile.

The sequences of *āsana* for the mental state of addicts and prisoners differ. I feel that disappointments, sorrow, negative attitude, too much money or poverty, dissatisfaction of family life, broken families, cause them to take to addiction and crime. Yet, we need to discuss with them first their basic

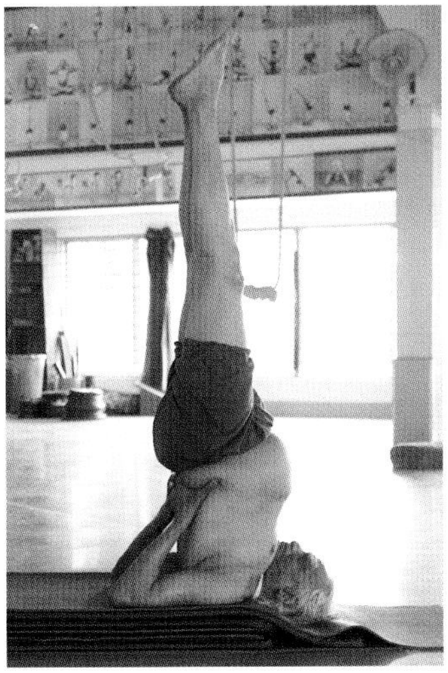

In rehabilitation plans, Gurujī may recommend asana that stimulate and refresh, such as Sālamba Sarvāṅgāsana.

requirements so that we plan the *āsana* or *prāṇāyāma* which are beneficial to them.

For the addicts, as I told you, I choose the *āsana* and *prāṇāyāma* which remove the emptiness, defeat and dejection in them. The standing *āsana*, inversions and backward extensions are very effective. Relaxing *āsana* like forward extensions do not help them much as their minds go towards depression. Therefore they need to be kept active.

Sometimes I make them do the standing *āsana* and backward extensions very fast to refresh their minds. *Āsana* such as *Ūrdhva Dhanurāsana*, *Viparīta Daṇḍāsana*, *Viparīta Chakrāsana* or *Adho Mukha Vṛkṣāsana*, *Pinca Mayurāsana*, exhilarate and bring cheerfulness in them. *Āsana* like *Sālamba Śīrṣāsana*, *Sālamba Sarvāṅgāsana* and *Setu Bandha Sarvāṅgāsana* sharpen their brain. Doing *Halāsana* and *Paścimottanāsana* repeatedly in quick succession acts like a bath as brainwashing which soon stimulates and freshens for better living and higher thinking. The *āsana* brings chemical changes. The smoker begins to enjoy fresh air, the addict no more likes dullness or dope. The stomach, the liver, and finally the entire body system reject alcohol."

From "Tune Yourself to the Music of Yoga", interview by Burjor Taraporewala and Sam Motivala for Eve's Weekly, *4–10.9.1982.*

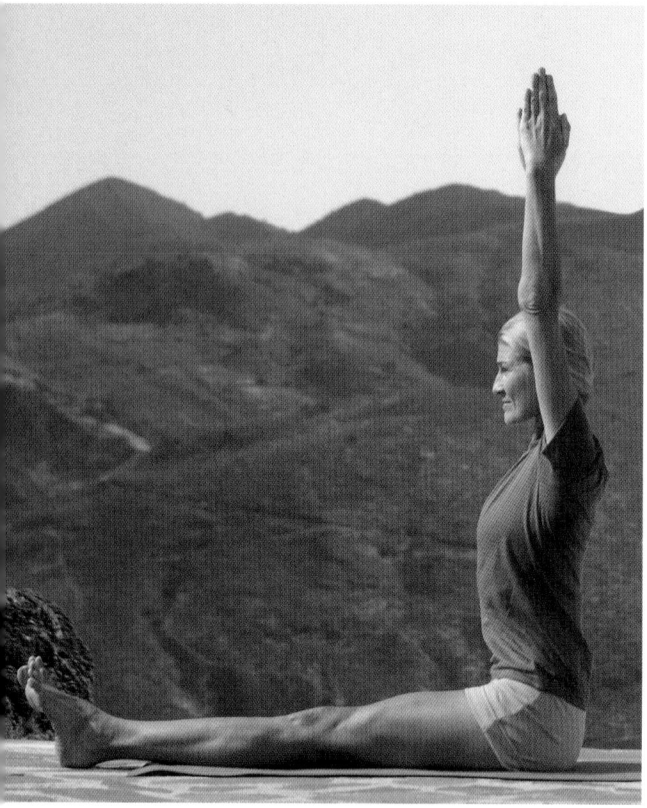

1 Sit in Dandasana (see pages 14–15). Extend both arms overhead until they are perpendicular to the floor and parallel to each other, palms facing inwards.

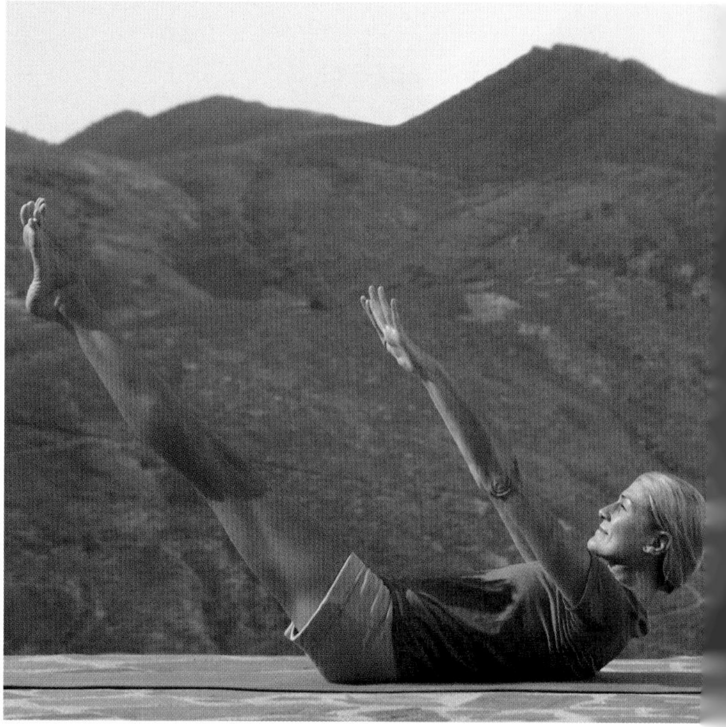

2 Exhale and begin to roll backwards, swinging your legs and hips up and over your head until your feet and arms touch the floor beyond your head.

Halasana to Paschimottanasana

Asana Sequence

"Repeated movements from *Halāsana* to *Paśchimottānāsana* bathe the brain with adequate oxygenated blood supply and sharpen the brain and mind to a considerable extent. *Prāṇāyāma*, too, helps in improving the memory, but when the body, brain, and nerves are tired, then one should stick to *āsana* only. They refresh fast."

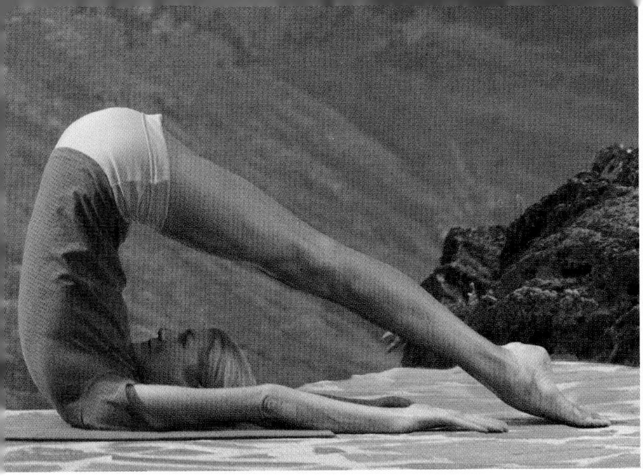

3 Press your toes into the floor, keep your knees tight, and lift your trunk. Extend your arms along the floor, palms facing upwards. Hold for a moment. This position is a variation of Halasana (see page 124).

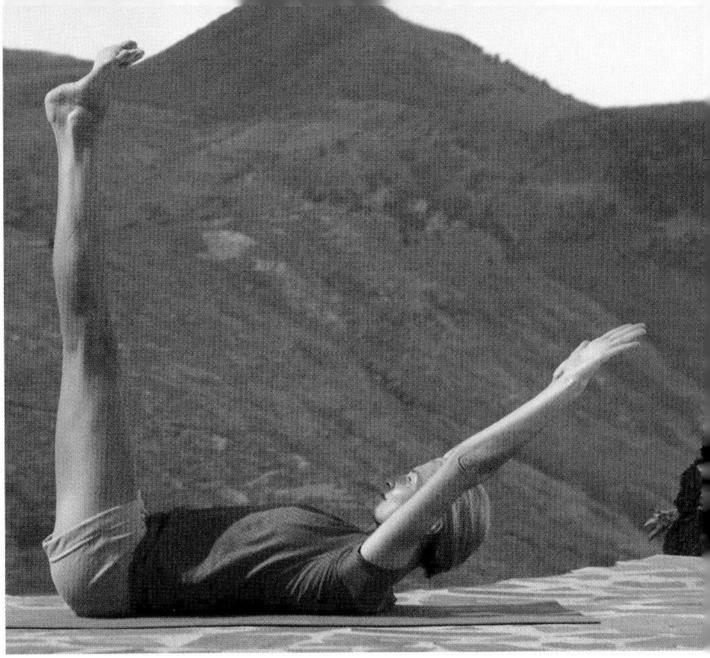

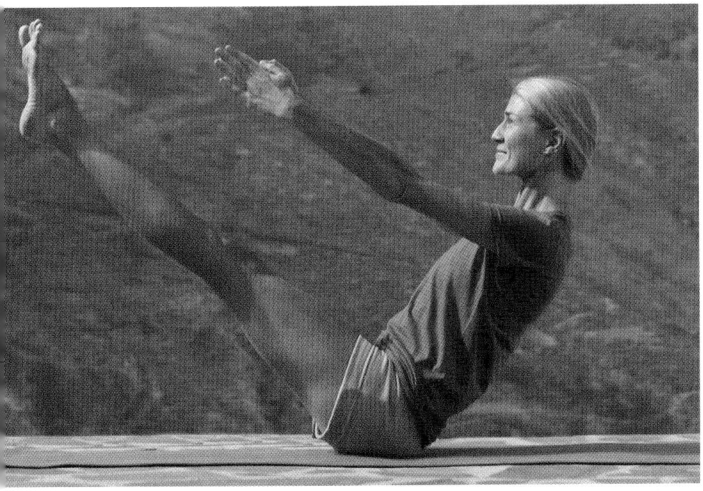

4 Exhale, lift your feet and legs, and begin to roll forwards, allowing forward momentum to lift your arms and torso.

5 Continue to roll forwards, keeping your arms, legs and spine extended.

6 When your legs and heels touch the floor, stretch your spine and arms over your legs into Paschimottanasana (see pages 218–19). Hold for a moment, then exhale and begin to roll backwards into Halasana and then again forwards into Paschimottanasana. Repeat until you feel refreshed.

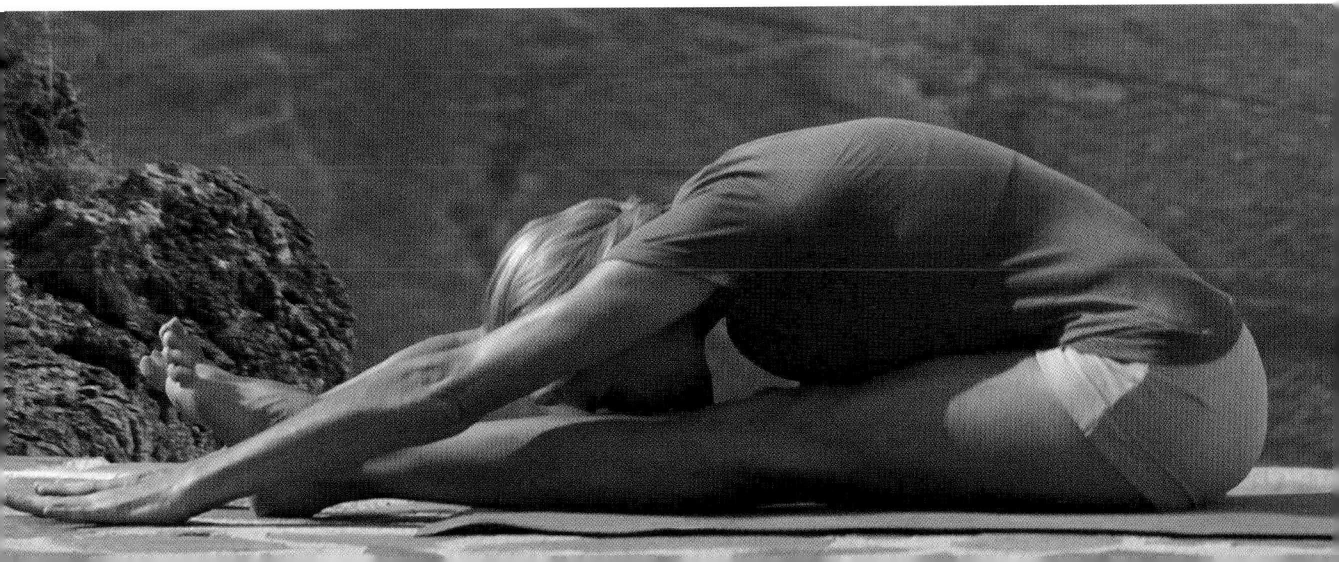

Yoga for Athletes

"Yogic techniques teach fast recovery from stiffness, heaviness, dullness, and fatigue."

"Athletics and all sports demand vigorous physical discipline to develop speed, strength, endurance, precision, and agility. While the muscular portion of the body is developed, very often the inner organs remain weak or stifled and the mind may actually be dulled. Athletes are unable to maintain supremacy in their fields for very long; while consumption of energy is at a maximum, the recuperative powers are hardly developed. Here it is yoga that can assist athletes....

The yogi's understanding and mastery of the body is far more intricate than that of the athlete. It recognizes five layers of the human body: the anatomical body, consisting of bones and muscles; the physiological layer, made up of the respiratory, nervous, circulatory, and alimentary systems; the psychological or emotional layer; the mental or intellectual inner layer, and finally the blissful state of being. No other system has mapped out with such precision the development of these various layers of the human being.

The usual repertoire of exercises for the athlete includes exercises for contracting and expanding the muscles. Weight-lifting, running, swimming, and playing games develop the anatomical structure of the body, but at the physiological or organic levels, attention is nil. We often have a huge bulk hung onto small, poorly developed internal organs. Yoga is not simply content with the external development of muscles. It believes in the proper communion of the internal organs and the anatomical structure of the body. Freedom and strength are given to the spleen, pancreas, liver, heart, kidneys, and all other organs by the same process of contraction and expansion that is normally used for the development of the muscles....

Also, the anti-gravitational positioning of the inner organs in the inverted *āsana,* such as standing on the head or on the shoulders, revitalizes the organs as the blood circulation is improved due to the change of gravitational pull.

Finally, the attention given to the absence of tension in the organs and to their response to the action of the muscles makes it much easier for those organs to go quickly to a state of relaxation and therefore to be quickly recharged by the energy generated by the practice of *āsana*. Also, elasticity is given to the intercostal muscles, rib joints, and spine as well as the lungs, and the breathing capacity is enhanced by the techniques known as *prāṇāyāma*. ”

"Even today many cricketers, athletes, runners, and sprinters are undergoing training at our Institute."

From "Yoga for Athletes", Poone Herald *Diwali Special Supplement, 21 October 1968.*

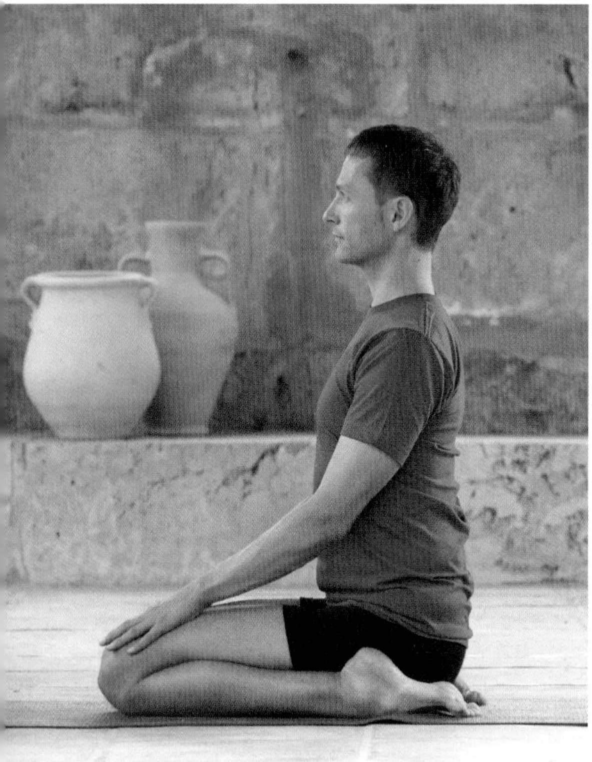

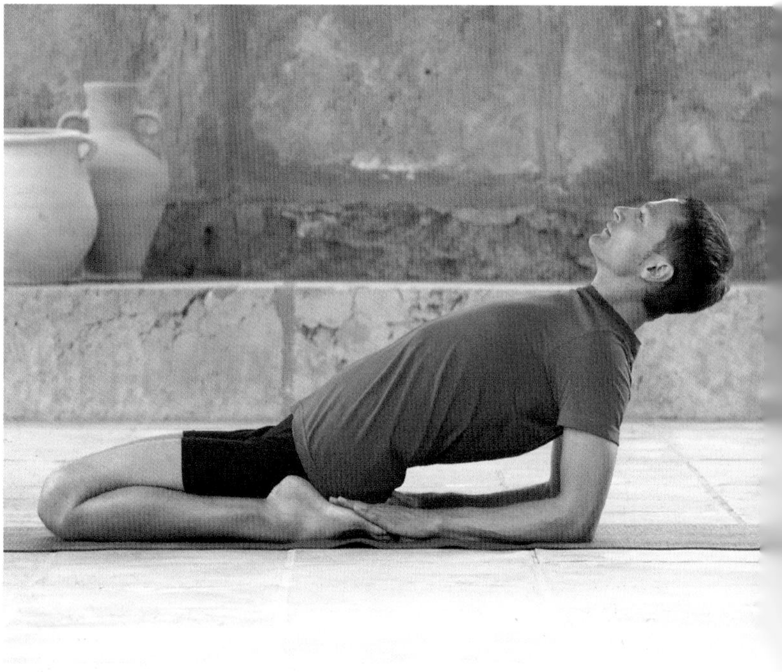

1 Sit in Virasana (see pages 136–37).

2 Exhale, lean back, and rest each elbow on the floor, palms on the soles of your feet. Lift your chest and extend your spine back and buttocks forwards.

Supta Virasana

Reclining Hero Pose

"Athletes and sports-persons consume more energy than normal in a very short time. This burning out of energy generates acids in the joints and muscles, bringing stiffness and fatigue. Yoga practices supply fresh blood for circulation, keeping the joints free from accumulation of acid and muscles free from fatigue. With the practice of *āsana*, the sports-persons begin to understand how to co-ordinate each and every action with the movement of the breath."

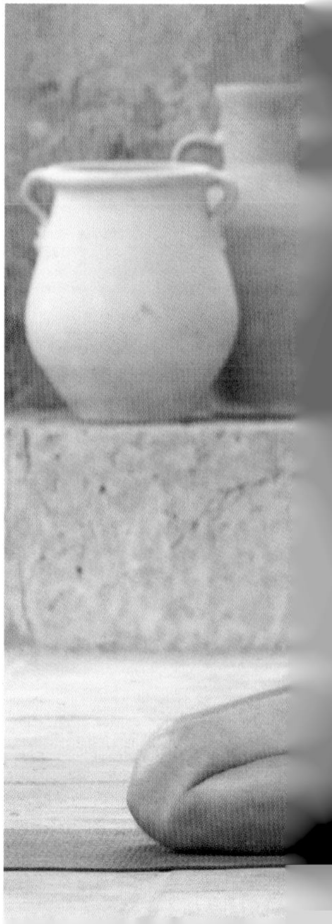

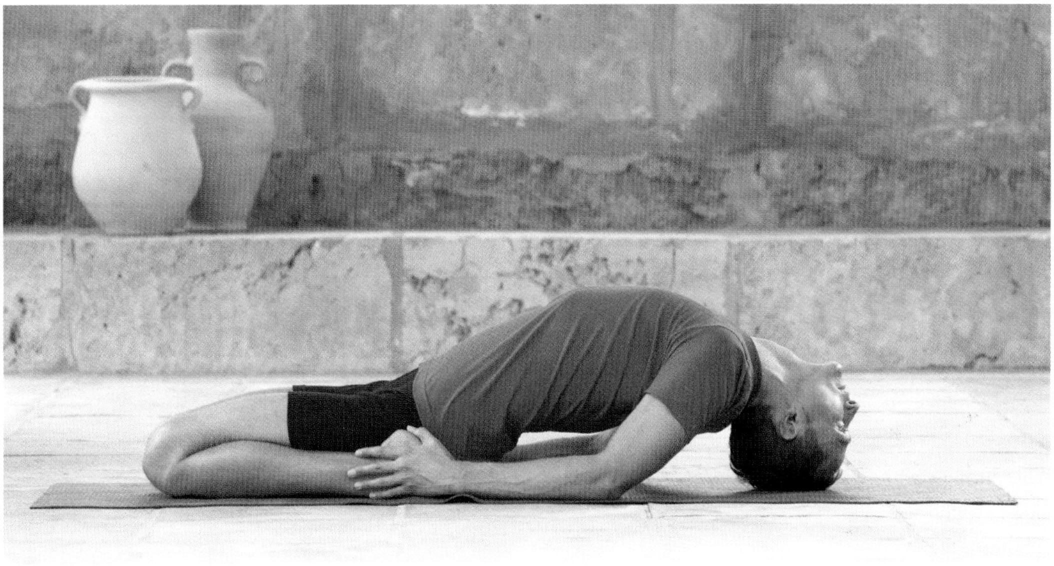

3 Lower yourself further, briefly placing the crown of your head on the floor. Gradually lower yourself until the back of your head and back rest on the floor.

4 Move your elbows to the sides and extend your spine fully. Stretch your arms overhead, palms up. Hold for 30-60 seconds. Take your hands to your ankles, lift your head and trunk, and support yourself on your elbows. Exhale, sit up, then straighten your legs into Dandasana (see pages 14-15).

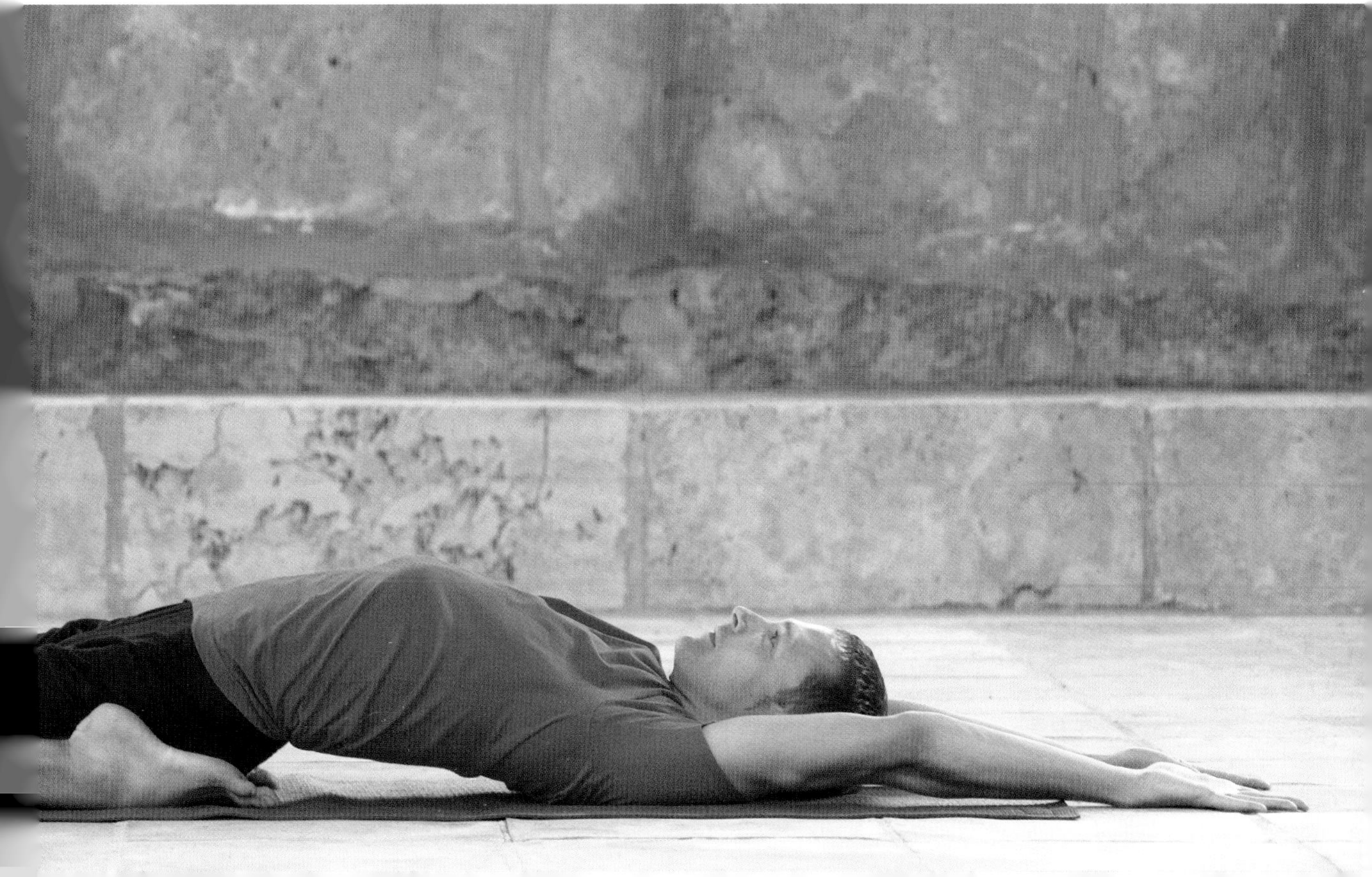

Baddha Konasana

Restrained Angle Pose

"*Yogāsana* help in bringing to our attention the weak parts of the body. They help in mobilizing the joints, increase the range of movements, bring efficiency in action and sharpness, correct the faults that occur in games, and keep one always fit and in a state of efficiency with minimum strain. They also lubricate the joints and keep movements and dynamics of the body at the optimum level."

1 Sit in Dandasana (see pages 14-15).

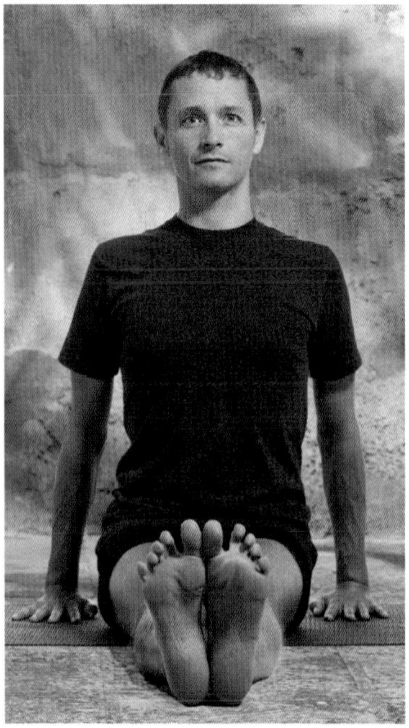

2 Bend your knees and bring the soles and heels of your feet together. Catch your feet near the toes and draw the heels towards your perineum. Widen your thighs and lower your knees towards the floor. Interlock your fingers, grip the feet, stretch the spine erect and gaze ahead. Hold for 30-60 seconds.

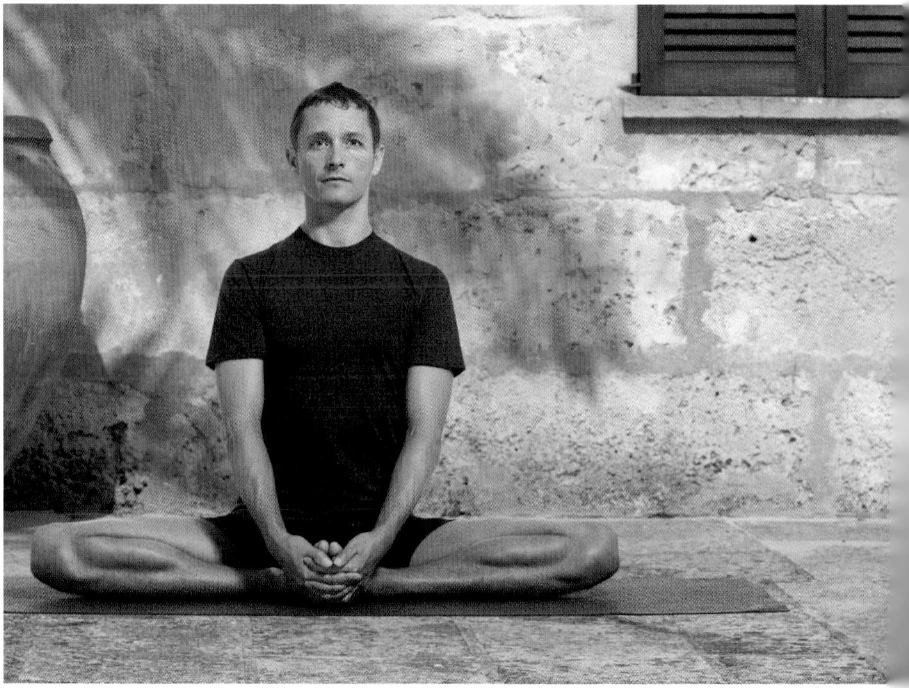

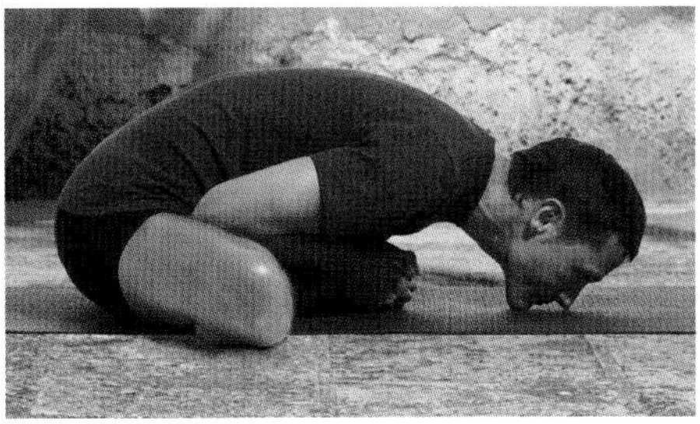

Baddha Konasana
viewed from the side.

3 Place your elbows on your thighs and press down. Exhale, bend forwards, and rest your head, nose, and lastly your chin on the floor. Hold for 30-60 seconds. Inhale, raise your trunk and finish in Dandasana.

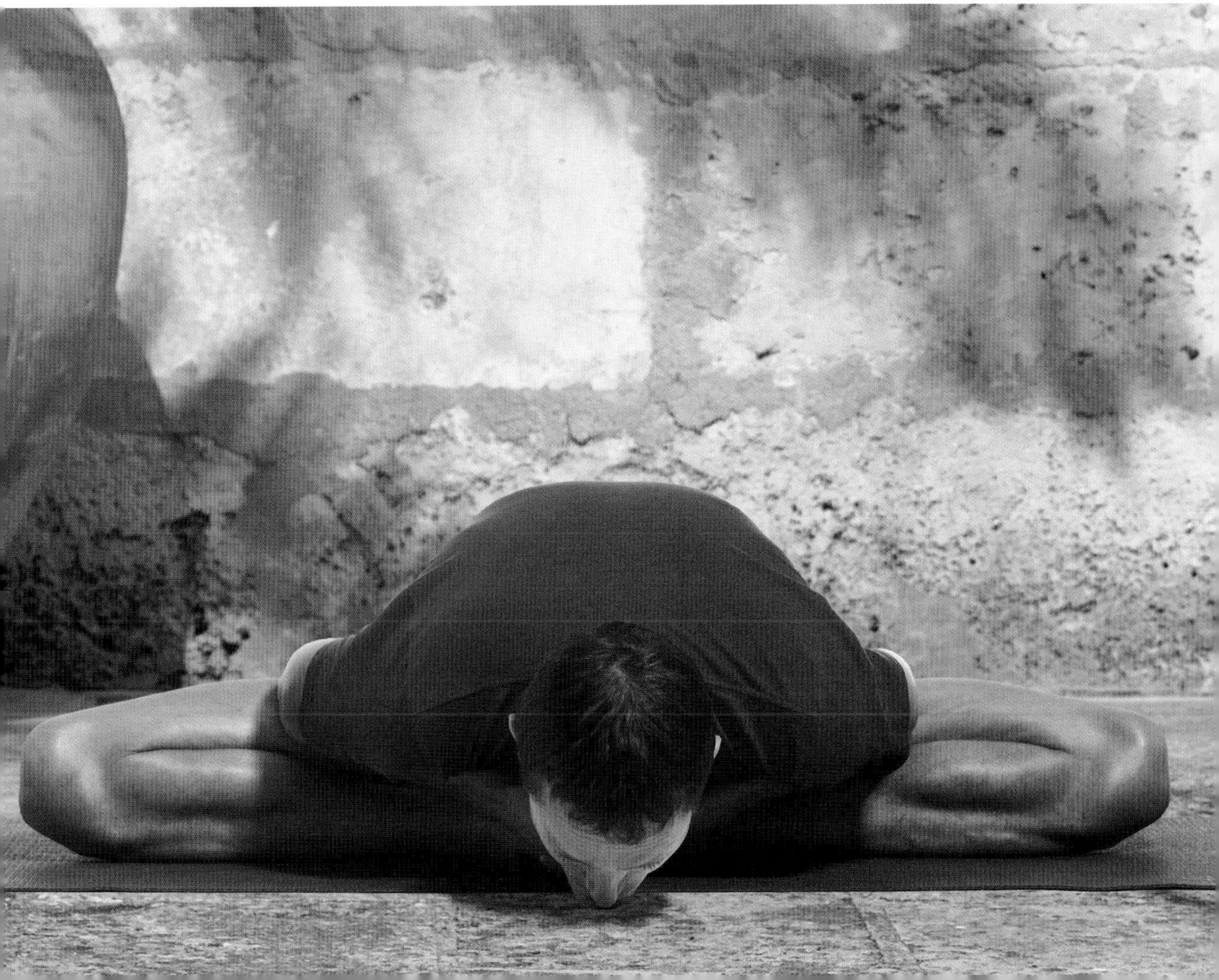

Yoga and Dance

“Yoga, being the root of all art, it is complementary and supplementary to dance. Practice of yoga develops a keen mind, alert eye, proportionate division of limbs, good features, and good voice. It brings agility, swiftness, and elegance in movement, repose, and reflection.

Yoga is a subjective expression of an experienced feeling. Dance is expression through the artful display of the emotions, gestures, and comportment of an experienced yogi.

Yoga is action. Outwardly it is static but dynamic within, whereas dance is motion and dynamic throughout.

Yoga is beauty in action and dance is beauty in motion.

Yoga has three types of movements – *tīvra* (intense), *madhyama* (medium), and *mṛdu* (soft). So, too, in dance there are *tāṇḍava* (vigorous), *lāsya* (soft and slow) with *abhinaya* (gesture, action, or emotional expression), *bhāva* (disposition and feeling), and *rasa* (the feeling or sentiment prevailing in a taste or a character).

As yoga has innumerable *āsana*, so are there *karaṇa* in dance, which are nothing but yogic *āsana*.

Yoga looks to the formless devoid of attributes or qualities (*nirguṇabrahma*). Dance looks at it with form and attributes (*saguṇabrahma*).

Yoga is a path of involution and renunciation – *nivṛtti mārga* – whereas dance is the path of evolution and acceptance of all creation – *pravṛtti mārga*. However, the paths of *karma*, *bhakti* and *jñāna* are blended beautifully in both the arts.

For a yogi it is important to treat the body as the temple of the soul and each movement as the *mantra* or the *japa*. Each adjustment is the *artha* or the meaning of the movement and each experience is *bhāvanā* or feeling. So also in dance.

Yoga develops a fine body, brings about a smiling face, a sweet voice, clear eyes, clean mind, firm legs, and abounding health. Dancers need all these to use the mouth for music, hands to convey meaning, eyes to express feelings, and feet for firmness and rhythm. So yoga is a great help for dance.

Yoga is a subjective presentation displaying position, gesture, and expression in the *āsana*, *prāṇāyāma* and *dhyāna*. It is an internal experience and feeling of integrating the body, the senses, the mind, and the intelligence with the self. Dance is an external expression of thoughts, passions, and actions. The six characteristics of desire, anger, ambition, love, pride, and jealousy are considered as the enemies for the growth of spiritual knowledge in yoga, and the yogi controls and sublimates them by friendliness (*maitri*), compassion (*karuṇā*), delight (*muditā*), and indifference (*upekṣā*). The above mentioned six characteristics are considered in dance as companions for expressing the varied sentiments of man's feelings. These six basic emotions are converted as *navarasa* into erotic (*śringāra*), comic (*hāsya*), pathetic (*karuṇā*), heroic (*vīra*), furious (*raudra*), fearful (*bhayānaka*), marvellous (*adbhuta*), revolting (*bibhatsa*), and peaceful or meditative (*śānta*). Yoga is a dynamic internal experience of oneself and dance imitates the inner experience of the yogi externally for one to see.

Thus, both yoga and dance glow from the immortal forms of the soul expressing themselves through the mortal frame – the body – the temple of the soul and the abode of God-consciousness. ”

From 'Yoga and Dance' December 1982, Aṣṭadaḷa Yogamālā *Volume 3, pp176–78.*

Natarajasana

King of the Dance Pose

"Is it a coincidence that the Lord of yoga is Lord Shiva – bestower of happiness – and the Lord of dance is the same Lord Shiva in the form of *Naṭarāja* – the king of dancers? Similarly, is it again a coincidence that Patañjali, the master of yoga, is also the master of dance and is considered as guru for both arts? Hence, as students of yoga and dance, we pay homage to Lord *Naṭarāja* and Patañjali, as both of them gave these arts, yoga and dance, for cultural growth and at the same time to savour the nectar of spiritual life."

Note: Because this is an advanced pose, no instructions are given. "Even if you do an advanced *āsana* like *Naṭarājāsana*, you have to feel that the mind is exactly even to that of the frame of the *āsana*. We've got about 700 muscles, 300 joints, so each and every part, the inner, the outer and the middle part have to be balanced in *Naṭarājāsana* accurately like *Taḍāsana*, or any other *āsana*, and that is, for me, spiritual practice."

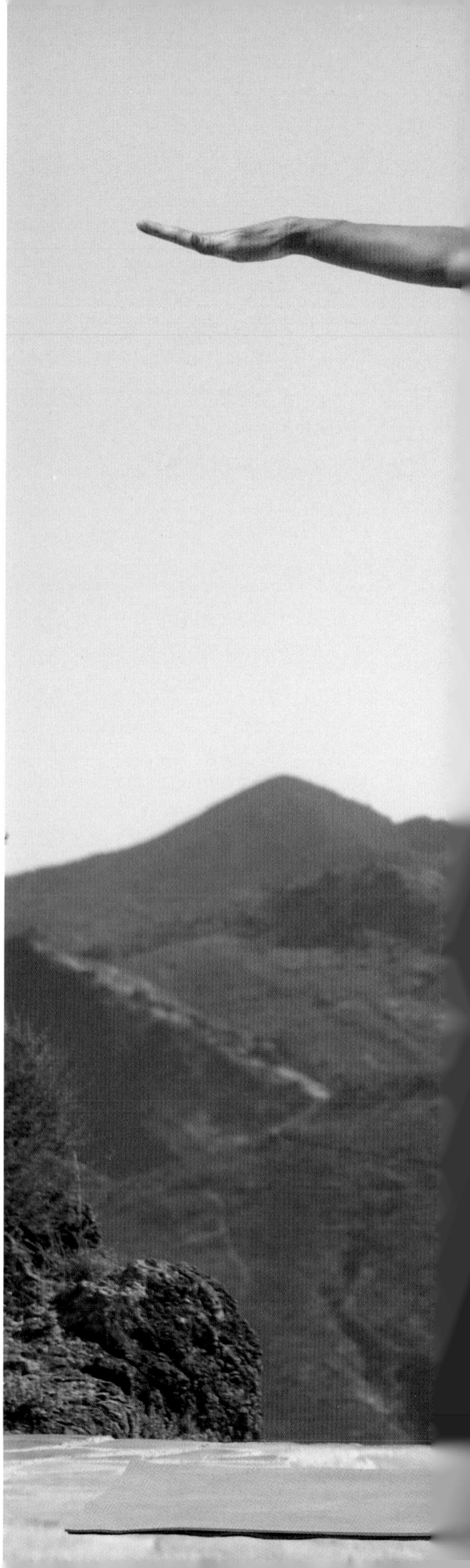

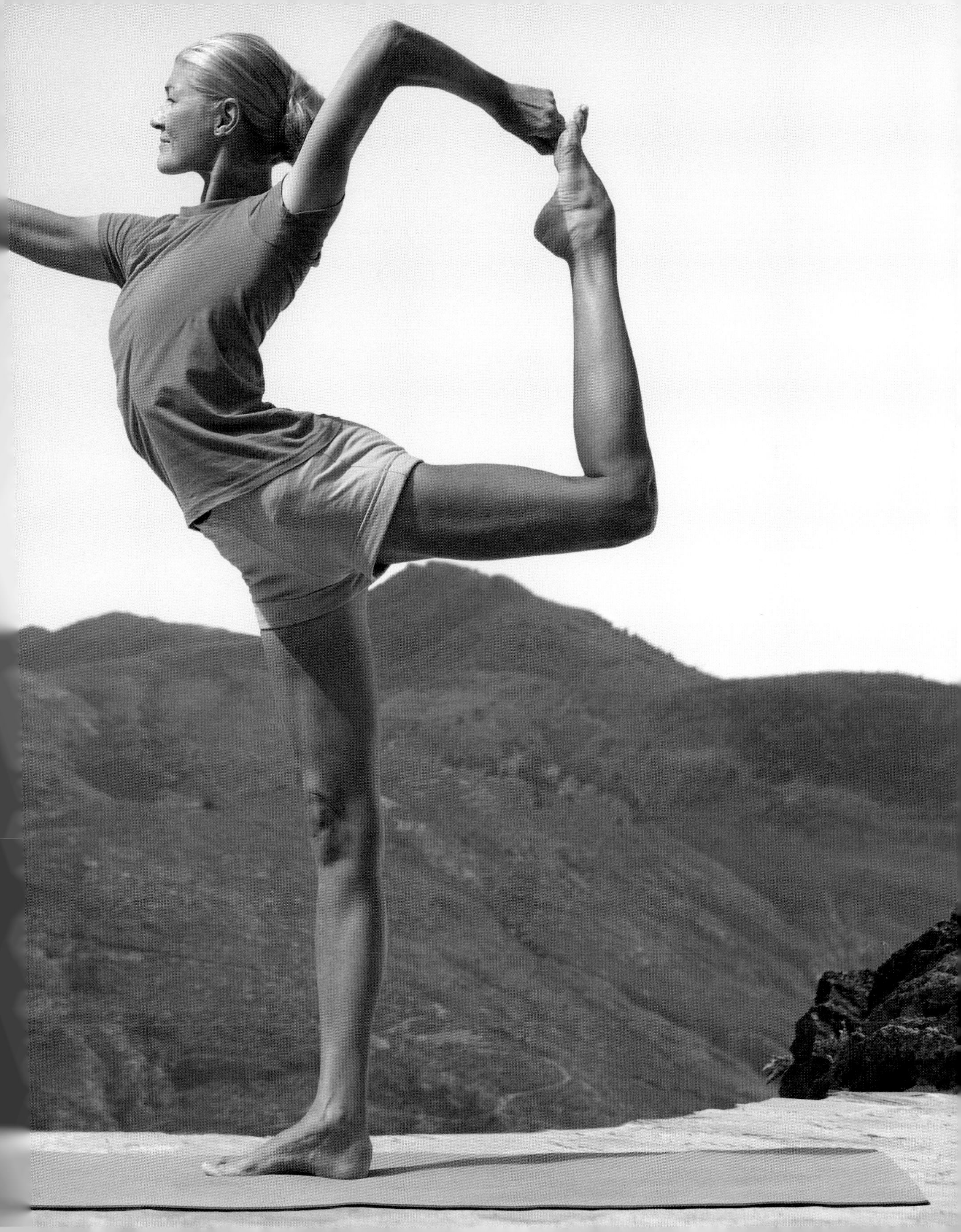

Yoga for Children

“In 1937, I was the pioneer to introduce yoga in schools and colleges, and at that time the other yogis said that yoga cannot be taught to the masses and it's wrong to do so. Now, the same people are wanting that yoga should be introduced in schools and colleges. I just laugh....

Children need competition, they need speed and variety. These are the three important things the youngsters demand. If you say go slowly in yoga, the child gets bored, you will never see that child in the class again. If you ask them to repeat, they say it is monotonous. In my classes, I take the same *āsana*, but I change the methodology and sequences in different ways, which they feel challenging, and they feel happy.

People who visit Pune have seen children from the age of six to the age of fifteen. We have once a week class on Sundays because other days they have school. Sunday is the only day which is a holiday for them, and children come to my class and never miss Sundays. I tell every-body, see how much interest is created in them. We play with them, and when necessary we admonish them. We as teachers join in competition. For instance, I may say, 'Let me see whether you are quick or I am quick.' Or as a teacher I may stand on the platform and tell them, 'I think you are all very young, you are going to do better than me.' I imitate as though I am stiff and I cannot do the *āsana*, and make them do it. Second time I say, 'Hey! You have all done very well, I will also compete with you. Let me see whether I can.' So I do a little better than them. I say, 'See, I am better than you, can you do better than me?' This way I create interest in them. What I take this Sunday I will not do next Sunday. I change in order to show a new

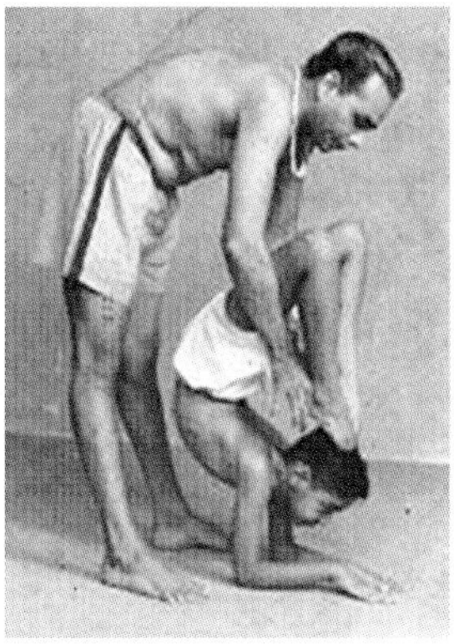

Guruji encourages his son Prashant in Vrschikasana.

variety every now and then. I make them do the same *āsana* in a new way each time. I adapt different sequences, I jump from top to bottom, bottom to top, middle to end, so that they are made to love doing that. It challenges not only their bodies but helps them to develop quickness, memory, intelligence, co-ordination, and synchronization in movements. If you take classes like that, I tell you, the child will enjoy yoga tremendously. ”

"Children want to know everything. They grasp fast. They have both one-channelled and all-pointed attention, and they should be encouraged to develop this faculty."

From "Meeting B.K.S.Iyengar", interview in London, May 1984, Yoga Today *(now* Yoga and Health, *UK) July and August 1984.*

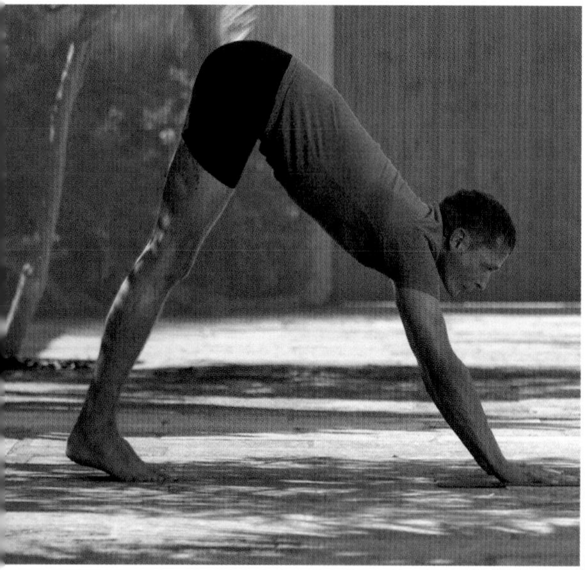

1 *Caution: This is not a sequence for beginners.* Stand erect 90cm (3ft) in front of your mat, then place your palms on the mat.

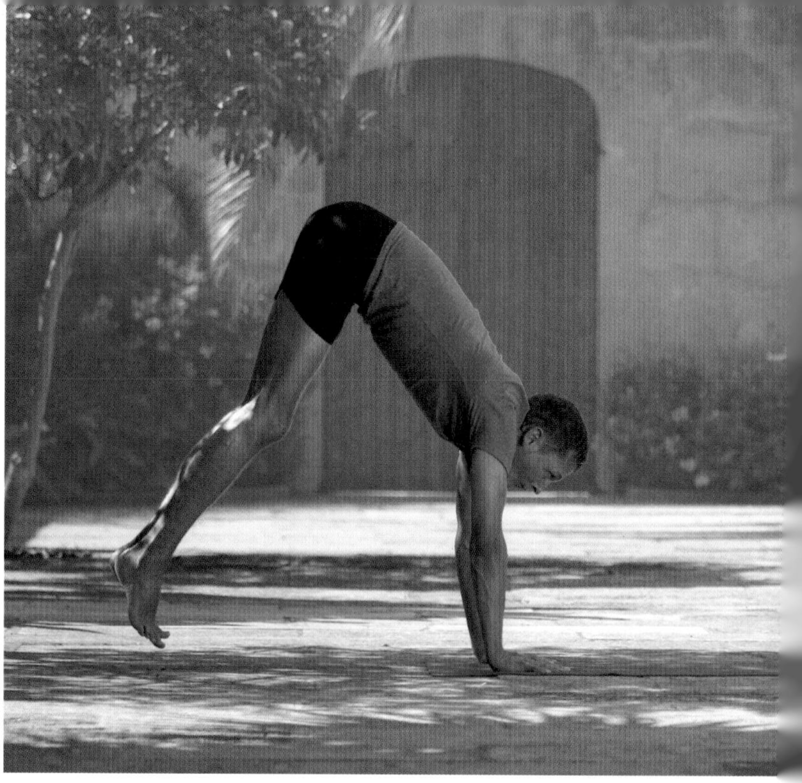

2 Exhale and swing both legs up, as if coming up into Adho Mukha Vrksasana (see pages 212–13).

Viparita Chakrasana

Reversed Wheel Pose

"Children have prolific energy. Their enthusiasm, courage, flexibility, and endurance keep them dynamically active. The varieties of *āsana* appear natural for them. First, let us channel their energy in *āsana*, so that when they reach adult age they do *prāṇāyāma* healthily."

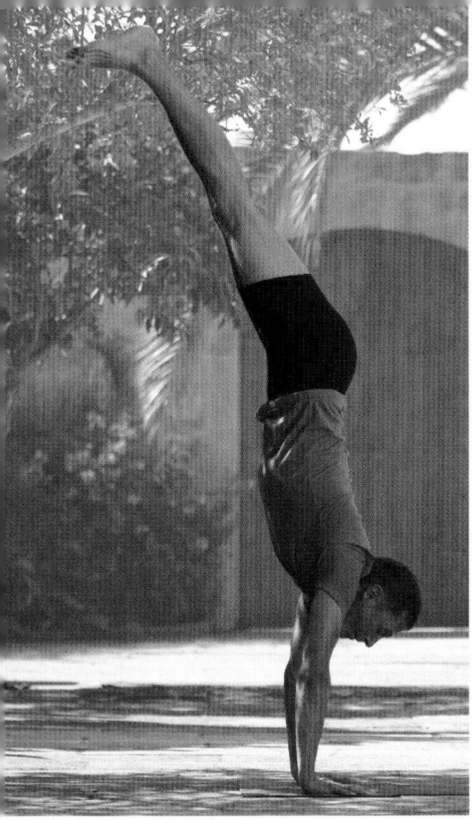

3 Keep extending your legs upwards until they are perpendicular to the floor.

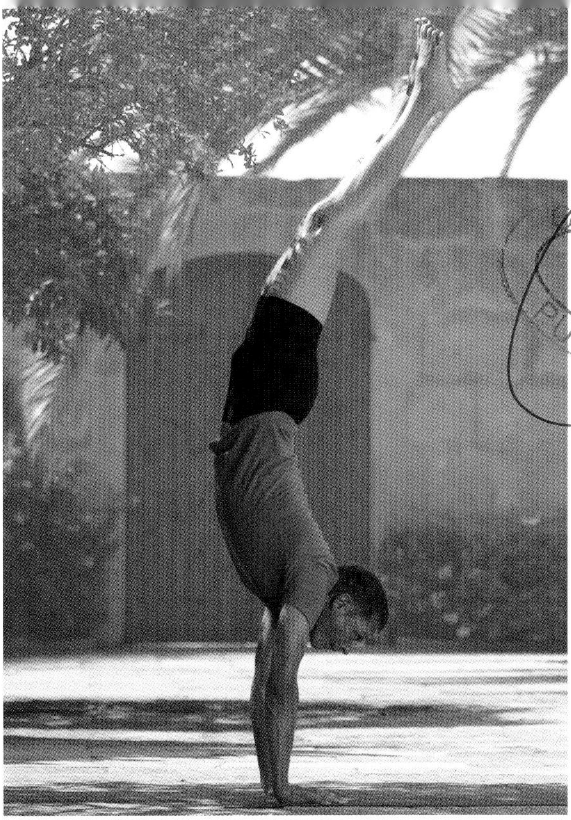

4 Start to bend your knees and arch your back as your legs come down beyond and behind your head.

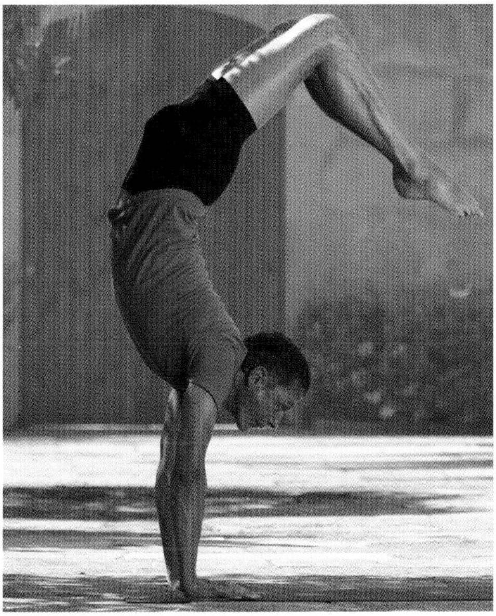

5 As you bring your legs down, contract your hips, extend your back up, stretch your ribs and abdomen and straighten your elbows. Unless you do this, you will sit on the floor with a bump.

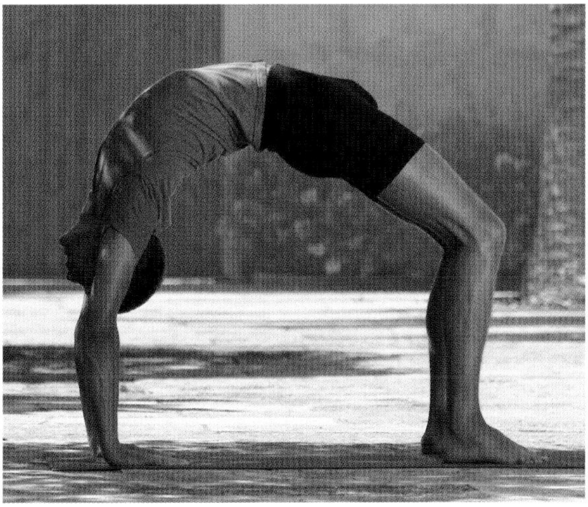

6 Land in Urdhva Dhanurasana (see pages 202–203). Come down as for this pose and rest. When you have mastered steps 1–6, learn the reverse swinging movement with a teacher, bringing your legs up and back in a reverse somersault. This is Viparita Chakrasana.

Glossary

A

abhyāsa constant, determined study or practice

ahiṁsā non-violence; the first ***yama***

ākāśa tattva ether element

ānandamaya kośa the blissful body of the Self, or ***ātman***

annamaya kośa the physical body of bones and muscles

aparigraha non-coveting; the fifth ***yama***

āp tattva water element

āsana posture; the third petal of ***aṣṭāṅga*** yoga

aṣṭāṅga yoga eight-petalled yoga; steps to self-realization through the practice of yoga

asteya non-stealing, the third ***yama***

ātman the Self

Āyurveda "knowledge of life"; ancient Indian system of healthcare

BC

bhakti yoga path of love or devotion

Brahma the Supreme Being, the Creator

brahmacarya continence; the fourth ***yama***

buddhi intelligence

cakra the seven energy centres within the spinal cord

citta consciousness; composed of mind, intelligence and ego

cognitive action done with knowledge by observation

conative external or physical action; pertaining to the exterior of the body or anatomical body

D

darśanas the six schools of Hindu philosophy

dhāraṇā complete attention of the consciousness on a single point or task; the sixth petal of ***aṣṭāṅga*** yoga

dhātu the seven elements that form the body

dhyāna mediation, or uninterrupted flow of concentration; the seventh petal of ***aṣṭāṅga*** yoga

dośa defects

GH

guru teacher; one who hands down a system of knowledge to a pupil

Gurujī respectful way to address a ***guru***

haṭha yoga the yoga of firmness and determined discipline

Haṭhayoga Pradīpikā treatise on yoga compiled by the sage Svatmarama in the 12th century

hiṁsā violence

Īśvara prāṇidhāna devotion to the Lord; the fifth ***niyama***

JKL

jāgrata wakeful state of consciousness

japa repetitive prayer

jñāna yoga the path of knowledge

kāraṇa śarīra cause body (one of three layers)

karma action

karma yoga path of action

kuṁbhaka retention of breath

kuṇḍalinī serpent energy

laya reflection

laya yoga the yoga of love and dissolution in the object of devotion

MN

madhyama nāḍī spinal cord, or central nervous system

manomaya kośa the psychological body and mind; includes the senses

mantra yoga the yoga of thoughtful prayer

merudaṇḍa spinal column

niyama individual discipline; the second petal of ***aṣṭāṅga*** yoga

P

pancakośa the body's five sheaths – ***annamaya kośa***, ***prāṇmaya kośa***, ***manomaya kośa***, ***vijñānamaya kośa*** and ***ānandamaya kośa***

Patañjali codifier of yoga; author of the ***Yoga Sūtras*** and treatises on grammar and medicine

prajñā consciousness, awareness

prakṛti nature

prāṇa energy

prāṇmaya kośa the physiological, or organic, body of vital organs

prāṇśakti life force or bio-energy (also known as ***jīvaśakti***)

prāṇāyāma control of breathing, the fourth petal of ***aṣṭāṅga*** yoga

pratyāhāra bringing the senses under control with the mind; the fifth petal of ***aṣṭāṅga*** yoga

pṛthvi tattva earth element

pūraka inhalation

RS

rājasic active, passionate; ***rajas*** is the ***guna***, or quality, of activity

rāja yoga the royal path of yoga

recaka exhalation

sādhaka seeker or aspirant

sādhanā practice or quest

samādhi when the body and senses are at rest, but the mind and reason are alert; the eighth and final petal of ***aṣṭāṅga*** yoga

samatvam equilibrium or balance

Sāṁkhyā one of six ***darśanas***, based on dualism

saṁskāra mental impression of the past

santoṣa contentment; the second ***niyama***

sāttvic pure, good, illuminated; ***sattva*** is the ***guṇa***, or quality, of goodness and purity

satya truth, the second ***yama***

śauca purity, the first ***niyama***

sthūla śarīra gross or external body (one of three layers)

sūkṣma śarīra subtle body (one of three layers)

supta supine

susupti sleep state of consciousness

sūtra aphoristic statement

svādhyāya study of the Self; the fourth ***niyama***

svapna dream state of consciousness

T

tāmasic inert or ignorant; ***tamas*** is the ***guṇa***, or quality, of darkness or ignorance

tapas ardour or austerity; the third ***niyama***

tapasvini a woman who has done much yoga and fervent penance

teja tattva fire element

UV

Upaniṣads section of the ***Vedas*** that discuss philosophy

vairāgya absence of worldly desires

vāyu tattva air element

Vedas the four most ancient and sacred collections of Hindu scripture

vedic relating to the Vedas and the era that produced them

veeṇā Indian plucked string instrument

vidyā intellect

vijñānamaya kośa the intellectual body or mental faculty

vikṛti "evolute"; matter assuming a form

Y

yama social discipline; ethical commandments for daily living; the first petal of ***aṣṭāṅga*** yoga

yoga control of the consciousness

Yogāchārya a master of yoga and teacher

yogasādhanā yoga practice

yogaśālā a place where yoga is taught

Yoga Sūtras collection of 196 aphorisms on yoga, attributed to Patañjali

Asana Index

Index

Citations

Citations for main extracts are detailed at the end of entries.

15 From "How I Learnt Pranayama", edited from Pranayama Symposium, interview by Neela Kamik, 15.12.1985, ***70 Glorious Years of Yogacharya BKS Iyengar****, published by Light on Yoga Research Trust (LOYRT).*

16 ***Ibid****, p65.*

20–21 From "On Astanga Yoga – Asana", ***Astadala Yogamala*** *Volume 7, p123.*

26 From "How Yoga Creates Joy in Life", interview by Dominique Umbert, ***Terre du Ciel****, December 94 – January 95.*

28 Quotation from "Yoga – A Divine Embroidery", interview by Zippy Wiener in the Library at RIMYI, 28.8.1997.

30 From "Meeting BKS Iyengar", interview in London, May 1984, ***Yoga Today*** *(now* ***Yoga and Health, UK****) July 1984 and August 1984.*

32 From "The Strength of Yoga", interview by Roger Raziel in Paris, 23 April 1984, published in ***Le Monde Inconnu*** *July 1984, and in* ***Victoria Newsletter****, May 1991.*

36 From "Yoga – Head to Toe", interview for BBC Radio 4 by Mark Tully in Pune, April 1999.

37 ***Ibid.***

38 ***Ibid****, pp318–19.*

40–41 From "Iyengar Looks Back", interview by Anne Cushman, ***Yoga Journal****, December 1997.*

42 From "Guidelines on Asana for Teachers", San Diego, 27.6.1990.

43 From "Adjustments in Practice", **Astadala Yogamala** Volume 7, pp313–14.

44 Ibid, p313.

46 Quotation from "Yoga Drsti (With yogic eyes)", cassette message played in centres across the world at B.K.S. Iyengar's 70th birthday celebrations 14.12.1988.

54 Quotation from "Evolution in Sādhanā", interview by Gabriella Giubillaro in Pune, January 1998, **Yogadhārā**, LOYRT, Mumbai, 2000.

55 Caption from "How Yoga Transformed Me", **Astadala Yogamala** Volume 1, p21.

56 From "Evolution in Sadhana", p203.

59 From "On Astanga Yoga – Pranayama", **Astadala Yogamala** Volume 7, p155.

61 Quotation from "How Yoga Transformed Me", p21.

Caption **ibid**, p20.

62 From "Yoga in General", **Astadala Yogamala** Volume 7, p39.

67 Quotation from "Yoga for Peace of Mind", **Astadala Yogamala** Volume 3, p25.

70 Quotation from "On Patanjali and Yoga", **Astadala Yogamala** Volume 6, p57.

72 From "Exchange of ideas between Mr Iyengar and Swami Radha", Victoria Yoga Center June 1992.

80 From "The Practical Psychology of Yoga", **Astadala Yogamala** Volume 7, p 261.

84 From Preface to **Astadala Yogamala** Volume 2, p22.

86 From "How Yoga Creates Joy in Life", interview by Dominique Umbert, **Terre du Ciel**, December 1994 – January 1995.

90 Quotation from "On Astanga Yoga – Asana", pp105–106.

91 Short quotation from "Yogasana: a search of the infinite in the finite body", **Yoga Rahasya**, Volume 2, no.1.

Caption quotation from "Anukrama Sadhana Sreni", talk given in Pune, 14.12.2001.

92 From "Yogasana: a search of the infinite in the finite body", p209.

94 Ibid, p211.

98 From "Alignment of Body and Mind with the Soul", interview by Carles Bruno, Jordi Marti and Patxi Lizardi, July 1991 in the Library at RIMYI, **Cuerpo Mente**, February 1994.

100 From "Yogasana: a search of the infinite in the finite body", p208.

102 Quotation from "What is Sthira Sukham Asnam?", talk given on Hanumān Jayanti day, 2007, Pune.

104 From "Reflections and Experiential Wisdom in Asana and Pranayama", talk on Patanjali Jayanti, 1998.

106 From "Yoga Described", **Yuva Bharati**, February, 1978.

108 From "A Path of Evolution and Involution", interview by Shirley Daventry French, Marlene Mawhinney and Kay Parry, October 1995 in the Library at RIMYI, **Victoria Yoga Centre Newsletter**, July/August 1997.

110 From "Adjustments in Practice", p284.

114 From "Reflections and Experiential Wisdom in Asana and Pranayama", p237.

116 From "Teaching Yoga: Vigour or Rigour", address at the Silver Jubilee of MDIIY (UK) November 1997.

120 From "Pearls of Yogic Wisdom", p257.

122 Quotation from "The Strength of Yoga", p186.

124 From "The Art of Teaching", interview by Shirley Daventry French, Leslie Hogya, Jim Rischmiller, Karen Fletcher, Caroline Coggins and Peter Thompson, **The Yoga Centre of Victoria Newsletter**, May and September 1986.

125 From "Jnana in Asana: Experiential Knowledge", message at American Iyengar Yoga Convention, San Diego, June 1990.

126 Quotation from "From Moha to Moksaa", talk given 14.12.1999.

127 Quotation from "On **Astanga** Yoga – **Asana**", p121.

128 From "Pearls of Yogic Wisdom", **Astadala Yogamala** Volume 1, p257.

130 From "Kayabrahma to Atmabrahma", **Astadala Yogamala** Volume 3, p40.

134 From "On Practice – Theory", **Astadala Yogamala** Volume 7, p357.

135 From "On Astanga Yoga – Asana", p112.

136 From "On Practice – Theory", p344.

138 From "How to Become a Yogi", interview by Rod Hayes, 'The Body Programme', Australian Broadcasting Corporation, September 1983. Transcribed and edited by Sandra Mulcahey, the **BKS Iyengar Association of Australasia Newsletter**, June 1985.

144 From "Salient Points About Practice and Teaching", **Astadala Yogamala** Volume 3, pp248–49.

148 From "On Astanga Yoga – Pranayama", pp140–41.

150 From "Mr Iyengar Meets the British Wheel of Yoga", **Yoga Today** November and December 1984.

154 From "Salient Points About Practice and Teaching", p249.

155 Ibid.

157 From "How I Learnt Pranayama", p65.

162 From "Iyengar Looks Back", p189.

166 From "Salient Points About Practice and Teaching", p247.

168 Short quotation from "Iyengar The Enigma", interview by Colonel D.I.M. Robbins, O.B.E, M.C, **Yoga and Health**, 7.1.89.

170 From "On My Practice", p251.

172 From "Suddhi Samyata Illumined Buddhi and Luminous Atman", B.K.S.Iyengar's message on Gurupurnima, 14.7.92.

177 Quotation from "One teacher or several teachers", **Astadala Yogamala** Volume 8, pp94–95.

178 From "Guidelines on **Asana** for Teachers", San Diego, 27.6.1990.

180 From "Adjustments in Practice", p291.

186 From Foreword to **Astadala Yogamala** Volume 3, p10.

188 Ibid, pp10–11.

190 From "Blood – a Gem", **Astadala Yogamala** Volume 8, pp201.

194 From "Cardiovascular Training Through Yoga", **Astadala Yogamala** Volume 8, p48.

196 From "Pearls of Yogic Wisdom", p251.

198 *Quotation from "Yoga – A Divine Embroidery", p153.*

Caption from "On Astanga Yoga – Asana", pp106-107.

202 *From "Yoga in General",* **Astadala Yogamala** *Volume 7, p25.*

206 *From "Yoga Destresses the Stress",* **Astadala Yogamala** *Volume 3, p114.*

212 *From "Yoga for Stress-free Life",* **Astadala Yogamala** *Volume 3, pp110–11.*

214 *From "A Subject of the Heart", interview by Cathy Boyer, Johanna Heckmann and Anne-Catherine Leter, August 1995.*

218 *Ibid, p65.*

222 *Introductory text from "The Grace of Consciousness in Asana", talk given at a course in Panchgani, November 1993.*

226 *From a speech given at a Nature Cure and Ayurveda conference, Karnataka Prakrtika Parisad, Bangalore.*

230 *From "The Art of Teaching", p253.*

234 *From "The Practical Psychology of Yoga",* **Astadala Yogamala** *Volume 7, p270–71.*

238 *From "The Importance of Yoga for Sports and Games",* **Astadala Yogamala** *Volume 3, p273.*

240 *Ibid, p272.*

244 *From "Yoga and Dance", December 1982,* **Astadala Yogamala** *Volume 3, pp176–77.*

Caption from "Yoga – Head to Toe", p289.

248 *From "On Astanga Yoga – Pranayama", p154.*

Acknowledgments

Author's Acknowledgments

To reach this pinnacle in my *sādhana*, I give credit and merit to my wife Smt. Ramāmaṇi, though it was my *Guru*, T. Krishnamacharya, who initiated me into yoga. I am filled with joy and wish to express my sense of gratitude to Dorling Kindersley for making my works and thoughts easily available to the lovers of philosophy and practitioners of yoga throughout the world.

Publisher's Acknowledgments

Dorling Kindersley would like to thank everyone at the Ramamani Memorial Yoga Institute (RMYI), Pune, for their assistance and expertise, especially Abhijata Sridhar and Stephanie Quirk. Dorling Kindersley would also like to thank the following: photographer John Freeman and his assistant Erin Eve; Judith Jones and Judi Sweeting for supervising the step-by-step sequence photography and advising on the step-by-step text; models Susie Brown and Mikey Hall; the Iyengar Institute, Maida Vale, London, and Yogamatters (www.yogamatters.com) for the kind loan of Iyengar Yoga props; Martin Gelgyn at Cortijo, and Karl Grant at La Pedra Redona for the locations; Sue Lightfoot for the index, and Peter Kirkham for proofreading; Tia Sarkar and Nita Patel for their editorial help.

Thanks to the Ramamani Memorial Yoga Institute for their permission to use photographs of B.K.S. Iyengar from their archives on pages 23, 69, 97, 103, 122, 132, 247

For further information see: www.dkimages.com

For more information on B.K.S. Iyengar Yoga visit www.bksiyengar.com

B.K.S. Iyengar's collected teachings can be found in *Aṣṭadaḷa Yogamālā*, Volumes 1–8, published by Allied Publishers Private Ltd., 13/14 Ali Road, New Delhi 11002, India.